Viktoriya Sereda (ed.)
War, Migration, Memory

Forum Transregionale Studien – Dossiers | Volume 4

Editorial

The "Forum Transregionale Studien – Dossiers" are bundles of texts on shared issues. They take their starting points in programmes, initiatives and events organised by the Forum Transregionale Studien or its partners.
The series is published by Forum Transregionale Studien e.V.

Viktoriya Sereda (Prof. Dr.) is a sociologist, head coordinator of the Virtual Ukraine Institute for Advanced Study (VUIAS), and senior advisor to the Prisma Ukraïna War, Migration, Memory research group that she initiated and directed at the Forum Transregionale Studien in 2022/23. Since 2020, she has also been a senior research fellow at the Institute of Ethnology of the National Academy of Sciences of Ukraine and professor in the department of Sociology at the Ukrainian Catholic University (Lviv, Ukraine). Her main areas of research include nationalism, migration and identity studies, memory studies, civil society, and urban sociology.

Viktoriya Sereda (ed.)

War, Migration, Memory

Perspectives on Russia's War Against Ukraine

[transcript]

This Dossier is an outcome of the collaborative work of the research group Prisma Ukraïna: War, Migration, Memory. Prisma Ukraïna is a research program at the Forum Transregionale Studien. The research program and group have been supported with funding by the Berlin Senate Department for Higher Education and Research, Health and Long-Term Care, Gerda Henkel Foundation, Marga und Kurt Möllgaard-Stiftung and ZEIT STIFTUNG BUCERIUS.

Senate Department for Higher Education and Research, Health and Long-Term Care | BERLIN

GERDA HENKEL STIFTUNG MARGA UND KURT MÖLLGAARD-STIFTUNG IM STIFTERVERBAND ZEIT STIFTUNG BUCERIUS

Bibliographic information published by the Deutsche Nationalbibliothek
The Deutsche Nationalbibliothek lists this publication in the Deutsche Nationalbibliografie; detailed bibliographic data are available in the Internet at https://dnb.dnb.de/

First published in 2025 by transcript Verlag, Bielefeld

transcript Verlag | Hermannstraße 26 | D-33602 Bielefeld | live@transcript-verlag.de

Cover layout: Maria Arndt, Bielefeld
Copy-editing: Natasha Klimenko, Mark Berman
Proofread: Alex Favalli, Martin Lochthofen
Printed by: Majuskel Medienproduktion GmbH, Wetzlar
https://doi.org/10.14361/9783839475874
Print-ISBN: 978-3-8376-7587-0 | PDF-ISBN: 978-3-8394-7587-4
ISSN of series: 2702-606X | eISSN of series: 2702-6078

Printed on permanent acid-free text paper.

In memory of Olha Labur (25 December 1972 – 28 September 2024), a dedicated scholar, generous colleague, and committed activist.

Contents

Representations

Experiences of Displacement

Minority Experiences

Authors

Dossiers

The following Dossiers have so far been published by Forum Transregionale Studien:

1/2020
Schindel, Estela, and Gabriel Gatti (eds.), *Social Disappearance: Explorations Between Latin America and Eastern Europe*, Dossiers, Forum Transregionale Studien, 1/2020, Berlin 2020. Open Access: https://perspectivia.net/receive/pnet_mods_00003944

2/2022
Alshaar, Nuha, Beate Ulrike La Sala, Jenny Rahel Oesterle, and Barbara Winckler (eds.), *The Humanities in the 21st Century: Perspectives from the Arab World and Germany*, Dossiers, Forum Transregionale Studien, 2/2022, Berlin 2022. Open Access: https://perspectivia.net/receive/pnet_mods_00005616

3/2022
Alshaar, Nuha, Beate Ulrike La Sala, Jenny Rahel Oesterle, and Barbara Winckler (eds.), *Al-insānīāt fī 'l-qarn al-ḥādī wa 'l-'ashrīn: wiǧhāt naẓar min al-ʿālam al-ʿarabī wa almānīā*, Dossiers, Forum Transregionale Studien, 3/2022, Berlin 2022. Open Access: https://perspectivia.net/receive/pnet_mods_00005617

4/2025
Sereda, Viktoriya (ed.), *War, Migration, Memory. Perspectives on Russia's War Against Ukraine*, Forum Transregionale Studien – Dossiers, 4/2025, transcript Verlag, Bielefeld 2025.

Introduction
War, Migration, Memory

Viktoriya Sereda and Andrii Portnov

Independent Ukraine emerged in 1991 as a result of the collapse of the Soviet Union. It has demonstrated *socio-cultural inclusiveness* through the automatic granting of citizenship to all those who lived in the country (regardless of ethnicity, language or religion), *political pluralism* through the regular change of power through democratic elections, and a clear propensity for *peaceful resolution of the most acute political conflicts*. The student Revolution on Granite of 1990, the Orange Revolution of 2004, and the Winter 2013/2014 Revolution of Dignity/Euromaidan – until 22 January 2014 – were fundamentally peaceful. Violence (including deaths) only started in early 2014 on the Maidan. Immediately after the victory of the Revolution of Dignity, Russia occupied Crimea and contributed to the outbreak of war in the Donetsk and Luhansk regions.

Since late February 2014, Ukraine has been at war, and on 24 February 2022, this war took on the character of a full-scale invasion. If not 2014, then certainly 2022 raised the question of rethinking the entire experience of Ukraine and Ukrainians before and after 1991. Was the full-scale war a belated and very high price to pay for the peaceful political transformation of the 1990s? Or should 2022 be considered the year of the final collapse of the Soviet Empire? And what socio-political factors allowed Ukrainian society to resist the military aggression of its neighbour? How does the war affect the historical memory of Ukraine or Europe in general?

These and other questions are addressed by the authors whose texts are collected in this Dossier. They testify to individual searches for the meaning of historical events and to the sincere motivation for the establishment of Ukrainian studies against the background of confusion and trauma imposed by the current Russian aggression. We should not forget for a second the context and circumstances of these inquiries: an ongoing military conflict in the centre of Europe, unprecedented in size and scope since the Second World War, a conflict that has taken on a genocidal character.[1]

1 As you, dear readers, read this book, you may find that some of the links provided by the authors are not accessible. This research was conducted by the authors under the circumstances of a brutal war. Ukrainian society faces daily missile attacks, affecting not only civilians but

This Dossier focuses on Ukraine in the context of Russian aggression since 2014. What distinguishes the Ukrainian case from other cases of Russian aggression in the region is that it is a long-term conflict with a changing character. Initially, Ukraine faced the occupation of Crimea and its incorporation into the legal body of the Russian Federation. The Russian military aggression in the eastern part of Ukraine did not lead to the immediate integration of these territories into Russia but instead resulted in the creation of the quasi-state entities of the 'DPR' (Donetsk People's Republic) and the 'LPR' (Luhansk People's Republic) in occupied parts of the Donetsk and Luhansk regions. On 12 February 2015, after many long negotiations between the leaders of France, Germany, Russia, and Ukraine, a 'package of measures for the implementation of the Minsk agreements' ('Minsk II') was signed by the Trilateral Contact Group on Ukraine. However, it did not achieve a stable ceasefire and did not prevent Russia's further aggression. The unprovoked Russian full-scale attack on Ukraine in February 2022 brought Ukraine to the attention of an international audience. War and mass displacement exposed millions of Ukrainians to new challenges. These challenges triggered intensive reinterpretations of the past – both the distant and the very recent – and a reevaluation of their memory and sense of belonging through the experiences they are going through.

Extreme events such as war and displacement create ruptures in sense-making narratives and, as suggested by Ryan Quinn and Monica Worline, "tend to strip people of identity, leaving them no sensible narrative to enact"[2]. People need plausible accounts of events to understand what is going on and how to respond through both individual and collective actions. Sense-making is an ongoing retrospective process grounded in personal experiences and is often linked to the construction of identity and a sense of belonging. In this process, history and the past turn into an important interpretive resource for one's attachment or alienation. The imagined past may consist of the memory of recently experienced events (e.g., 'after the beginning of the war'), which is later linked to selected symbolic markers, events, or figures from the past that help explain current events or legitimise individuals or their actions.

The essays of this Dossier aim to reach beyond the politics of history and examine how collective and individual memories and people's sense of belonging are reshaped when used to interpret the shocking realities of the current war. Additionally, they investigate how memory is mobilised on a personal and collective level to

also critical infrastructure and cultural and academic institutions. Due to destruction, relocation, or power outages, servers may be temporary or permanently inaccessible. Additionally, information is a valuable resource targeted by hackers (as seen in the case of the 'My War' online project) or subject to concealment (as with official Russian statistics on the number of internally displaced persons and migrants).

2 Ryan W. Quinn and Monica C. Worline, "Enabling Courageous Collective Action: Conversations from United Airlines Flight 93", *Organization Science* 19/4, 2008, 497–516, here 501.

deal with the ruptures and threats posed by this war in an attempt to explain what is happening. The main research questions addressed in this volume are not new. Scholars have been working on similar issues for a long time and have developed several explanatory schemes.[3] For example, Peter Gatrell's work on refugees during the First World War illustrates how the outbreak of war can dramatically change the established landscape of social and national identities. He argues that the new category of 'refugee' created by the war suddenly became an important social category and a factor of identity. For millions of people, it outweighed many of their previous statuses and identities, influencing not only their perceptions of themselves but also their destinies.[4]

The reaction of Ukrainian society to all these challenges is quite complex, and this makes our task even more complicated and demanding. Scholars working on the region often simplified the complex transformations in Ukrainian society after 1991 and after 2014 (including the functions of memory and attitudes towards the past) into a binary of East-West divisions, a conflict of two identities (ethnic vs. civic),[5] or two models of historical memory (national vs. Soviet).[6] A more complex

3 Janet S. Watson, *Fighting Different Wars: Experience, Memory, and the First World War in Britain*, Cambridge: Cambridge University Press, 2004; Sune Haugbolle, *War and Memory in Lebanon*, Cambridge: Cambridge University Press, 2010; Stephan Milich, Friederike Pannewick, and Leslie Tramontini (eds.), *Conflicting Narratives: War, Trauma and Memory in Iraqi Culture*, Wiesbaden: Reichert Verlag, 2012; Hariz Halilovich, "Reclaiming erased lives: archives, records and memories in post-war Bosnia and the Bosnian diaspora", *Archival Science* 14/3, 2014, 231–247; and Katrin Stoll, "Transcending the divide between history and memory: Szymon Datner's practical Holocaust historiography in the early post-war period", *Holocaust Studies: A Journal of History and Culture* 21, 2015, 4–23.

4 Peter Gatrell, *A Whole Empire Walking: Refugees in Russia during World War I*, Bloomington: Indiana University Press, 1999.

5 Samuel P. Huntington, "The Clash of Civilizations?", *Foreign Affairs* 72/3, 1993, 22–49; Andrew Wilson, "The Donbas Between Ukraine and Russia: The Use of History in Political Disputes", *Journal of Contemporary History* 30/2, 1995, 265–289; Mykola Rjabtschuk, *Die reale und die imaginierte Ukraine*, Berlin: Suhrkamp, 2005; Valeriy Khmelko, "Iz-za chego politikam udaetsia raskalyvat Ukrainu", *Vechernii Lugansk* 24, 2006; Ivan Katchanovski, "East or West? Regional Political Divisions in Ukraine since the 'Orange Revolution' and the 'Euromaidan'", paper prepared for the Annual Meeting of the American Political Science Association in Washington, DC, 28–31 August, 2014; Taras Kuzio, "Competing Nationalisms, Euromaidan, and the Russian-Ukrainian Conflict", *Studies in Ethnicity and Nationalism* 15/1, 2015, 157–169; Andrew Wilson, *The Ukrainians: Unexpected Nation*, New Heaven-London: Yale University Press, 2015; and Bruno De Cordier, "Ukraine's Vendée War? A look at the 'resistance identity' of the Donbass insurgency", *Russian Analytical Digest* 198, 2017, 2–6.

6 Viktoriya Sereda, "Regional Historical Identities in Ukraine: Case Study of Lviv and Donetsk", *Naukovi Zapysky: Natsional'nyy universytet "Kyyevo-Mohylyans'ka Akademiya", Sotsiolohichni nauky* 20, 2002, 26–34; Viktoriya Sereda, "Rehional'ni vymiry ukrayinskoho sotsiumu istorychne mynule ta natsionalni identychnosti", *Ahora. Ukrayina–rehional'nyy vymir* 3, 2006, 29–41; Serhey Makeev and Anzhela Patrakova, "Rehional'na spetsyfikatsiya sotsiokul'turnykh

analysis of the variety of Ukrainian experiences in different parts of the country and on the national level could provide a more accurate picture.[7] Accordingly, the essays in this Dossier consider multifaceted issues such as: how to differentiate between models of nation-building in Ukraine before the war (for example, in ethnic and civil regards); how do different perceptions of the nation interact in 2022; how do discourses of decommunisation and decolonisation figure into this interaction; what is the impact of war on the perception and prospects of Ukraine's ethnic diversity; what are shifts in the linguistic of religious landscapes, gender roles, and many more.

Changes in Ukrainian society can be studied in various contexts and perspectives – local, regional, national, and global – and focus on certain topics. This Dossier combines two approaches: Through a variety of case studies and themes, it offers a multi-scalar perspective on the transformational effects of war; on the macro-level, it considers how war influences memory and its politics. While the perspectives on the transformational effects of war provide insights of and into shifts of memory and symbolic representations, experiences of dislocation, and the repercussions of war on minority groups, the focus on memory considers how war influences discussions on the politics of memory in official discourses, in the educational system or in the media in Ukraine, in the region and the world. Through this approach, some issues, such as the Polish-Ukrainian "memory wars", are marginalised, while others, like the frameworks of understanding and commemoration of the Second World War, are reassessed. The essays reflect how the war fuels an antagonism between pro-Ukrainian and pro-Russian versions of historical and cultural memory. They address and illustrate the shifts in writing styles and in identities of Ukrainian writers. In

---

vidminnostey v Ukrayini", *Sotsiolohiya: teoriya, metody, marketynh* 3, 2004, 109–125; Volodymyr Kravchenko, "Fighting the Shadow: The Soviet Past in the Historical Memory of Contemporary Ukrainian Society (RUS)", *Ab Imperio* 2, 2004, 329–369; Oleksandr Hrytsenko, *Prezydenty i pamyat': Polityka pamyati prezydentiv Ukrayiny (1994–2014), pidgruntya, poslannya, realizatsiya, rezul'taty*, Kyiv: KIS, 2017; and Georgiy Kasianov, *Memory Crash*, Budapest: Central European University Press, 2022.

7 Serhii Plokhy (ed.), *The Future of the Past: New Perspectives on Ukrainian History*, Cambridge: Harvard Ukrainian Research Institute, 2016; Julie Fedor, Markku Kangaspuro, Jussi Lassila, and Tatiana Zhurzhenko (eds.), *War and Memory in Russia, Ukraine and Belarus*, New York: Palgrave Macmillan, 2017; André Liebich, Oksana Myshlovska, and Viktoriia Sereda, "The Ukrainian Past and Present: Legacies, Memory and Attitudes", in: Oksana Myshlovska and Ulrich Schmid, *Regionalism without Regions. Reconceptualizing Ukraine's Heterogeneity*, Budapest: Central European University Press, 2019, 67–134; Barbara Törnquist-Plewa and Yuliya Yurchuk, "Memory politics in contemporary Ukraine: Reflections from the postcolonial perspective", *Memory Studies* 12/6, 2019, 699–720; Natalia Kudriavtseva, "Contested names in the toponymic landscapes of post-soviet space", *Ideology and Politics Journal* 1/15, 2020, 4–10; and Andrii Portnov, *Poland and Ukraine: Entangled Histories, Asymmetric Memories*, Berlin: Forum Transregionale Studien, 2020.

relation to war-induced migration, the politics of counting displaced or gendered experiences of war are analysed: How does war (re)define roles and divisions within Ukrainian society? Another avenue of exploration delves into the ways different media outlets narrate and represent wartime realities. What, for example, are the main markers of victory and resistance? Which symbols (including famous literary characters, religious or territorial imaginaries) are employed to mobilise certain identities, to create a sense of belonging, or to draw new lines of division? Moreover, media coverage of events or situations in the occupied territories at times significantly depends on an editorial perspective, on state policy, or on military conditions that restrict journalists' personal access to information. The case study of Mariupol illustrates how media messages (which are often prone to propaganda distortions and information restrictions) result in a multitude of perspectives and representations of the event and its participants. These narratives later might have a strong impact on the postwar reintegration of Ukrainian society. Moreover, several texts focus on the community level and explore the socio-cultural aspects of refugees' adaptation, shifts in collective memories and identities, motives for returning or prolonging their stay, new forms of self-aid and self-organisation, and on topics that become salient or silenced in closed social media channels.

This volume uses a cross-sectional approach to discuss the transforming impact of war on minority groups (ethnic, religious, or people diagnosed with cancer). In this collection, readers are presented with an exploration into the process of reclaiming the history of Crimea and Crimean Tatars through the lens of a single family's narratives. It illustrates how minority groups use family memories to create narratives of belonging to a community or a particular space.

Studies focusing on the personal level look at how war transforms individual communicative and cultural memories and people's experience of time, for example, when the natural flow of biographical time is disrupted by a 'before and after the beginning of the war'. How do people reference to certain symbolic markers, events or historical figures, redefine their identities, legitimise, explain current events, or make a nostalgic escape from reality? References to the past might also help overcome the traumas of the present. These phenomena are discussed in this volume in contributions analysing personal stories of common Ukrainians posted by the witnesses of war on the "My War" platform or narrated by Ukrainian refugees in Poland and Germany during the in-depth interviews conducted by the authors.

The first section on War and Memory begins with an examination of memory. Roman Holyk introduces the question of competing historical memories through the use of symbols of the World Wars I and II to interpret the ongoing war in Ukraine. Ihor Dvorkin reviews the newest Ukrainian history textbooks as indicators of current ideological trends. Denys Shatalov analyses the Ukrainian official rhetoric of war and illustrates the scale of the challenge of Ukrainian competition with the Russian Federation over the Victory of 1945, while simultaneously seeking a consistent dissociation from Soviet experience and symbolism. Olha Polishchuk writes about nonfiction personal stories on the "My War" platform in an effort to better understand "the current collective trauma of Ukrainians caused by Russian aggression in 2022". The text by Olha Haidamachuk deals with another important concept: the tonality of archives. The author discusses this on the basis of interviews conducted with forcibly displaced people. She also touches upon the exceptionally important discourse of decolonization. The widespread reference to it in current Ukrainian discussions reflects both an attempt to legitimately join the already established Western mainstream and, at the same time, an attempt to deconstruct it and give the desired legitimacy to "Ukrainian voices".

Among the tests on representations in the second section, Alina Mozolevska draws attention to the unprecedented visualisation of the current war and offers an interesting analysis of its geographic imagery. Yuliya Yurchuk contributes to the discussion on postsecularity and analyses the application of religious imagery and symbols in wartime Ukraine. Oleksandr Zabirko created a careful and thoughtful analysis of the rhetorical strategies for naming the enemy. In his analysis, he engages literary works and films, from Tolkien's "The Lord of the Rings" to Romero's "Night of the Living Dead" and comes to an important conclusion about the significance of situations where Russian and Ukrainian war rhetoric reinforce each other. No less important is his conclusion that the constant exchange and cultural negotiation between the state and society "reveals the highly decentralised structure of Ukrainian war rhetoric". Tetiana Shestopalova focuses on the attempts of Ukrainian writers from Donbas to rethink the issue of being a Russian-speaking person and author and discusses the choice of language as a factor of cultural and political security. An equally complex, painful, and controversial topic is touched upon in the article by Yuliia Soroka, who analyses Ukrainian, Russian, and English-language media reports on Mariupol produced in Spring 2022. Soroka emphasises the importance of the spectrum of perceptions of the character of occupation and assessments of the behaviour of the population of the occupied territories, both by the international media and within Ukrainian society.

The third section of the Dossier addresses experiences of displacement. The opening text by Lidia Kuzemska discusses the challenges in obtaining accurate data on the displacement of Ukrainians to Russia since the full-scale invasion in February 2022. She draws on the "politics of numbers" concept and illustrates how intentional efforts to inflate or lower displacement figures can serve political agendas. The essay by Olena Strelnyk explores the complex and contradictory nature of gender transformations in the context of Russia's war and the related forced displacement in Ukraine. The war challenges and reinforces traditional gender roles, particularly regarding men as 'protectors' and women as the 'protected.' Gender expectations shape the divergent attitudes of the Ukrainian population towards forcibly displaced refugees and internally displaced persons (IDPs).

The following three essays delineate the experiences of Ukrainian refugees residing in Poland and Germany, detailing their adjustment within their newfound host communities and elucidating how displacement transforms their notions of belonging. Ivan Kozachenko's research shows how Ukrainian refugees in Poland reevaluate their sense of national belonging to Ukraine, marked by the shifting role of the Ukrainian language and the heroisation of resistance. He describes an attenuation of the pro-Russian 'supranational' identity and an increased criticism towards the Soviet past and its mythology. Participants assign blame to both Putin's regime and the Russian people for the invasion and deliberately distance themselves from the Russian language, culture, and literature. Concurrently, Poland is viewed favourably and closer in terms of culture and geography as an effect of the support and welcome. Natalia Zaitseva-Chipak's text assesses the potential for future return migration of Ukrainian refugees to postwar Ukraine and focuses on the motivations guiding individuals' decisions. She advocates for a qualitative approach and reveals two distinct behavioural strategies of displaced people: those who put their lives on hold, awaiting the end of the war before returning, and those leveraging opportunities in Germany to improve their future prospects. Factors that influence the decision to stay or return encompass social connections and status, language proficiency, educational opportunities, and perceived social or medical security, as well as emotional motivations such as family reunification, homesickness, or the intensity of national identity. Taisiia Ratushna examines another aspect of displaced communities: their self-aid practices. She explores how displaced Ukrainians use social media platforms, particularly Telegram channels, to share information, seek assistance, and connect with others in similar situations. Ratsushna also explores key communication topics over time and offers insights into the processes of adaptation and integration, as well as community building and isolation.

The text of the fourth section on minority experiences by Denys Brylov and Tetiana Kalenychenko examines ongoing transformations of religious identities in Ukraine during the last decade and especially after Russia's full-scale aggression. Ukraine's religious landscape is often mistakenly described by external viewers as predominantly Orthodox. However, in Ukraine, over one-third of all believers resist aligning themselves with specific denominations and affiliations with specific religious institutions. This has visible regional variances, steadily decreasing from west to east.[8] The authors describe how the Russian invasion not only caused a profound internal crisis within the once biggest Orthodox denomination, the Ukrainian Orthodox Church of the Moscow Patriarchate, but also how the increasingly salient

8 Religious Pluralism Story Map, *Mapa. Digital Atlas of Ukraine*, 2019, https://harvard-cga.maps.arcgis.com/apps/MapSeries/index.html?appid=9d7160c9e77a4f7bbd0384fe60eb3e2a [accessed 18.06.2024].

position of a national component over a religious one constitutes a major transformation within Ukrainian religious communities. The following two essays uncover the experiences of two ethnic minority groups – Roma and Crimean Tatars – who are becoming more visible and acknowledged as part of the Ukrainian political nation. Mykola Homanyuk and Janush Panchenko illustrate how one notable incident reported in the media (an alleged theft of a Russian tank by Romani individuals from the village of Lyubymivka in the Kherson region) made not only a substantial impact on the Roma community but also may overcome negative stereotypes towards their perception as Ukrainian Roma within Ukrainian society and the nation at large. A rather personal essay by Emine Ziyatdinova recounts the experiences of three generations of Crimean Tatar women – the author's grandmother, mother, and herself – spanning from 1937 to 2022. It brings attention to the difficulties faced by Crimean Tatars in reclaiming their history, from the 1937–1938 repressions, the 1944 deportations to the ongoing struggle to preserve the Crimean Tatar language and culture. The essay questions the historical narratives imposed by Russian and Soviet authorities and the current occupation. She argues that the inclusion of ethnic and other minority groups into the idea of Ukrainian statehood remains potentially fragile if only measured in terms of position and contribution during wartimes. The last text of the Dossier brings to attention another invisible group – cancer patients. Olha Labur discusses the severe effects of the Russian invasion of Ukraine on the oncological care system of Ukraine, including the destruction of medical infrastructure and the termination of cancer treatments. The text analyses the intersection of war and cancer, highlighting the militarisation of the cancer-related media space through the use of military vocabulary and metaphors in discussing cancer, drawing parallels between the two fronts – the war with Russia and the battle against cancer. She also explores the experiences of cancer patients who became refugees, leaving Ukraine to seek treatment abroad. Their stories reflect the temporary nature of the 'window of opportunities' in accessing medications, innovative treatments, and the high cost of care, as well as the prominent role of voluntary organisations in overcoming those difficulties.

All texts collected in this Dossier were written by Ukrainian scholars under the duress of war and displacement.[9] Many of the authors base their contributions on interviews they conducted on social media and online resources. We think that, individually and together, the essays underline the need for a nuanced understanding and invite more research into the evolving consequences of the Russian war in Ukraine, for Ukraine, for Europe, and for its neighbouring regions. The identification of key questions and research problems related to War, Migration, and Memory through a Ukrainian prism is the basic idea of our publication. We consider this collection to be a significant step towards establishing the intellectual legitimacy of

9 All texts of this Dossier underwent a double blind peer review process.

Ukrainian voices as well as a contribution to the search for an appropriate comparative framework, methodological perspectives, and, ultimately, a new analytical language for describing our part of Europe.

Acknowledgements

This publication emerged from a web of various institutional and intellectual impulses. One was Prisma Ukraïna – Research Network Eastern Europe, initiated in 2014 by Andrii Portnov (Professor of Entangled History of Ukraine, European University Viadrina and Co-Director of the Viadrina Center of Polish and Ukrainian Studies) and hosted at the Forum Transregionale Studien since the beginnings. Prisma Ukraïna is based on the cooperation of scholars from various institutions in and around Berlin.[10] The central idea of the program is to look at Ukraine not as an object but as a site and a prism for questions that are relevant to Europe and its neighbouring regions. Prisma Ukraïna probes the idea of open area studies and analyses questions in and of Ukraine by employing Ukrainian and regional expertise and transregional comparisons. With funding from the Land Berlin and private foundations, it invites scholars from Ukraine and neighbouring countries for fellowships and arranges workshops and transregional academies held in Berlin, Dnipro, Sofia, or Warsaw on themes such as history and memory, the politics of history or the shadows of empires.

Based on these legacies and networks, and in reaction to Russia's full-scale invasion, a new interdisciplinary research group of Ukrainian scholars in Ukraine and Germany, Prisma Ukraïna: *War, Migration, Memory*, was constituted in summer 2022 based on the ideas of Viktoriya Sereda and the experience of the Forum Transregionale Studien in arranging decentral college-like groups of scholars. Sereda was appointed as a Senior Fellow of the Forum Transregionale Studien for the years 2022–2023 to direct the research group. The main idea of the research group has been to investigate the transformational effects of war and dislocation on people's memory, history, and sense of belonging. The change of memory, historiography, perhaps even of history itself in times of upheaval certainly raises questions and interest not only in Ukraine or Eastern Europe but also in its former west, north,

10 Centre Marc Bloch, Deutsche Gesellschaft für Osteuropakunde (DGO), Europa-Universität Viadrina Frankfurt (Oder), Osteuropa-Institut, Freie Universität Berlin, Institut für Slawistik, Humboldt-Universität zu Berlin, Institut für Sozialwissenschaften, Humboldt-Universität zu Berlin, Institut für Slawistik, Universität Potsdam, Leibniz-Zentrum für Literatur- und Kulturforschung, Berlin, Zentrum für Zeithistorische Forschung, Potsdam, Deutsches Historisches Institut Warschau, Wissenschaftskolleg zu Berlin, Zentrum für Osteuropa- und internationale Studien (ZOiS).

and south as well. The research group currently consists of ten Ukrainian academics in Ukraine and at their places of refuge in Germany and Switzerland.

The first phase (2022–2023) of Prisma Ukraïna: *War, Migration, Memory* was realised with funding from the Berlin Senate Department for Higher Education and Research, Health, and Long-Term Care. The ZEIT STIFTUNG BUCERIUS and the Marga and Kurt Möllgaard Foundation provided funding for sur-place or non-resident fellowships for scholars in Ukraine affected by the war. The support of the Forum, the Land of Berlin, and the two foundations enabled the group to conduct their individual and collaborative research projects through fellowships and academic events. For instance, in October 2022, the first larger hybrid workshop for the project, "Studying Migration and Memory in Times of War", organised at the Forum, brought together the Ukrainian members of the group, other Ukrainian scholars displaced in Germany with similar research foci, and scholars from different German and Austrian institutions and foundations researching memory or displacement to discuss methodological questions. The Fellows also broadened their network and thematic insights during the monthly online Prisma Ukraïna seminar, "Rethinking East European Studies in Times of Upheaval", chaired by Andrii Portnov. In February 2023, the "Prisma Ukraïna Book Talk" series was launched, where scholars discussed their recently published books on Ukraine or other topics related to the project. All public and hybrid events provided opportunities for networking and connecting across disciplines, countries, and regions during times of war and displacement. All these activities helped us and the contributors to this Dossier to generate new research questions, crystallise conceptual frameworks or research designs, and opened avenues for reciprocal learning and knowledge sharing. We are grateful to the Forum Transregionale Studien, its staff, and all donors for their support of the project activities and for the publication of this volume, as well as to all participants and authors for their involvement in this fruitful exchange of ideas. The vibrant, international environment of the Forum further enabled the Fellows to develop comparative perspectives due to the exchange of ideas and experiences on currently debated questions in the fields of science policy, epistemology, and ethics, among other things.

A major part of the contributions to this volume emerged from the work of our *War, Migration, Memory* research group. All its members contributed to this volume. First, we had to adjust the umbrella topic of "War, Migration, Memory" to provide for individual research and for cohesion between an interdisciplinary group of scholars (coming from history, sociology, philosophy, anthropology, social linguistics, arts, and religious studies) in a way that provided meaning to all participants. It was important to find issues that are relevant not only for Ukrainian scholars or German academia but also for scholars from other regions of the world to stimulate a multivocal discussion and mutual rethinking instead of 'dialogical' structures or ways of 'monological informing' by a particular side or a particular group of experts.

One of the unexpected effects of the project was that all scholars, irrespective of their disciplinary approach, felt that it was important to record and document the experiences of their compatriots and the changes in their society concerning the war. We discussed the significance of records and archival materials for an understanding of past events and felt responsible for the collection of data and documentation of current history. As one Fellow wrote in a feedback, “everything is unfolding in front of us, and it is important to record and understand it”. In their personal accounts published on the TRAFO – Blog for Transregional Research and in feedback form, many Fellows admitted that the war either made them radically shift their focus or return to problems they studied earlier. War brought about a new sense of relevance. The collaborative work and publications of the group members were facilitated by the science communication and administrative team at the Forum Transregionale Studien, namely Tamara Beresh, Natasha Klimenko, Simon Kötschau, Sophie Schmäing, and Judith Sieber. We highly appreciate their considerate editorial expertise, the respectful and engaged cooperation, and their administrative support. Based on the principle of non-hierarchical openness, the project members defined the focus, structure, and content of their work and collaboration. They discussed ideas and themes in seminars and workshops and shared them on Trafo-Hub, the Forum's virtual communication platform. The research group members developed the concept for this volume in cooperation with the editor and suggested additional external contributors. We would like to thank all those involved for the invaluable discussions and the respectful and productive collaboration on this volume. Many thanks to all authors, Fellows, and the Forum Transregionale Studien, especially Georges Khalil, for their continuous support and mindful feedback. Many more people made this publication possible. We are grateful to Mark Berman and Natasha Klimenko for thoroughly copy-editing the articles, as well as to Alex Favalli and Martin Lochthofen for proofreading the contributions to this volume.

This volume is a result of these ongoing collaborative efforts. It is published during the second phase of the project (2024–2025), which itself is another result of our joint work, made possible on the basis of a renewed research agenda developed collectively by the members of the group and the generous funding by the Gerda Henkel Foundation, which supports the research group with individual stipends for the Ukrainian researchers and additional funds for academic events and science communication. The Berlin Senate Department for Higher Education and Research, Health, and Long-Term Care provides funding for personnel costs for the Forum, whose staff, inspiration, and support we would like to acknowledge with gratitude.

Bibliography

De Cordier, Bruno, "Ukraine's Vendée War? A look at the 'resistance identity' of the Donbass insurgency", *Russian Analytical Digest* 198, 2017, 2–6.

Fedor, Julie, Markku Kangaspuro, Jussi Lassila, and Tatiana Zhurzhenko (eds.), *War and Memory in Russia, Ukraine and Belarus*, New York: Palgrave Macmillan, 2017.

Gatrell, Peter, *A Whole Empire Walking: Refugees in Russia during World War I*, Bloomington: Indiana University Press, 1999.

Halilovich, Hariz, "Reclaiming erased lives: archives, records and memories in post-war Bosnia and the Bosnian diaspora", *Archival Science* 14/3, 2014, 231–247.

Haugbolle, Sune, *War and Memory in Lebanon*, Cambridge: Cambridge University Press, 2010.

Hrytsenko, Oleksandr, *Prezydenty i pamyat': Polityka pamyati prezydentiv Ukrayiny (1994–2014), pidgruntya, poslannya, realizatsiya, rezul'taty*, Kyiv: KIS, 2017.

Huntington, Samuel P., "The Clash of Civilizations?", *Foreign Affairs* 72/3, 1993, 99–118.

Kasianov, Georgiy, *Memory Crash*, Budapest: Central European University Press, 2022.

Katchanovski, Ivan, "East or West? Regional Political Divisions in Ukraine since the 'Orange Revolution' and the 'Euromaidan'", paper prepared for the Annual Meeting of the American Political Science Association in Washington DC, 28–31 August 2014.

Khmelko, Valeriy, "Iz-za chego politikam udaetsia raskalyvat Ukrainu", *Vechernii Lugansk* 24, 2006.

Kravchenko, Volodymyr, "Fighting the Shadow: The Soviet Past in the Historical Memory of Contemporary Ukrainian Society (RUS)", *Ab Imperio* 2, 2004, 329–369.

Kudriavtseva, Natalia, "Contested names in the toponymic landscapes of post-soviet space", *Ideology and Politics Journal* 1/15, 2020, 4–10.

Kuzio, Taras, "Competing Nationalisms, Euromaidan, and the Russian-Ukrainian Conflict", *Studies in Ethnicity and Nationalism* 15/1, 2015, 157–169.

Liebich, André, Oksana Myshlovska, and Viktoriya Sereda, "The Ukrainian Past and Present: Legacies, Memory and Attitudes", in: Oksana Myshlovska and Ulrich Schmid, *Regionalism without Regions. Reconceptualizing Ukraine's Heterogeneity*, Budapest: Central European University Press, 2019, 67–134.

Makeev, Serhey, Alla Patrakova, "Rehional'na spetsyfikatsiya sotsiokul'turnykh vidminnostey v Ukrayini", *Sotsiolohiya: teoriya, metody, marketynh* 3, 2004, 109–125.

Milich, Stephan, Friederike Pannewick and Leslie Tramontini (eds.), *Conflicting Narratives: War, Trauma and Memory in Iraqi Culture*, Wiesbaden: Reichert Verlag, 2012.

Plokhy, Serhii (ed.), *The Future of the Past: New Perspectives on Ukrainian History*, Cambridge: Harvard Ukrainian Research Institute, 2016.

Portnov, Andrii, *Poland and Ukraine: Entangled Histories, Asymmetric Memories*, Berlin: Forum Transregionale Studien, 2020.

Quinn, Ryan W. and Monica C. Worline, "Enabling Courageous Collective Action: Conversations from United Airlines Flight 93", *Organization Science* 19/4, 2008, 497–516.

Religious Pluralism Story Map, Mapa. Digital Atlas of Ukraine, 2019, https://harvard-cga.maps.arcgis.com/apps/MapSeries/index.html?appid=9d7160c9e77a4f7bbd0384fe60eb3e2a [accessed 18.06.2024].

Rjabtschuk, Mykola, *Die reale und die imaginierte Ukraine*, Berlin: Suhrkamp, 2005.

Sereda, Viktoriya, "Rehional'ni vymiry ukrayinskoho sotsiumu istorychne mynule ta natsionalni identychnosti", *Ahora. Ukrayina–rehional'nyy vymir*, 3, 2006, 29–41.

Sereda, Viktoriya, "Regional Historical Identities in Ukraine: Case Study of Lviv and Donetsk", *Naukovi Zapysky: Natsional'nyy universytet "Kyevo-Mohylyans'ka Akademiya", Sotsiolohichni nauky* 20, 2002, 26–34.

Stoll, Katrin, "Transcending the divide between history and memory: Szymon Datner's practical Holocaust historiography in the early post-war period", *Holocaust Studies: A Journal of History and Culture* 21, 2015, 4–23.

Törnquist-Plewa, Barbara and Yuliya Yurchuk, "Memory politics in contemporary Ukraine: Reflections from the postcolonial perspective", *Memory Studies* 12/6, 2019, 699–720.

Watson, Janet S., *Fighting Different Wars: Experience, Memory, and the First World War in Britain*, Cambridge: Cambridge University Press, 2004.

Wilson, Andrew, *The Ukrainians: Unexpected Nation*, New Heaven-London: Yale University Press, 2015.

Wilson, Andrew, "The Donbas Between Ukraine and Russia: The Use of History in Political Disputes", *Journal of Contemporary History* 30/2, 1995, 265–289.

War and Memory

Memories of the War and the War of Memories

Roman Holyk

War, as a tectonic fracture of social life, is the source of such deep and all-consuming experiences that they become a key constituent of individual and collective memories. War, as socially organised violence, is also viewed differently. Some authors consider humans to be "the most dangerous animal" in whom natural aggressiveness is combined with intelligence and the ability for social organisation.[1] Paradoxically, (and known to these observers,) the dark side of this capacity for social cooperation is how often it is used to promulgate conflict. This makes humans ready for violence and war. At the same time, from this point of view, war as violence is dehumanisation, evolutionary degeneration, and a regression of humanity. War opponents claim that war is not socially and sociobiologically inevitable and that the forms and methods of resolving armed conflict are determined by culture and the ideas different societies have about what war is[2]. Collective, cultural, individual, and communicative memories of war are determined by both public discourse and an individual reaction to war as an upheaval in social life and an event with widespread physical destruction.[3]

1 David Livingstone Smith, *The Most Dangerous Animal: Human Nature and the Origins of War*, New York: St. Martin's Press, 2007.

2 Brian R. Ferguson, "Ten Points on War", *Social Analysis* 52/2, 2008, 32–49.

3 This is both an integrative memory and a confrontational memory, a memory of one's own traumatic experiences and a memory that glorifies and idealises armed confrontation, a memory that condemns war, a memory of fear, and a memory traumatised and stigmatised by history. The collective and cultural memory of the war, as well as the individual memory of the participants in the war, can be described as a pathophysiological phenomenon. This is a damaged, injured, deformed, and lacunar memory, from which the most traumatic moments have been erased or torn. However, the individual memory of the war can also be filled with traumatic experiences that lead to psychopathology, which must be pushed out to the subconscious after the war. War provokes real/physical and virtual injuries, and individual or social amnesia or the deformation of consciousness and thinking. For more, see: William A. White, *Thoughts of a Psychiatrist on the War and After*, New York: Paul B. Hoeber, 1919. For an individual, the impressions of war are often chaotic, and it is the collective cultural memory of the war that organises and directs this individual memory, in the process selecting it. This is how the 'immediate' and 'short-term' vis-à-vis the distanced, long-term, and remote memory of the war appears. Radically different versions of the war give rise to either a war of memo-

Modern and Postmodern War Memories: Ukrainian and Russian Contexts

Modern Ukrainian and Russian personal/direct and collective/mediated/constructed memories of war have a long tradition.[4] The modern Russian tradition of heroising war dates back to at least Leo Tolstoy's novel *War and Peace* (*Voina i mir*, 1865–1869) or Mikhail Lermontov's poem "Borodino" (1837). In the formation of this tradition, texts that depict key events and images from the First World War,[5] the Revolution of 1917, and the postrevolutionary Civil War in Russia played an important role.[6] These and other texts and films[7] laid the foundation for the Russian as well as the Soviet perception of war in the 20th century. In Ukrainian historical memory, the First World War and the Civil War were seen with the established division of 'own'/'ours' ('*svoihk*') and 'foreign'/'theirs' ('*chuzhykh*') in Russian and Ukrainian memories of the wars of the 20th century.[8]

---

ries of different communities, or a shared memory of one community. Both can become tools of information warfare, and both (ideally) need reconciliation, coordination, and correlation.

4 Julie Fedor, Markku Kangaspuro, Jussi Lassila, Tatiana Zhurzhenko (eds.), *War and Memory in Russia, Ukraine and Belarus*, London: Palgrave Macmillan, 2017.

5 In a rare instance, NATO Secretary General Jens Stoltenberg compared Russia's war in Ukraine from 2022 to 2023 (and in particular Bakhmut in 2023) with the events of World War I: "Russia is throwing waves of soldiers against the Ukrainian defense lines in a way we haven't seen since the First World War". Justina Ilkevičiūtė, "'Russia is constantly planning for new offensives' – interview with NATO chief Stoltenberg", *Lithuanian Radio and Television (LRT)*, 28 February 2023, https://www.lrt.lt/en/news-in-english/19/1923076/russia-is-constantly-planning-for-new-offensives-interview-with-nato-chief-stoltenberg/ [accessed: 28.02.2023].

6 Sheila Fitzpatrick, "The Civil War as a Formative Experience", in: Abbot Gleason, Peter Kenez, and Richard Stites (eds.), *Bolshevik Culture: Experiment and Order in the Russian Revolution*, Bloomington: Indiana University Press, 1985, 57–76.

7 For literary texts, see, for example, Dmitry Furmanov's *Chapaev* (1923) and Mikhail Bulgakov's *Belaya gvardiya* (*The White Guard*, 1925). For films, see, for example, *Chapayev* (1934) by Georgi and Sergei Vasilev and *Neulovimye mstiteli* (*The Elusive Avengers*, 1967) by Edmond Keosayan.

8 This imagination formed through non-Soviet visions of war refugees in the works of Katria Hrynyevycheva or the representations of extreme experience of prisoners of war (POWs) in the works of Osyp Turyansky (e.g., *Poza mezhamy boliu*, *Beyond the Pain*, 1989), as well as through the image of the anti-Soviet 'national revolution' of 1917–1921 in interwar Western Ukrainian artistic texts. In Ukrainian Soviet literature and culture, the idea of the 'Great October Socialist Revolution' and the Civil War took various forms: from the romantic *Vershnyky* (*The Riders*, 1935) by Iurii Ianovskii to *Arsenal* (1929) and *Shchors* (1939) by Oleksandr Dovzhenko. Here, as in Russian socialist literature, the image of one's own (Ukrainian Soviet and Russian Soviet) soldier was formed. This soldier defeats the enemies of the Soviet government and working people, such as the 'Denikinians', 'Vrangelovians', 'Petlyurians', and 'Makhnovians'. In Ukrainian non-Soviet literature, on the contrary, Ukrainian Sich Riflemen became heroes, fighting first against the Russian Imperial Army, and then, together with the army of the Ukrainian People's Republic (and in particular under the leadership of Simon Petliura) against the Communists/Bolsheviks.

In the Soviet Union, there was an attempt to form an official Ukrainian and Russian war memory according to the same model to potentially form a common Soviet historical memory. At the same time, the Russian Soviet image of the Second World War[9] was constructed along the lines of the mythology of the 'Great Patriotic War', which became even more ideological and controversial when compared to Ukrainian Soviet literature that depicted the war in a similar, but slightly different way.[10] Already in this memory model, the dichotomy of the 'Ukrainian and Russian Soviet soldier' and their antipodes of the 'German fascist occupier', 'Nazi', and 'fascist' was established. The image of a Soviet intelligence officer – as seen in Vladimir Basov's film *The Shield and the Sword* (*Shchit i mech*, 1968) and Yulian Semyonov's *Seventeen Moments of Spring* (*Semnadtsat mgnovenii vesny*, 1973) – also became significant for Soviet historical memory.[11] Subsequently, the figures of postwar counterintelligence agents from the USSR and Eastern Bloc countries were added to it. These later figures fought with 'capitalist intelligence' agents (from Western Europe and the USA) or hunted Nazis (as in Semyonov's *TASS is Authorised to Declare…*, *TASS upolnomochen zayavit…*, 1984, and *Confrontation*, *Protivostoyanie*, 1985). Negative depictions of anti-Soviet partisans who fought against the Red Army in Western Ukraine also featured, unsur-

9 See texts such as *Vasili Tyorkin* (1941–1945) by Aleksandr Tvardovsky, *Semnadtsat mgnovenii vesny* (*Seventeen Moments of Spring*, 1973) by Yulian Semyonov, and *Zhizn i sudba* (*Life and Fate*, 1959) by Vasiliy Grossman.

10 See, for example, the romanticised *Praporonostsi* (*The Standard Bearers*, 1946–1948) by Oles Honchar or *Bytva za nashu Sovetskuiu Ukraynu* (*Ukraine in Flames*, 1943) by Oleksandr Dovzhenko.

11 The memory of the Second World War is central when describing the war in Ukraine in 2022. Russian propaganda created the image of the 'Ukrainian neo-Nazis' who could attack Russia, like the German Nazis who once attacked the USSR. In the Ukrainian imagination, on the contrary, Putin's Russian Federation is identified with Hitler's Germany, and simultaneously with the repressive Stalinist USSR. For example, the Russians fighting at Bakhmut and Soledar are associated with the strategically meaningless losses of Soviet soldiers in the Battles of Rzhev in World War II. See: Artur Levchenko, "Ia zahynuv pid Bakhmutom. Rosiiany bilshe ne mozhut povtoryty" ("I Died Near Bakhmut: The Russians Can No Longer Repeat"), *Zaxid.Net*, 2023, https://zaxid.net/ya_zaginuv_pid_bahmutom_n1556155 [accessed: 31.07.2024]. Less often, the Russo–Ukrainian War of 2022 is contextualised in the memory of other wars of the late 20th and early 21st centuries. It has been compared with the wars in Syria and Afghanistan (by the Prime Minister of Hungary, Viktor Orban), as well as with the Yugoslav Wars. See: Rob Myers, "The War in Ukraine Through Some Memories of the Yugoslav *Wars*", *Insurgent Notes: Journal of Communist Theory and Practice*, 29 December 2022, http://insurgentnotes.com/2022/12/the-war-in-ukraine-through-some-memories-of-the-yugoslav-wars/ [accessed: 31.07.2024]; and Rod Dreher, "Viktor Orban: West Is 'In A War With Russia'", *The American Conservative*, 26 January 2023, https://www.theamericanconservative.com/viktor-orban-we-are-in-a-war-with-russia/ [accessed: 31.07.2024].

prisingly, in Soviet discourse.[12] These stereotypes were reactualised in post-Soviet Russian, and partly also in Ukrainian, cultural memories. Meanwhile, based on the cultural memories of émigrés, positive representations of Ukrainian anti-Communist partisans/rebels who fought against the Soviets/Russians for the independence of Ukraine were incorporated into post-Soviet Ukrainian cultural discourse.[13] But Soviet images of the Second World War, as the Great Patriotic War, and its heroes also remained on Ukrainian television screens and in Ukrainian culture and places of memory.[14] Lastly, the general scheme of the reception of the interaction between Soviet Ukraine and Russia as parts of the USSR in peacetime and wartime that was fixed in Soviet memory was also visibly present.[15]

Ukrainian post-Soviet memory of the war developed in different directions during different periods. Ukrainian memory politics oscillated between 'war' and 'peace' vis-à-vis their main contender, Russian collective memory.[16] Post-Soviet Ukrainian memory of the war was more heterogeneous, containing both anti-Soviet (which opponents called nationalist and anti-Russian) and pro-Soviet (which

---

12 In the Soviet discourse, they were described as 'Banderites'/'Nazi allies' or 'Ukrainian bourgeois nationalists', and both were associated with the surname of the leader of the Organisation of Ukrainian Nationalists (OUN), Stepan Bandera, and with the idea of the 'bandit' and the 'criminal'. See, for example, the propagandistic texts of Yaroslav Galan or Volodymyr Belyaev as well as Yuriy Ilyenko's *Bilyi ptakh z chornoiu oznakoiu* (*The White Bird Marked with Black*, 1971) or Timofyi Levchuk's *Duma o Kovpake* (*The Poem of Kovpak*, 1973, 1975, 1977) film series.

13 See the novels *Braty hromu* (*Brothers of Thunder*, 2009) by Mykhailo Andrusiak and *Vohnenni stovpy* (*Pillars of Fire*, 2006) by Roman Ivanychuk as well as the films *Zalizna sotnya* (*The Iron Hundred*, 2004) and *Neskorenyy* (*The Undefeated*, 2000) by Oles Yanchuk.

14 Tatiana Zurchenko, "Shared Memory Culture? Nationalizing the 'Great Patriotic War' in the Ukrainian–Russian Borderlands", in: Małgorzata Pakier and Joanna Wawrzyniak (eds), *Memory and Change in Europe: Eastern Perspectives*, Oxford: Berghahn, 2016, 169–192.

15 Serhy Yekelchyk, *Stalin's Empire of Memory: Russian–Ukrainian Relations in the Soviet Historical Imagination*, Toronto: University of Toronto Press, 2004.

16 Oleksandr Hrytsenko, *Prezydenty i pamiat. Polityka pamiati prezydentiv Ukrainy (1994–2014): pidgruntia, poslannia, realizatsiia, rezultaty. (Presidents and Memory: The Policy of Memory of the Presidents of Ukraine (1994–2014): Background, Message, Implementation, Results*), Kyiv: K.I.S., 2017; Oksana Shevel, "The Politics of Memory in a Divided Society: A Comparison of Post-Franco Spain and Post-Soviet Ukraine", *Slavic Review*, 1, 2011, 137–164; Andriy Portnov, "Memory Wars in Post-Soviet Ukraine (1991–2010)", in: Uilleam Blacker, Alexander Etkind, and Julie Fedor (eds.), *Memory and Theory in Eastern Europe*, New York: Palgrave Macmillan, 2013, 233–254; Anna Wylegała and Małgorzata Głowacka-Grajper (eds.), *The Burden of the Past: History, Memory, and Identity in Contemporary Ukraine*, Bloomington: Indiana University Press, 2020; and Tatiana Zhurzhenko, "Legislating Historical Memory in Post-Soviet Ukraine", in: Eleazar Barkan and Ariella Lang (eds.), *Memory Laws and Historical Justice*, London: Palgrave Macmillan Cham, 2022, 97–130.

opponents called retrograde and pro-Russian) divisions. This also led to the regionalisation of memory in Ukraine.[17] At the same time, the Soviet/Russian paradigm of memory remained very influential, especially on the level of mass culture. This was facilitated by both a shared Russo–Ukrainian mass media communicative space – which existed substantially until at least 2014 and continued in diminished form until 2022 – and by Russo–Ukrainian bilingualism – which was a channel for the formation of hybrid Russo–Ukrainian memories.[18] The struggle between different types of memory provoked sharp discussions around topics like, for example, the Holodomor (1932–1933)[19] and figures and movements from Ukrainian history from the 1920s onward (e.g., Stepan Bandera, Roman Shukhevych, the Organisation of Ukrainian Nationalists, and the Ukrainian Insurgent Army).[20] Eventually, the events of the Orange Revolution (2004–2005) and the Revolution of Dignity/Euromaidan (2013–2014) became sites for the wars of memory as well. In the latter case, pro-Ukrainian Maidan positions (centred around nodes like the Warriors of Light/the Order of the Heavenly Hundred – i.e., activists who died on the Maidan in 2014)[21] confronted the pro-Russian anti-Maidan stance in Kyiv.

---

17 Viktoriya Sereda, "Regional Historical Identities and Memory", in: Yaroslav Hrytsak, Andrii Portnov, and Victor Susak (eds.), *Lviv-Donetsk: sotsialni identychnosti v suchasnii Ukraini. Ukraina Moderna. Spetsialnyi vypusk* (*Lviv-Donetsk: Social Identities in Modern Ukraine. Modern Ukraine, Special issue*), Lviv-Kyiv: Krytyka, 2007, 160–209; and Roman Holyk, "'Tsentr ukrainskoho Skhodu' y 'Natsionalnyi Piemont': 'donbaski' siuzhety halytskoi kulturnoi pamiati" ("The 'Centre of the Ukrainian East" and 'National Piedmont': The 'Donbas' Plots of Galician Cultural Memory), in: Mykola Lytvyn (ed.), *Mizh viinoiu i sobornistiu. Sotsiokulturna intehratsiia ta adaptatsiia pereselentsiv z Donbasu ta Kpymu. Zakhidnoukpainskyi vektor* (*Between War and Unity: The Sociocultural Integration and Adaptation of Immigrants from the Donbas and Crimea, the Western Ukrainian Vector*), Lviv: I. Krypyakevych Institute of Ukrainian Studies, 2017, 89–144.

18 Marco Puleri, *Ukrainian, Russophone, (Other) Russian: Hybrid Identities and Narratives*, Berlin: Peter Lang, 2020.

19 Georhii Kasianov, *Danse macabre: holod 1932–1933 rokiv u politytsi, masovii svidomosti ta istoriohrafii (1980-ti–pochatok 2000-kh)* (*Danse macabre: The Famine of 1932–1933 in Politics, Mass Consciousness, and Historiography (1980s–early 2000s)*, Kyiv: In-t istorii Ukrainy NAN Ukrainy and Nash chas, 2010. The Holodomor, which in historical memory appears as a kind of undeclared war of the Soviet authorities against the Ukrainian peasantry, is also a demonstrative example of historical trauma in the Ukrainian collective memory before the Second World War. Iryna Starovoyt, "Traumatic memories: from Holodomor to Maidan", in: Rob van der Laarse et al. (eds.), *Religion, state, society, and identity in transition: Ukraine*, Oisterwijk: Wolf Legal Publishers, 2015, 219–240.

20 For the discussions surrounding the name of Stepan Bandera in relation to traumatic memories of the events of 1939–1944 and the first postwar years in Western Ukraine, see: Yhor Balynskyi, Yaroslav Hrytsak, and Taryk Syryl Amar (eds.), *Strasti za Banderoiu: statti ta esei* (*Passions for Bandera: Articles and Essays*), Kyiv: Hrani-T, 2010.

21 In certain contexts, the Heavenly Hundred were contrasted with the Russian Immortal Regiment, originally intended to record the memory of the myth of the Great Patriotic War.

The Memory of the Russo-Ukrainian War from 2014 to 2023

In 2014, Russia's hybrid war in Ukraine highlighted the conflict between pro-Ukrainian and pro-Russian versions of historical and cultural memory.[22] In the occupied territories of Ukraine (Crimea and the Donbas), Russians and pro-Russian organisations began to fashion new local variants of Russian memory to describe the formation of the so-called 'Luhansk and Donetsk People's Republics'.[23] On the Ukrainian side, the collective consciousness and memories of events from 2014 onwards developed in the opposite direction.[24] During this period, each party tried to encode the other in cultural memory as the aggressor and perpetrator of war crimes. Accordingly, both sides published books on war crimes in the Donbas, which became tools in the wars of memories and perceptions. Russian propagandists, in particular, manipulatively used the name of the Organization for Security and Co-operation in Europe (OSCE) to construct a picture of the 'atrocities of the Ukrainian army'.[25] But this confrontation of memories eventually became 'frozen', with neither side able to claim new ground – just like in the physical war in Eastern Ukraine.

Subsequently, some Ukrainian politicians and businesspeople began to promote the idea of a relatively quick forgetting of the war (and a displacement of its trau-

---

22 Ultimately, the ideologies of Russian Orthodoxy, nationalism, and totalitarianism became the foundations of this war. See: Taras Kuzio, *Putin's War Against Ukraine: Revolution, Nationalism, and Crime*, Toronto: Chair of Ukrainian Studies, 2017; and Taras Kuzio, *Russian Nationalism and the Russian–Ukrainian War: Autocracy – Orthodoxy – Nationality*, London and New York: Routledge, 2022.

23 This included St. George ribbons as signs of the Great Victory over fascism and the cults of the 'heroes' of the so-called Donetsk People's Republic (DNR) and Luhansk People's Republic (LNR) (e.g., Mikhail Tolstykh "Givi" and Arsen Pavlov "Motorola") and of Crimea (the 'little green men' or 'polite people', i.e., disguised Russian military personnel). These symbols have been placed in opposition to those of the 'antiheroes' (e.g., 'Ukrainian occupiers' or 'dills', 'fascists', 'the Kyiv junta', and 'the Kyiv regime').

24 The hybrid war in Eastern Ukraine was associated with the figures of 'cyborgs' (i.e., the defenders of the Donetsk Airport), with the tragic events near Ilovaisk and Debaltseve (i.e., the encirclement and destruction of the Ukrainian military there), with the shooting down of Malaysia Airlines Flight 17 and the Russian Buk missile system, and with the figures of Russian antiheroes (e.g., 'separatists' or 'separs' and 'colorados' or 'Colorado beetles').

25 For the Russian side, see: The Foundation for the Study of Democracy, *War Crimes of the Armed Forces and Security Forces of Ukraine: torture and inhumane treatment*, report, April 2016, https://www.osce.org/files/f/documents/e/7/233896.pdf [accessed: 24.02.2023]. For the European and Ukrainian side, see: Małgorzata Gosiewska et al., *Report: Russian War Crimes in Eastern Ukraine in 2014*, report, *Ji-Magazine*, 2015, https://ji-magazine.lviv.ua/engl-vers/2015/Russian_War_Crimes_in_Eastern_Ukraine_in_2014.pdf [accessed: 31.07.2024].

matic memories).[26] However, the war of memories continued. The continuation of hostilities was evident in Russian school textbooks, which reinterpreted the history of Ukraine in a neocolonial style, preparing readers not for peace but for war.[27]

Russia's full-scale invasion of Ukraine on 24 February 2022 opened a new stage in this battle of memories. In Ukrainian discourse, the definitions of this event were unambiguous: it was called 'Russian aggression' and 'war'. By contrast, the Russian media declared the invasion a 'special military operation for the denazification and demilitarisation of Ukraine'. The ideological preparation for the Russo–Ukrainian War was an eight-year-long propagation of false and misleading images about the Ukrainian people and government by the Russian government for the Russian public. These images included the tropes of 'Ukrainian neo-Nazis and nationalists',[28] who precipitated 'the illegal coup in Kyiv in 2014' and 'the Kyiv regime'; the topics of 'the genocide of Russians in the Donbas' and the 'militarisation of Ukraine by NATO countries'; and talking points about the 'aggressive West' (i.e., Europe and the USA), the 'threat of creating a nuclear bomb in Ukraine', and, lastly, the 'artificiality' of Ukrainian statehood and Ukrainians as a people in general. On an unofficial level, the negative stereotypes of a Ukrainian as a '*Khokhol*' (a derogatory name for a Ukrainian, from the early modern Russian "khohol" – a tuft of hair on a shaved head) with little intrinsic worth and of Ukraine as the '*Khokhlands*' (a country of *Khokhls*) was promulgated. To this negative image of Ukrainians the ideas of 'good Little Russians' and 'good Little Russia' were added, which reside next to 'Novorossiya'. In general, the period starting in 2014 became a time of a war of words and concepts, which Ukrainian intellectuals tried to win and explain to Western readers.[29]

---

26 Anton Troianovski, "A Ukrainian Billionaire Fought Russia. Now He's Ready to Embrace It", *The New York Times*, 13 November 2019, https://www.nytimes.com/2019/11/13/world/europe/ukraine-ihor-kolomoisky-russia.html [accessed: 31.07.2024].

27 Vitalii Yaremchuk and Andrii Smirnov, *Analitychnyi ohliad "Istoriia Ukrainy v rosiiskykh shkilnykh pidruchnykakh z istorii" (An Analytical Review of "the History of Ukraine in Russian School History Textbooks")*, Kyiv: Almenda, 2023.

28 This attitude appeals to the memory of the Great Victory over German fascism in the Great Patriotic War and, in particular, to the campaign against Germany. The slogan of Russian propagandists is: "We can repeat it!" This idea is also visible in the inscriptions on Russian equipment and ammunition, such as, for example, "To Berlin!". Such slogans are in opposition to the interpretation of wars adopted in Ukraine and Europe: "Never again". Oleksii Polegkyi, "'Never again' vs. 'We can repeat it': Russians will pay any price to restore the glory of Soviet victory in WWII", *Forum for Ukrainian Studies*, 11 June 2022, https://ukrainian-studies.ca/2022/06/11/never-again-vs-we-can-repeat-it-russians-will-pay-any-price-to-restore-the-glory-of-soviet-victory-in-wwii%ef%bf%bc/ [accessed: 31.07.2024].

29 Andriy Kulakov et al. (eds.), *Words and Wars: Ukraine facing Kremlin propaganda*, Kyiv: KIC, 2017.

On the other side, Ukrainians called the aggression 'Putin's attack', and coined terms such as 'Ruscism'/'Rucsianism' and 'Ruscist'/'Ruscianist' (combining 'Russian' with 'fascism'), 'Putinists', and 'Pushkinists'.[30] As a result, in Ukrainian discourse, Russian troops began to be depicted in dehumanised (e.g., 'pig-dogs') or ethnographised (e.g., '*lapti* legs'[31]) ways, as monstrous, hybrid creatures. This could also take the form of literary monsters (e.g., orcs or goblins), while Russia could be shown as Mordor and its leaders as 'Saurons'. These images stemmed from J.R.R. Tolkien's *The Lord of the Rings*. Additionally, Russia's leaders could also be presented as 'Voldemorts', based on the villain from J.K. Rowling's *Harry Potter* series.[32]

The Russo–Ukrainian War of 2022 also became a war of visual symbols. These symbols included Russian identification signs in the form of special letters: Z, O, V, X, and A.[33] The Ukrainian side saw in Russian visual symbols the distinguishing marks of the troops of Nazi Germany.[34] To counter the Russian imagery, the Ukrainian army began using the sign of the cross, among other symbols, relying on its obvious religious significance. The linguistic context for the war of visual sym-

30 In this discourse, 'Putinists' are supporters of Russian President Vladimir Putin. Fans of the Russian poet Alexander Pushkin and supporters of the Russian language, and Russian literature and culture in general, are called 'Pushkinists' in the Ukrainian military lexicon.

31 *Lapti* are archaic footwear made of tree bark, which in Ukrainian discourse, in contrast to the Ukrainian analogues of *lychaks*, are considered a marker of Russian peasant culture and Russian national identity.

32 Serhy Yekelchyk, "Naming the War: Russian aggression in Ukrainian Official Discourse and Mass Culture", *Canadian Slavonic Papers* 64/2–3, 2022, 232–246.

33 Julia Khrebtan-Hörhager and Evgeniya Pyatovskaya, "The Banality of Putin's Propaganda: A Dangerous Déjà vu", *Forum for Ukrainian Studies*, 26 September 2022, https://ukrainian-studies.ca/2022/09/26/the-banality-of-putins-propaganda-a-dangerous-deja-vu/ [accessed: 31.07.2024].

34 For example, the Ukrainian media discourse associates 'V' with the slogan "*Deutschland siegt an allen Fronten*" ("Germany is Victorious on All Fronts"), which appeared on famous landmarks including the Eiffel Tower and the Palais Bourbon in occupied Paris. 'Z', meanwhile, is associated with the emblems of the 4th SS Polizei Panzergrenadier Division, among other Nazi groups. Oleksandr Bekker, "Z — natsystskyi symvol samoznyshchennia Rosii" ("Z is the Nazi Symbol of Russia's Self-Destruction"), *ArmiiaInform* (*ArmyInformation*), 17 March 2022, https://armyinform.com.ua/2022/03/17/z-naczystskyj-symvol-samoznyshhennya-rosiyi/ [accessed: 31.07.2024].

bols became the spelling/orthographic war with Russia and its supporters on mass media and social networks.[35]

The Ukrainian memories of the war from 2022 to early 2023 are fixed in significant events, concepts, words, material objects, and figures.[36] These include air raid alarms, shelters, mobilisation, roadblocks, the ban on the departure of men abroad, the mass appearance of refugees, Russian 'tags' on military objects, the tracking of Russian agents/collaborators, rocket attacks (at first on military targets, and then on civil infrastructure), and, as a result of the rockets, blackouts, the destruction of thousands of civilian houses, and the devastation of important Ukrainian cultural sites. Russian war crimes, such as the genocide in Bucha, Hostomel, and Irpin,[37] as well as the mass burials in Mariupol, became important elements of the war memories. Russia used the simulacrum of the 'genocide of Russians and Russian speakers in the Donbas' as a pretext for the war. To counteract this damage, Ukraine is trying to establish in world memory the historical and geographical chain of Russian

35 This is expressed through writing the country's name and the names of its political leaders with lowercase letters. There is also a virtual struggle over the name 'Russia' and the ethnonym 'Russians'. Some of the Ukrainian narratives represent Russians retrospectively as 'Muscovites' and the country itself as 'Moscovia' (the Western name of present-day Russia and its inhabitants until the 18th century). The names 'Russia' and 'Russians' are described as 'stolen' ethnonyms or the former self-names of current Ukrainians. In response to the aggression, Ukrainians want to push names associated with Russia out of their memory, language use, and everyday life: the former 'Moscow' sausage became the 'Stolychna' or 'Chernihivska' sausage, 'Russian' cheese became 'Smetankovyji' cheese, and 'Borodino' bread became 'Trypilia' bread. Yuliia Semenets, "'Kovbasa "Moskovska" pishla vslid za korablem', – kazhut pokuptsiam chernihivski prodavtsi" ("'"Moskovska" Sausage Followed the Ship', Chernihiv Sellers Tell Customers"), *Texty.org.ua*, 18 July 2022, https://texty.org.ua/fragments/107271/kovbasa-moskovska-pishla-vslid-za-korablem-kazhut-pokuptsjam-chernihivski-prodavtsi/ [accessed: 31.07.2024].

36 Kateryna Topolyuk, "Rik nezlamnosti. Yak tse bulo dlia Lvova" ("The Year of Indomitability: How It Was for Lviv"), *032 Sayt mista Lvova* (*032 Website of the City of Lviv*), 24 February 2023, https://www.032.ua/news/3553072/rik-nezlamnosti-ak-ce-bulo-dla-lvova [accessed: 31.07.2024]; and Antonina Kostyk, "Yak mynuv rik povnomasshtabnoi viiny dlia Lvova: spohady, foto, tsyfry" ("How the Year of the Full-Scale War Passed for Lviv: Memories, Photos, Numbers"), *Tvoie misto* (*Your City*), 2023, https://tvoemisto.tv/exclusive/yak_mynuv_pershyy_den_povnomasshtabnogo_vtorgnennya_u_lvovi_ta_kudy_letily_rakety_144240.html [accessed: 31.07.2024].

37 These are cities and towns in the Kyiv Oblast. In very recent Ukrainian discourse and memory, they are considered 'hero cities' and 'cities of the mass murder of Ukrainians by the Russian Army'.

war crimes: Chechnya (1999–2009), Ukraine (2014), Syria (2015), and, again, Ukraine (2022).[38]

Weapons became another object of collective memory. On the one hand, this includes Russian missiles (in particular the Kalibr and Kinzhal/Dagger missiles) and Iranian drones (the Shahed), and on the other hand, Turkish Bayraktar drones, American portable antitank missile complex Javelins, and portable antiaircraft missile complex Stingers (and, subsequently, the Norwegian Advanced Surface-to-Air Missile System (NASAMS), the American High Mobility Artillery Rocket System (HIMARS), and German Leopard tanks). Another area of memory is the narratives of heroism and courage during the siege of Mariupol, and particularly of Azovstal.[39] Additionally there are 'memories of triumph', the liberation of part of the occupied territories (particularly Kherson[40]), and the concept of 'cotton'[41] – that is, strikes on Russian military facilities – all of which were established in mass culture. President of Ukraine Volodymyr Zelenskyy, Commander-in-Chief of the Armed Forces of Ukraine Valerii Zaluzhnyi, and, for some time, even former Advisor of the Office of the President Oleksiy Arestovych became iconic figures inhabiting this memory. Next to them appeared an animal hero, the literal and figurative 'bravest military dog Patron'.[42] The war also caused the appearance of new linguistic formulas and slogans, such as "Ukrainians will resist [the Russian aggression]", "say

38 Ministry of Culture and Information Policy of Ukraine, *Russia's War Crimes All Over the World: From Chechnya to Syria*, report, https://mkip.gov.ua/files/pdf/%D0%B7%D0%BB%D0%BE%D1%87%D0%B8%D0%BD%D0%B8_eng.pdf [accessed: 31.07.2024].

39 Azovstal (literally meaning 'Azov steel') is the name of the metallurgical plant in Mariupol (a Ukrainian city in the south of the Donetsk Oblast), which in 2022 became a battleground between Ukrainian defenders and the Russian military that surrounded it.

40 Kherson is an oblast in Southern Ukraine that in Ukrainian collective memory is often associated with watermelons, although the name itself refers to the ancient Greek/Byzantine name 'Khersones'.

41 This is due to the homography of the Russian words *khlopók* (meaning a short sound of impact, clapping, or a flash of gas less powerful than an explosion) and *khlópok* (meaning cotton). The Ukrainian military lexicon began to ironically call the Russian military discourse's references to explosions in the occupied territories of Ukraine and at Russian military facilities 'cotton'. This was present in internet memes.

42 Patron is the nickname of a dog that sniffed out explosives. This dog is presented as the mascot of the State Emergency Service of Ukraine and a symbol of the indomitability of the Ukrainian people in the fight against the Russian military. Patron the dog also became the hero of a recent Ukrainian song.

'*palianytsia*'!"[43], "to go with the Russian (war) ship",[44] "good evening, we are from Ukraine",[45] and "everything will be Ukraine".[46] In European and American memory, these expressions corresponded to conceptions of fearless Ukrainians: "Be brave, like Ukrainians".[47]

In stories about the full-scale Russo–Ukrainian War of 2022, even ordinary concepts and common things (e.g., 'earth', 'bus', 'thunder', 'lightning', 'lamp', 'letter', 'bear') acquired new connotations dependent, in some cases, on individual, in others, on collective perception.[48] Some of these connotations already had a certain semantic or semantic-symbolic tradition: for example, the bear as an archetype of Russia. However, even well-established references have been transformed under the influence of direct, day-to-day military conflict.

New Ukrainian heroes represent difficult terrain for collective memory. Here, 'heroic memory' and 'tragic memory' collide. On the one hand, there are soldiers who performed heroic feats (such as the pilot, the Ghost of Kyiv); on the other hand, there are those who perished in the war. New places of memory are associated with the latter, including the numerous new military cemeteries (e.g., the reactivated Mars Field near the Lychakiv Cemetery in Lviv[49]), which testify to the scale of the losses.

---

43 In Ukrainian, *palianytsia* is a type of bread. It is believed that this lexeme is difficult to articulate for those who use only the Russian language. Such words play the role of a 'shibboleth' – that is, a differential linguistic feature of a certain ethnonational community that are difficult to pronounce by the representatives of another community.

44 The phrase comes from the (obscene) expression of a soldier – a defender of the Ukrainian island Zmiinyi in the Black Sea and Odesa Oblast – who answered the representatives of the Russian cruiser Moskva, who offered the Ukrainians to surrender, "Russian warship, go fuck yourself".

45 The phrase, taken from a single of the musical group DakhaBrakha, which was distributed as early as 2021, became an unofficial military salute after the Russian aggression in 2022.

46 According to one version, this phrase was coined in 2014 or 2015 by representatives of the pro-Ukrainian forces of the Luhansk Oblast as a counterweight to the pro-Russian/separatist slogan "Everything will be Donbas!". The Ukrainian phrase was supposed to simultaneously signify the Ukrainian ownership of the territories occupied by the Russian Federation and be a substitute for the phrase "everything will be fine!".

47 This concept is reflected in the French book of the Ukrainian philosopher Konstantin Sigov. Konstantin Sigov, *Le courage de l'Ukraine* (*The Courage of Ukraine*), Paris: Éditions du Cerf, 2023.

48 For example, a bus as a place of rescue from Russian shells and as a transport to the Ukrainian checkpoint as a symbol of security. Ostap Slyvynskyi (ed.), *Slovnyk vijny* (*Dictionary of the War*), Kyiv: Vivat, 2023, p.14.

49 'Mars Field' or the 'Field of Mars' is an example of the changes in memory policy and memory places in 20th-century Eastern Europe. This military cemetery was established in Lviv/Lemberg during WWI for the burial of soldiers of the Austro–Hungarian Empire. After WWII, it was sovietised, the remains of Austrian soldiers were exhumed, and representatives of the Soviet Army and NKVD/MGB troops were buried in their place. After February

Part of the Russo–Ukrainian War is also a war of monuments and toponyms. On the territory occupied by the Russians, monuments and memorial signs related to Ukrainian history and culture are being removed from public places, and Ukrainian place names are changed to Russian ones. In a certain way, this mirrors the Ukrainian de-Sovietisation of cities and villages.[50] Meanwhile in Ukraine, monuments to Russian figures are also dismantled, and streets and squares named after famous Russians are renamed. Increasingly, this war becomes a war of languages, literatures, and cultures.[51]

The Russo–Ukrainian War contributes to the de-Russification of Ukrainian cultural and historical memory. Based on this new memory, novel Ukrainian identities are being formed, although it is still difficult to say which of them will become dominant. On the one hand, these identities are based on an almost total opposition of Russian identity in terms of language and culture (e.g., a Ukrainophone identity, or one based on the Ukrainian as opposed to the Russian language), religious denomination (e.g., the Orthodox Church of Ukraine and Ukrainian Greek Catholic Church versus the Russian Orthodox Church or the Ukrainian Orthodox Church of the Moscow Patriarchate), and ideology (e.g., the 'Ukrainian identity' against the '*russikiy mir*' (the 'Russian World'). On the other hand, a Russophone identity is also forming in Ukraine. This is ideologically, or even confessionally, opposed to a Russian identity, but relates to it through the Russian language and the inclusion of at least some Russian culture. This 'Ukrainian Russian culture' is still in the process of differentiating itself from 'Russian Russian culture'. At the same time, there are also other hybrid identities that combine Ukrainian and Russian linguistic and cultural identification in different configurations and to varying degrees. Each of these identities appeals to one or the other's cultural memory.

As long as the war has not ended, the memory of it is incomplete as well. Rather, the changing fortunes of war on the front and at home ensure that cultural and collective memory of the war is and will remain fragmented and internally differentiated. This manifests through internal migration and refugees. Particularly from 2014 to 2023, this occurred with the image of the migrant from Eastern Ukraine in the public discourses in the west of the country.[52] This was a reflection of the general

---

2022, instead of representatives of the Soviet armed forces, current Ukrainian soldiers who died in battles against the Russian Army began to be buried in the Field of Mars.

50 There are even discussions about renaming the occupied cities to their former Soviet names (e.g., Luhansk to Voroshilovograd).

51 Some people demanded the complete removal of the Russian language and Russian classics from school curricula. This would include the works of Pushkin, Tolstoy, and Fyodor Dostoyevsky, whom Ukrainian critics satirically call 'Tolstoyevsky'.

52 A significant portion of Internally Displaced Persons (IDPs) are perceived as 'us' and 'patriotic' figures who survived the occupation and whose memory recorded the horror of all-out urban battles. Some of them also internalised the new local identity despite their difficult

trends in the development of Ukrainian cultural and historical memory. On the one hand, this demonstrated the desire for reconciliation and the formation of an integrated and whole 'national memory'; on the other hand, it showed regionalisation and the opposition of different types of memory.

Because the Russo–Ukrainian War is ongoing, the memory of it is still an unfinished, dynamic, and unstable collection of different structures. Theoretically, the memories of the war in Ukraine can be imagined as a system divided into several zones. First are the memories of those who survived full-scale combat operations in the centre, east, and south of Ukraine. This may also be divided into several possible segments: the memories of soldiers engaged in direct combat; the memories of civilians who witnessed battles and war crimes; the memories of refugees/migrants or of those who remained; and the memories of those who survived the Russian occupation or captivity (among the military) as compared to those who were continuously in the territories controlled by Ukraine. War memories are also stratified according to gender and age. This can be broken up into the memories of women, men, and children.[53] Memories may also be differentiated based on professions, be it of politicians, writers, scientists, clergy members, military personnel, or energy workers (who restored the infrastructure destroyed by Russian strikes), or on types of dwellings, such as the memories of the residents of cities, towns, or villages, among other configurations.

---

living conditions in the cities of Western Ukraine. Ivan Stanislavskyi, "Novyi dim v staromu hurtozhytku. Yak pereselentsi zi Skhodu namahaiutsia vlashtuvaty svoie zhyttia u Lvovi Ivan Stanislavskyi" ("A New Home in an Old Dormitory: How IDPs from the East Are Trying to Organise Their Lives in Lviv"), *LB.ua*, 22 June 2022 https://lb.ua/society/2022/06/22/520803_noviy_dim_staromu_gurtozhitku_yak.html [accessed: 31.07.2024]. However, there are also cases where IDPs are seen as the Other, as people with a Soviet or post-Soviet memory and belonging to the 'Russian world'. In 2022, the situation changed, as the bearers of the different representations of Ukrainian memory were now seen as victims of the same war. Kateryna Sadlovska,and Anastasiia Yarmolovska, "Pereselenka z Mariupolia pratsiuie pediatrom u Lvovi" ("A Migrant from Mariupol Works as a Paediatrician in Lviv"), *Suspilne novyny* (*Public News*), 04 February 2023, https://suspilne.media/370849-pereselenka-z-mariupola-pracue-pediatrom-u-lvovi/ [accessed: 31.07.2024]; Olena Danylo and Kateryna Sadlovska, "Brat znyk bezvisty. Rozpovid mariupolky, yaka evakuiuvalasia z mista u veresni" ("Brother is Missing: The Story of a Mariupol Woman who Evacuated from the City in September"), *Suspilne novyny* (*Public News*), 15 January 2023, https://suspilne.media/358548-brat-znik-bez visti-rozpovid-mariupolki-aka-evakuuvalasa-z-mista-u-veresni/ [accessed: 31.07.2024]; and Kateryna Rodak, "Bilshist pereselentsiv na Lvivshchyni namahaiutsia hovoryty ukrainskoiu, – opytuvannia" ("Most of the Immigrants in the Lviv Try to Speak Ukrainian, According to a Survey"), *Zaxid.net*, 31 May 2022, https://zaxid.net/bilshist_pereselentsiv_na_lvivshhini_n amagayutsya_govoriti_ukrayinskoyu___opituvannya_n1543703 [accessed: 31.07.2024].

53 Aleksandra Boroń and Agnieszka Gromkowska-Melosik, *Ukraińskie uchodźczynie wojenne. Tożsamość, trauma, nadzieja* (*Ukrainian Female War Refugees: Identity, Trauma, Hope*), Kraków: Oficyna Wydawnicza Impuls, 2022.

All these memories differ territorially. The war memories of the civilian population of Western Ukraine are, to a certain extent, 'cold' and somewhat distant from the war.[54] In the 'hot' memories of Ukrainian soldiers on the frontline, the war is an image of real battles, weapons, enemies, and the lives and deaths of other soldiers or civilians. The 'memories of the front' largely differ from 'rear memories'. The memories of those who survived the occupation are ones that incorporate stories about Russian soldiers and their power, collaborators, the disoriented population, destruction, looting, murders, death threats, evacuations, and difficult material conditions (e.g., a lack of light, gas, water, food, etc.). All these memories are currently in the (unstable) deep structures of collective memory, and not on the surfaces of culture or literature.[55] On the Russian side, meanwhile, the perception of the war that started in 2022 is not very clear for various reasons (including totalitarian control over public opinion).[56]

---

54 This memory contains images of missile attacks, the victims and heroes from among the military (and their burial ceremonies), as well as book and television depictions of the war. It also holds images from heroic songs of the First World War, which gained popularity after February 2022, such as "Oi u luzi chervona kalyna" ("Oh, the Red Viburnum in the Meadow"), first published in 1875 and given a modern treatment in 1914 by Stepan Charnetsky to honour the Sich Riflemen of WWI.

55 They are partially reflected in academic tests, in the diaries and memories of the historian Vladyslav Verstyuk (*Dumky z pidvalu, Thoughts from the Cellar*, 2022) from Hostomel and Vorzel, in Valeriy Smoliy's reflections *Istorik i viina* (*The Historian and the War*, 2022), and in the studies of the first year of the confrontation (e.g., *Nad prirvoiu. 200 dniv rosiiskoi viiny, Over the Abyss: 200 Days of the Russian War*, 2022, by Volodymyr Horbulin and Valentyn Badrak). Other memoirs, diaries, interviews (as well as the documentary film *Hod, The Year*, 2023, by Dmytro Komarov) that form the overall picture of the aggression on 24 February 2022 and the following days and months record the images of 'indomitable' Ukrainian men and women, the monthly public speeches of the President of Ukraine during the war, and the chronicle of events (Olexandr Krasovytskyi series *Dvanadtsiat misiatsiv viiny. Khronika podii. Promovy ta zvernennia Prezydenta Volodymyra Zelenskoho (Twelve Months of War. Chronicle of events. Speeches and addresses of President Volodymyr Zelenskyi*, 2023). Attempts to fictionalise the memory of the war remain a problem. In the first steps, such intentions were perceived as conjunctures, and they were abandoned. However, later, even adventure books about the war appeared, such as the work of Andrii Kokotyukha *Taimer viiny. Dovha komendantska hodyna* (*War Timer. Long Curfew*, 2023). Some of the visual productions – including the film *Zvychainyi rashyzm* (*Ordinary Rashism*, 2023) by Ihor Piddubny, as a response to Mikhail Romm's film *Obyknovennyi fashizm* (*Ordinary Fascism*, 1965) – began to shape the image of the Russian enemy-aggressor in the cultural memory of Ukrainians. Currently, the (often pessimistic) memory from the fronts of war (the 'memory of losses') is rare in publications, because it is inconsistent with the optimistic memory of the rear (the 'memory of victories'). Despite everything, all memories are still a mosaic and partially 'closed', although in this, as in other war memories, 'post-memory' zones are already forming.

56 State propaganda portrays the heroism of Russian troops in the fight against neo-Nazis in works such as the book *Krasnye linii* (*Red Lines*, 2023) by Ivan Solovyov (its cover is decorated

The modern war of memories in the context of the Russo–Ukrainian War has at least three possible analogies in or can be based on three possible models stemming from European events in the 20th century, as well as their aftermath. The first is the case of the First World War and the interwar period. In 1918, a conflict arose in European collective memories between the memories of the victors (the Entente countries) and the memories of the vanquished (especially Germany and Austria). Initially, the memories of the victors dominated and shaped European historical and political discourse, but in the 1930s, resulting from the growing influence of Germany and its allies, these memories weakened and found a powerful opponent

with the Z symbol iconic for Russian propaganda). For the majority of Russians, the 'special operation in Ukraine' is a 'close distant war' or a 'distant close war'. For more, see: Svetlana Erpyleva, Natalia Savelyeva (eds.) *The War Near and Far. How Russians Perceive the Invasion of Ukraine February 2022 through June 2022*, Amsterdam: Lmverlag 2023. It is symptomatic that the Russian authorities tried to suppress these materials of the Laboratory of Public Sociology|Public Sociology Laboratory (*Laboratoriya publichnoy sotsiologii*) from the Russian collective memory: after the representatives of this organisation were called "foreign agents" (*inostrannye agenty*), the website of the Laboratory stopped working, and reports related to the Russian-Ukrainian war became unavailable. Ukrainian media also offer their visions of the collective memory of Russians. On the one hand, they describe it sarcastically as a memory of '*Chmobikes*' ('partially mobilised' Russians), whom the family sends to their deaths in order to receive material compensation and buy a new Russian car. Ihor Berezhanskyi, "Na novii 'Ladi' — do syna na kladovyshche: rosiianam pokazaly 'pliusy' vid zahybeli ditei na viini z Ukrainoiu" ("In the New 'Lada' to Their Son's Gravesite: The Russians Were Shown the 'Benefits' of the Death of Children in the War with Ukraine"), *Televiziinoi sluzhby novyn (TSN) (Television news service)*, 19 July 2022, https://tsn.ua/ato/na-noviy-ladi-do-sina-na-kladovische-rosiyanam-pokazali-plyusi-vid-zagibeli-ditey-na-viyni-z-ukrayinoyu-2113738.html [accessed: 31.07.2024]. In other cases, the focus is on released bandits who do not have sufficient motivation, engage in looting, and commit war crimes. At the same time, in the interviews of captured Russians for Ukrainian media, their memory appears as that of victims of 'Z-propaganda', who do not orient themselves in the situation and mechanically follow orders. *Lviv Media*, "Stoiaty v oboroni i vse: ekskliuzyvne interviu osliploho u boiu polonenoho rosiianyna" ("Standing in Defence and That's It: An Exclusive Interview with a Russian Prisoner of War Who Went Blind in Battle"), 07 October 2022, https://lviv.media/viyna/57011-stoyati-v-oboroni-i-vse-eksklyuzivne-intervyu-osliplogo-u-boyu-polonenogo-rosiyanina/ [accessed: 31.07.2024]; and Alina Haievska, "'Pryvezly na miasokombinat': polonenyi na Kharkivshchyni — pro prymusovu mobilizatsiiu v samonazvanii 'DNR'" ("'They Brought Me to a Meat-Packing Plant': A Prisoner in the Kharkiv Oblast Talks about Forced Mobilisation in the Self-Proclaimed 'DNR'"), *Suspilne novyny (Public News)*, 04 June 2022, https://suspilne.media/246704-privezli-na-masokombinat-polonenij-na-harkivsini-pro-primusovu-mobilizaciu-v-samonazvanij-dnr/ [accessed: 31.07.2024]. Such interviews are not always a manifestation of a real memory of the war. The same POW, returning to Russia, may publish the opposite version of events and their assessments. The 'truthfulness' of either version may be relative.

in the form of the memories of the defeated. The collective memories of the defeated constitute the second possible memory model. Ultimately, the signing of the Franco–German Armistice of 22 June 1940 (the surrender of France at the beginning of the Second World War) in the Compiègne Wagon became a symbolic destruction of the memories of the Armistice signed in the same carriage on 11 November 1918 (the surrender of Germany at the end of the First World War). It is no coincidence that in contemporary historical discourse, there is a desire to compare and look for analogies between the Russian Federation (whose leaders cultivate the memory of the 'greatness of the USSR' and the trauma of its collapse) and Nazi Germany (whose representatives also instrumentalised past humiliations and the need for revenge).

At the same time, both sides of the Russo–Ukrainian War also appeal to the defeat of Nazi Germany in the Second World War. This represents the third possible memory model and trajectory for the developments of memory culture. The Ukrainian and Russian sides both appeal to the memory of the victory over fascism in ways that mirror each other. Russian propaganda portrays contemporary Ukraine as analogous to Nazi Germany and fascist Italy, implying that 'Ukrainian Nazism/fascism' is exported from the West, and particularly from Germany. Crucially, the Russian Federation emphasises the German–Soviet War and Nazi Germany's attack on the USSR on 22 June 1941. On the other side, Ukrainians, using terms like 'Ruscism' and 'Ruscianism', denote contemporary Russian ideology and the country itself as heirs of Hitler's Germany and Mussolini's Italy. One ideology of contemporary Western Europe – that is, the European Union – is considered to be based on the model of reexamining, overcoming, and reconciling German and French memories of the Second World War. There are currently, however, no such prospects for reconciliation in the memory war between Ukraine and Russia. This would require democratic systems and peaceful attitudes in both states and societies. In Ukraine and Russia, elements of all three models can be combined, and the prospects for the current war of memories depend on how the Russo–Ukrainian War ends.

Conclusions

Each war memory, and the war of different types of memory within these war memories, exemplifies contradictions. On the one hand, war is perceived as a heroic act that mobilises society. On the other hand, it is a tragedy that destroys, deforms, injures, or completely devastates collective and individual memories. Wars can take different forms, can be fought under different slogans, use different strategies and tactics, and be fair or unfair, but at their core lies the destruction of one society by another. Each memory of a war is different, because, significantly, it represents a radically opposite view depending on which side of the front it is based and in which cultural tradition it is grounded. However, in their depths (or 'denotative' levels), these memories directly or indirectly record the same thing: the destruction, death, and suffering of some people, caused, as a rule, by the simple and, at the same time, terrible actions of other people. One of the thematic centres of such memory is, naturally, violence.[57]

Simultaneously, such memories, like the war itself, collect and transform large numbers of events, actions, reactions, and emotions of entire societies involved in the armed conflict. In this sense, such memories are 'pandemonium'. This makes the memories of the war into a kind of drama,[58] which encapsulates the situation of a person during a war. Nonetheless, the memory of the current Russo-Ukrainian War also contains everydayness and the 'banality of evil' (as coined by Hannah Arendt).[59] However, the case of Ukrainian collective memories during the Russo–Ukrainian armed conflict since 2014 shows that even militarised, non-pacifist memory can become both a weapon and a factor of social integration and peace, or at least in the sense of the resistance of the aggressor. Everything depends on the society, historical situation, cultural context, emotion, and ultimate intentions of those who form and use such memories.

Bibliography

Balynskyi, Yhor, Yaroslav Hrytsak, and Taryk Syryl Amar (eds.), *Strasti za Banderoiu: statti ta esei* (*Passions for Bandera: Articles and Essays*), Kyiv: Hrani-T, 2010.

Bekker, Oleksandr, "Z — natsystskyi symvol samoznyshchennia Rosii" ("Z is the Nazi Symbol of Russia's Self-Destruction"), *ArmiiaInform* (*ArmyInformation*),

57 This has already been shown in the cases of Syria and Ukraine. See: Ismail Salwa, *The Rule of Violence: Subjectivity, Memory and Government in Syria*, Cambridge: Cambridge University Press, 2018.

58 Oksana Kuzmenko, *Dramatychne buttia liudyny v ukrainskomu folklori: kontseptualni formy vyrazhennia (period Pershoi ta Druhoi svitovykh voien)* (*Dramatic Human Existence in Ukrainian Folklore: Conceptual Forms of Expression (during the Time of the First and Second World Wars)*), Lviv: Institute of Ethnology of the National Academy of Sciences of Ukraine, 2018.

59 Ali Omar Forozish, "The Banality of Evil, the Ukraine War and Russia's Strategic Goals", *Fair Observer*, 19 June 2022, https://www.fairobserver.com/world-news/the-banality-of-evil-the-ukraine-war-and-russias-strategic-goals/ [accessed: 31.07.2024]. One can also speak about the 'banality of the banality of evil'. It is interesting that this thesis is illustrated by the painting of the anonymous Banksy (*The Banality of the Banality of Evil*, 2013), who in 2022 visited Ukraine incognito and left seven murals on the destroyed walls of Ukrainian cities. One of these murals is the symbolic image of a boy tackling a large adult judoka who looks like Vladimir Putin. This image, like others, also became part of the memory of the war in Ukraine.

17 March 2022, https://armyinform.com.ua/2022/03/17/z-naczystskyj-symvol-samoznyshhennya-rosiyi/ [accessed: 16.07.2024].

Berezhanskyi, Ihor, "Na novii "Ladi" — do syna na kladovyshche: rosiianam pokazaly "pliusy" vid zahybeli ditei na viini z Ukrainoiu" ("In the New 'Lada' to Their Son's Gravesite: The Russians Were Shown the 'Benefits' of the Death of Children in the War with Ukraine"), *Televiziinoi sluzhby novyn* (*TSN*) (*Television news service*), 19 July 2022, https://tsn.ua/ato/na-noviy-ladi-do-sina-na-kladovische-rosiyanam-pokazali-plyusi-vid-zagibeli-ditey-na-viyni-z-ukrayinoyu-2113738.html [accessed: 16.07.2024].

Boroń, Aleksandra, and Agnieszka Gromkowska-Melosik, *Ukraińskie uchodźczynie wojenne. Tożsamość, trauma, nadzieja* (*Ukrainian Female War Refugees: Identity, Trauma, Hope*), Kraków: Oficyna Wydawnicza Impuls, 2022.

Danylo, Olena, and Kateryna Sadlovska, "Brat znyk bezvisty. Rozpovid mariupolky, yaka evakuiuvalasia z mista u veresni" ("Brother is Missing: The Story of a Mariupol Woman who Evacuated from the City in September"), *Suspilne novyny* (*Public News*), 15 January 2023, https://suspilne.media/358548-brat-znik-bezvisti-rozpovid-mariupolki-aka-evakuuvalasa-z-mista-u-veresni/ [accessed: 16.07.2024].

Dreher, Rod, "Viktor Orban: West Is 'In A War With Russia'", *The American Conservative*, 26 January 2023, https://www.theamericanconservative.com/viktor-orban-we-are-in-a-war-with-russia/ [accessed: 16.07.2024].

Erpyleva, Svetlana, Savelyeva, Natalia (eds.), *The War Near and Far. How Russians Perceive the Invasion of Ukraine February 2022 through June 2022*, Amsterdam: Lmverlag, 2023.

Fedor, Julie, Markku Kangaspuro, Jussi Lassila, Tatiana Zhurzhenko (eds.), *War and Memory in Russia, Ukraine and Belarus*, London: Palgrave Macmillan, 2017.

Ferguson, Brian R., "Ten Points on War", *Social Analysis* 52/2, 2008, 32–49.

Fitzpatrick, Sheila, "The Civil War as a Formative Experience", in: Abbot Gleason, Peter Kenez, and Richard Stites (eds.), *Bolshevik Culture: Experiment and Order in the Russian Revolution*, Bloomington: Indiana University Press, 1985, 57–76.

Forozish, Ali Omar, "The Banality of Evil, the Ukraine War and Russia's Strategic Goals", *Fair Observer*, 19 June 2022, f

Foundation for the Study of Democracy, *War Crimes of the Armed Forces and Security Forces of Ukraine: torture and inhumane treatment*, report, April 2016, https://www.osce.org/files/f/documents/e/7/233896.pdf [accessed: 16.07.2024].

Gosiewska, Małgorzata, et al., *Report: Russian War Crimes in Eastern Ukraine in 2014*, report, *Ji-Magazine*, 2015, https://ji-magazine.lviv.ua/engl-vers/2015/Russian_War_Crimes_in_Eastern_Ukraine_in_2014.pdf [accessed: 16.07.2024].

Haievska, Alina, "'Pryvezly na miasokombinat': polonenyi na Kharkivshchyni — pro prymusovu mobilizatsiiu v samonazvanii 'DNR'" ("'They Brought Me to a Meat-Packing Plant': A Prisoner in the Kharkiv Oblast Talks about Forced Mobilisation in the Self-Proclaimed 'DNR'"), *Suspilne novyny* (*Public News*), 04

June 2022, https://suspilne.media/246704-privezli-na-masokombinat-polonenij-na-harkivsini-pro-primusovu-mobilizaciu-v-samonazvanij-dnr/ [accessed: 16.07.2024].

Holyk, Roman, "'Tsentr ukrainskoho Skhodu' y 'Natsionalnyi Piemont': 'donbaski' siuzhety halytskoi kulturnoi pamiati" ("The 'Centre of the Ukrainian East" and 'National Piedmont': The 'Donbas' Plots of Galician Cultural Memory), in: Mykola Lytvyn (ed.), *Mizh viinoiu i sobornistiu. Sotsiokulturna intehratsiia ta adaptatsiia pereselentsiv z Donbasu ta Kpymu. Zakhidnoukpainskyi vektor* (*Between War and Unity: The Sociocultural Integration and Adaptation of Immigrants from the Donbas and Crimea, the Western Ukrainian Vector*), Lviv: I. Krypyakevych Institute of Ukrainian Studies, 2017, 89–144.

Hrytsenko, Oleksandr, *Prezydenty i pamiat. Polityka pamiati prezydentiv Ukrainy (1994–2014): pidgruntia, poslannia, realizatsiia, rezultaty. (Presidents and Memory: The Policy of Memory of the Presidents of Ukraine (1994–2014): Background, Message, Implementation, Results*), Kyiv: K.I.S., 2017.

Ilkevičiūtė, Justina, "'Russia is constantly planning for new offensives' – interview with NATO chief Stoltenberg", *Lithuanian Radio and Television (LRT)*, 28 February 2023, https://www.lrt.lt/en/news-in-english/19/1923076/russia-is-constantly-planning-for-new-offensives-interview-with-nato-chief-stoltenberg/ [accessed: 16.07.2024].

Kasianov, Georhii, *Danse macabre: holod 1932–1933 rokiv u politytsi, masovii svidomosti ta istoriohrafii (1980-ti–pochatok 2000-kh)* (*Danse macabre: The Famine of 1932–1933 in Politics, Mass Consciousness, and Historiography (1980s–early 2000s)*, Kyiv: In-t istorii Ukrainy NAN Ukrainy and Nash chas, 2010.

Khrebtan-Hörhager, Julia, and Evgeniya Pyatovskaya, "The Banality of Putin's Propaganda: A Dangerous Déjà vu", *Forum for Ukrainian Studies*, 26 September 2022, https://ukrainian-studies.ca/2022/09/26/the-banality-of-putins-propaganda-a-dangerous-deja-vu/ [accessed: 16.07.2024].

Kostyk, Antonina, "Yak mynuv rik povnomasshtabnoi viiny dlia Lvova: spohady, foto, tsyfry" ("How the Year of the Full-Scale War Passed for Lviv: Memories, Photos, Numbers"), *Tvoie misto* (*Your City*), 2023, https://tvoemisto.tv/exclusive/yak_mynuv_pershyy_den_povnomasshtabnogo_vtorgnennya_u_lvovi_ta_kudy_letily_rakety_144240.html [accessed: 16.07.2024].

Kulakov, Andriy, et al. (eds.), *Words and Wars: Ukraine facing Kremlin propaganda*, Kyiv: KIC, 2017.

Kuzio, Taras, *Russian Nationalism and the Russian–Ukrainian War: Autocracy – Orthodoxy – Nationality*, London and New York: Routledge, 2022.

Kuzio, Taras, *Putin's War Against Ukraine: Revolution, Nationalism, and Crime*, Toronto: Chair of Ukrainian Studies, 2017.

Kuzmenko, Oksana, *Dramatychne buttia liudyny v ukrainskomu folklori: kontseptualni formy vyrazhennia (period Pershoi ta Druhoi svitovykh voien)* (*Dramatic Human Exis-

tence in Ukrainian Folklore: Conceptual Forms of Expression (during the Time of the First and Second World Wars)), Lviv: Institute of Ethnology of the National Academy of Sciences of Ukraine, 2018.

Levchenko, Artur, "Ia zahynuv pid Bakhmutom. Rosiiany bilshe ne mozhut povtoryty" ("I Died Near Bakhmut: The Russians Can No Longer Repeat"), *Zaxid.Net*, 2023, https://zaxid.net/ya_zaginuv_pid_bahmutom_n1556155 [accessed: 16.07.2024].

Lviv Media, "Stoiaty v oboroni i vse: ekskliuzyvne interviu osliploho u boiu polonenoho rosiianyna" ("Standing in Defence and That's It: An Exclusive Interview with a Russian Prisoner of War Who Went Blind in Battle"), 07 October 2022, https://lviv.media/viyna/57011-stoyati-v-oboroni-i-vse-eksklyuzivne-intervyu-osliplogo-u-boyu-polonenogo-rosiyanina/ [accessed: 16.07.2024].

Livingstone Smith, David, *The Most Dangerous Animal: Human Nature and the Origins of War*, New York: St. Martin's Press, 2007.

Ministry of Culture and Information Policy of Ukraine, *Russia's War Crimes All Over the World: From Chechnya to Syria*, report, https://mkip.gov.ua/files/pdf/%D0%B7%D0%BB%D0%BE%D1%87%D0%B8%D0%BD%D0%B8_eng.pdf [accessed: 19.02.2023].

Myers, Rob, "The War in Ukraine Through Some Memories of the Yugoslav Wars", *Insurgent Notes: Journal of Communist Theory and Practice*, 29 December 2022, http://insurgentnotes.com/2022/12/the-war-in-ukraine-through-some-memories-of-the-yugoslav-wars/ [accessed: 16.07.2024].

Polegkyi, Oleksii, "'Never again' vs. 'We can repeat it': Russians will pay any price to restore the glory of Soviet victory in WWII", *Forum for Ukrainian Studies*, 11 June 2022, https://ukrainian-studies.ca/author/oleksii-polegkyi/ [accessed: 16.07.2024].

Portnov, Andrii, "Memory Wars in Post-Soviet Ukraine (1991–2010)", in: Uilleam Blacker, Alexander Etkind, and Julie Fedor (eds.), *Memory and Theory in Eastern Europe*, New York: Palgrave Macmillan, 2013, 233–254.

Puleri, Marco, *Ukrainian, Russophone, (Other) Russian: Hybrid Identities and Narratives*, Berlin: Peter Lang, 2020.

Rodak, Kateryna, "Bilshist pereselentsiv na Lvivshchyni namahaiutsia hovoryty ukrainskoiu, – opytuvannia" ("Most of the Immigrants in the Lviv Try to Speak Ukrainian, According to a Survey"), *Zaxid.net*, 31 May 2022, https://zaxid.net/bilshist_pereselentsiv_na_lvivshhini_namagayutsya_govoriti_ukrayinskoyu___opituvannya_n1543703 [accessed: 16.07.2024].

Sadlovska, Kateryna, and Anastasiia Yarmolovska, "Pereselenka z Mariupolia pratsiuie pediatrom u Lvovi" ("A Migrant from Mariupol Works as a Paediatrician in Lviv"), *Suspilne novyny* (*Public News*), 04 February 2023, https://suspilne.media/370849-pereselenka-z-mariupola-pracue-pediatrom-u-lvovi/ [accessed: 16.07.2024].

Salwa, Ismail, *The Rule of Violence: Subjectivity, Memory and Government in Syria*, Cambridge: Cambridge University Press, 2018.

Semenets, Yuliia, "'Kovbasa "Moskovska" pishla vslid za korablem', – kazhut pokuptsiam chernihivski prodavtsi" ("'"Moskovska" Sausage Followed the Ship', Chernihiv Sellers Tell Customers"), *Texty.org.ua*, 18 July 2022, https://texty.org.ua/fragments/107271/kovbasa-moskovska-pishla-vslid-za-korablem-kazhut-pokuptsjam-chernihivski-prodavtsi/ [accessed: 16.07.2024].

Sereda, Viktoriya, "Regional Historical Identities and Memory", in: Yaroslav Hrytsak, Andrii Portnov, and Victor Susak (eds.), *Lviv-Donetsk: sotsialni identychnosti v suchasnii Ukraini. Ukraina Moderna. Spetsialnyi vypusk (Lviv-Donetsk: Social Identities in Modern Ukraine. Modern Ukraine, Special issue)*, Lviv-Kyiv: Krytyka, 2007, 160–209.

Shevel, Oksana, "The Politics of Memory in a Divided Society: A Comparison of Post-Franco Spain and Post-Soviet Ukraine", *Slavic Review*, 1, 2011, 137–164.

Sigov, Konstantin, *Le courage de l'Ukraine* (*The Courage of Ukraine*), Paris: Éditions du Cerf, 2023.

Slyvynskyi, Ostap, (ed.), *Slovnyk vijny* (*Dictionary of the War*), Kyiv: Vivat, 2023.

Stanislavskyi, Ivan, "Novyi dim v staromu hurtozhytku. Yak pereselentsi zi Skhodu namahaiutsia vlashtuvaty svoie zhyttia u Lvovi Ivan Stanislavskyi" ("A New Home in an Old Dormitory: How IDPs from the East Are Trying to Organise Their Lives in Lviv"), *LB.ua*, 22 June 2022 https://lb.ua/society/2022/06/22/520803_noviy_dim_staromu_gurtozhitku_yak.html [accessed: 16.07.2024].

Starovoyt, Iryna, "Traumatic memories: from Holodomor to Maidan", in: Rob van der Laarse et al. (eds.), *Religion, state, society, and identity in transition: Ukraine*, Oisterwijk: Wolf Legal Publishers, 2015, 219–240.

Topolyuk, Kateryna, "Rik nezlamnosti. Yak tse bulo dlia Lvova" ("The Year of Indomitability: How It Was for Lviv"), *032 Sayt mista Lvova* (*032 Website of the City of Lviv*), 24 February 2023, https://www.032.ua/news/3553072/rik-nezlamnosti-ak-ce-bulo-dla-lvova [accessed: 16.07.2024].

Troianovski, Anton, "A Ukrainian Billionaire Fought Russia. Now He's Ready to Embrace It", *The New York Times*, 13 November 2019, https://www.nytimes.com/2019/11/13/world/europe/ukraine-ihor-kolomoisky-russia.html [accessed: 16.07.2024].

White, William A., *Thoughts of a Psychiatrist on the War and after*, New York: Paul B. Hoeber, 1919.

Wylegała, Anna, and Małgorzata Głowacka-Grajper (eds.), *The Burden of the Past: History, Memory, and Identity in Contemporary Ukraine*, Bloomington: Indiana University Press, 2020.

Yaremchuk, Vitalii, and Andrii Smirnov, *Analitychnyi ohliad "Istoriia Ukrainy v rosiiskykh shkilnykh pidruchnykakh z istorii"* (*An Analytical Review of "the History of Ukraine in Russian School History Textbooks"*), Kyiv, 2023.

Yekelchyk, Serhy, "Naming the War: Russian aggression in Ukrainian Official Discourse and Mass Culture", *Canadian Slavonic Papers* 64/2–3, 2022, 232–246.

Yekelchyk, Serhy, *Stalin's Empire of Memory: Russian–Ukrainian Relations in the Soviet Historical Imagination*, Toronto: University of Toronto Press, 2004.

Zurchenko, Tatiana, "Legislating Historical Memory in Post-Soviet Ukraine", in: Eleazar Barkan and Ariella Lang (eds.), *Memory Laws and Historical Justice*, London: Palgrave Macmillan Cham, 2022, 97–130.

Zurchenko, Tatiana, "Shared Memory Culture? Nationalizing the 'Great Patriotic War' in the Ukrainian–Russian Borderlands", in: Małgorzata Pakier and Joanna Wawrzyniak (eds), *Memory and Change in Europe: Eastern Perspectives*, Oxford: Berghahn, 2016, 169–192.

Coverage of the Second World War in School Textbooks on the History of Ukraine

Before and After Euromaidan

Ihor Dvorkin

After Ukraine gained independence in 1991, national and post-Soviet historical narratives coexisted in the country's political, scientific, and educational spheres. However, the events of Euromaidan and the beginning of the Russo–Ukrainian War in 2014 – particularly after the legislative changes of 2015, known as the 'decommunisation laws' – shifted the situation in favour of a national approach. These events significantly impacted the politics of memory and historical politics in Ukraine. Textbooks and curricula on the history of Ukraine now largely reflect the changes in the perception and interpretation of historical events since 2014. Furthermore, alternations and additions have been made to the interpretation of the Second World War in the newest generation of Ukrainian textbooks, which were published in 2018. Lastly, the full-scale Russian invasion influenced the latest updates to school curricula, which were implemented in 2022.

Nancy Popson points out that "textbooks are the main educational tool by which the values and norms of the political and social system are transmitted to young members of society".[1] Textbooks also play a crucial role in reflecting the national master narrative. According to Georgiy Kasianov, the national master narrative is "a systematized, canonical version of a nation's past which claims the status and power of the universal norm".[2] In Ukraine, national history textbooks are written based on narratives approved by the Ministry of Education and Science, which undergo significant updates over time to reflect the state's memory politics. In this regard, textbook authors do not have absolute freedom in their work; they are bound by school programmes and the changes that these programmes undergo.

1 Nancy Popson, "The Ukrainian History Textbook: Introducing Children to the 'Ukrainian Nation'", *Nationalities Papers: The Journal of Nationalism and Ethnicity* 29/2, 2001, 325–350, here 326.

2 Georgiy Kasianov, "National Master Narrative: Vicissitudes of Method", *AREI: Journal for Central and Eastern European History and Politics* 1, 2022, 108–127, here 110.

Ukrainian and Western researchers have deeply researched Ukrainian history textbooks.[3] This has included the influence of the events of 2014 on textbook writing as well as the writing of history textbooks in the context of war (after 2014).[4] Lina Klymenko, for instance, has studied the Second World War in previous generations of Ukrainian school textbooks, and has examined and compared Second World War narratives in Belarussian, Russian, and Ukrainian textbooks.[5] Adding to this scholarship, my article analyses textbooks on the history of Ukraine that were published before and after 2014 and reflect changes in the analysis and interpretation of the Second World War. These 'new' textbooks focus more on previously ignored or under-evaluated topics. More specifically, this analysis examines the shifts in the politics of memory, new approaches to selecting visual material, the choice of historical sources presented in the books, the topics of individual book sections, terminology, and other relevant factors.

This article compares the textbooks of two generations: those from 2011/2012 and those from 2018. The books from 2018 are currently used in schools. In this study, I only draw examples from a selection of textbooks and am not able to cover all of them. All the current school textbooks are available online.[6] At the time of writing this article, the newest textbooks have not yet been released, but the 2022 history curriculum updates are available. Lastly, this article considers only textbooks on the history of Ukraine (world history, for example, is taught as a separate subject). Within this study, I see textbooks on national history as sources that "contain an ex-

---

3 Popson, "The Ukrainian History Textbook".

4 In the case of the influence of the events of 2014 on textbooks, see: Marta Studenna-Skrukwa, "What history? What homeland? The nationalization of history in the school education before the breakthroughs in 2014–15 and after", in: Tomasz Stryjek and Joanna Konieczna-Sałamatin (eds.), *The Politics of Memory in Poland and Ukraine: From Reconciliation to De-Conciliation*, London: Routledge, 2022, 85–103. In the case of the influence of the war that started in 2014 on textbooks, see: Kateryna Pryshchepa, "Nation-building and school history lessons in Ukraine after 2014", in: Tomasz Stryjek and Joanna Konieczna-Sałamatin (eds.), *The Politics of Memory in Poland and Ukraine: From Reconciliation to De-Conciliation*, London: Routledge, 2022, 120–135.

5 For previous generations of Ukrainian textbooks, see: Lina Klymenko, "World War II in Ukrainian School History Textbooks: Mapping the Discourse of the Past", *Compare: A Journal of Comparative and International Education* 44/5, 2014, 756–777. For the comparative study, see: Lina Klymenko, "Narrating the Second World War: History Textbooks and Nation Building in Belarus, Russia, and Ukraine", *Journal of Educational Media, Memory, and Society* 8/2, 2016, 35–57.

6 For examples of relevant eleventh-grade textbooks on the history of Ukraine, see: Instytut modernizatsiyi osvity (Institute of the Modernisation of Education), "4. Istoriia Ukrainy 11 klas" ("4. The History of Ukraine for the 11th Grade"), https://lib.imzo.gov.ua/yelektronn-vers-pdruchnikv/11-klas/4-storya-ukrani-11-klas/ [accessed: 31.07.2024].

pression of the self-image of the nation-state, characterized by the representation of national history, which students are required to acquire".[7]

Memory Politics

The first generation of the textbooks that I analyse – those from 2011/2012 – were published during the presidency of Viktor Yanukovych (2010–2014). Memory politics during the office of Yanukovych's predecessor, Viktor Yushchenko (2005–2010), typically contained anti-Soviet elements. The goal of memory politics during that period was to unite Ukrainians through the reconciliation of memories around the Second World War. Meanwhile, memory politics under Yanukovych showed a partial return to the 'Soviet' model of commemorating the war, which fell close to Russian commemoration.[8] The 2018 textbooks were published during Petro Poroshenko's presidency (2014–2019). After Euromaidan, Yanukovych's rule ended and Russian aggression against Ukraine started. At this point, memory politics changed significantly at state and legal levels. In 2015, the government adopted several laws that consolidated the state's view of the Second World War. Particularly important was the Law of Ukraine "On the perpetuation of the victory over Nazism in the Second World War of 1939–1945", which justified the change

> considering the fact that during the Second World War of 1939–1945, the National Socialist (Nazi) and Communist totalitarian regimes committed numerous crimes against humanity, war crimes and crimes of genocide on the territory of Ukraine, as a result of which Ukraine and the Ukrainian people suffered huge losses, [and] noting the world-historical significance of the victory over Nazism in the Second World War of 1939–1945.[9]

7 Eckhardt Fuchs and Marcus Otto, "Introduction Educational Media, Textbooks, and Postcolonial Relocations of Memory Politics in Europe", *Journal of Educational Media, Memory, and Society* 5/1, 2013, 1–13, here 3.

8 Barbara Törnquist-Plewa and Yuliya Yurchuk, "Memory politics in contemporary Ukraine: Reflections from the postcolonial perspective", *Memory Studies* 12/6, 2019, 699–720, here 704.

9 Petro Poroshenko, "Pro uvichnennya peremohy nad natsyzmom u Druhiy svitoviy viyni 1939–1945 rokiv" ("On the Perpetuation of the Victory over Nazism in the Second World War of 1939–1945"), Verkhova Rada Ukrainy (Ukraine's Verkhova Rada), 09 April 2015, https://zakon.rada.gov.ua/laws/show/315-19#Text [accessed 31.07.2024] [author's trans.].

The Shift of the Second World War Paradigm in Textbooks

Existing since the Soviet period, the term 'Great Patriotic War' – the name of the World War II–era German–Soviet armed conflict of 1941–1945 – remained in Ukrainian textbooks for a long time following Ukrainian independence (including in the textbooks of 2011/2012). After a brief break from the term, it returned in 1995 to the new national narrative.[10] It was used much less during the term of Yushchenko, but in 2011, it reappeared in textbooks. Sociological research has shown a widespread use of the term in the last decade. For example, in 2011, more than 66 percent of Ukrainians used Great Patriotic War, while about 29 percent preferred WWII.[11] However, after Euromaidan, the term Great Patriotic War was banished from Ukrainian legislation and, afterward, from new Ukrainian textbooks for the tenth grade, which were issued in 2018.[12]

The textbooks of 2011/2012 have a conception of the Great Patriotic War that is somewhat altered as compared to the Soviet period. The Ukrainian version of the Great Patriotic War pays more attention to the feat and suffering of 'ordinary people' and the significant mistakes of the military and state leaders during the war.[13] Usually, the first page of the corresponding section of the textbook carries the main message that the authors want to present. The illustrative material of these pages is also important for the presentation of the main information. In a textbook from 2012, the topic section begins with images of Soviet patriotic posters and photographs.[14] A version of the same textbook that was revised in 2018, however, contains the image of a contemporary Ukrainian poster depicting red poppies and the recent slogan used during Ukrainian celebrations of Victory Day, "We honour. We Prevail. 1939–1945".[15] Notably, the Ukrainian Institute of National Memory proposes using these new symbols for the purposes of education and commemoration. The symbols were inspired

10 Andrii Portnov, *Istoriyi dlya domashnogo vzhytku: Eseyi pro polsko-rosijsko-ukrayinskyj trykutnyk pamyati (Histories for Home Use: Essays on the Polish–Russian–Ukrainian Triangle of Memory)*, Kyiv: Krytyka, 2013, 174.

11 Ibid., 167.

12 UNIAN, "Rada zaminyla u zakoni Velyku Vitchyznyanu vijnu na Drugu svitovu" ("The Rada Replaced the Great Patriotic War with the Second World War in the Law"), 14 November 2017, https://www.unian.ua/politics/2242759-rada-zaminila-u-zakoni-veliku-vitchiznyanu-viynu-na-drugu-svitovu.html [accessed 31.07.2024].

13 Portnov, *Istoriyi dlya domashnogo vzhytku*, 174.

14 Olena Pometun and Nestor Hupan, *Istoriya Ukrayiny: Pidruchnyk dlya 11 klasu zagalnoosvitnix navchalnyx zakladiv (A History of Ukraine: A Textbook for the 11th Grade of Secondary Schools)*, Kharkiv: Sycyya, 2012, 5.

15 Olena Pometun and Nestor Hupan, *Istoriya Ukrayiny: Pidruchnyk dlya 10 klasu zakladiv zagalnoyi serednoyi osvity (A History of Ukraine: A Textbook for the 10th Grade of General Secondary Education Institutions)* Kyiv: Orion, 2018, 193 [author's trans.].

by European commemoration practices. If in 2012 the textbooks present war and victory as heroic, then the later books focus on memorialising the victims of the war. This is evidenced by a quote from a well-known Ukrainian historian, researcher, and Holocaust educator, Anatolii Podolskyi, which is on the first page of the section on WWII in Olena Pometun's and Nestor Hupan's 2018 textbook: "Ukraine should join the European perception of war as a tragedy. We are not responsible for the past. We are responsible for the memory of the past".[16]

My analysis of the 2011–2018 textbooks reveals that their main topics include the German–Soviet Nonaggression Pact, the inclusion of part of the territory of what is now Ukraine into the Soviet Union in 1939–1940 (previously this was part of Poland and Romania), the German–Soviet military confrontation on the territory of Ukraine, and the Soviet and Ukrainian national resistance movements. In the most recent textbooks, the general schema has not changed significantly. However, in some cases, new aspects of the 'old' problems and/or new topics that were previously ignored or mentioned without evaluative judgements have been added. Below, I discuss these changes in detail.

The German-Soviet Nonaggression Pact

Traditionally, the section of the textbook dedicated to WWII begins with the German–Soviet Nonaggression (also known as the Molotov–Ribbentrop) Pact of 1939. Both generations of textbooks present the pact negatively – however, the accents change. In the newer generation of textbooks, we can see the impact of current events and recent changes in memory politics. Notable is the appearance of the term 'aggressor state', used broadly in modern legislation and rhetoric.[17] In the new textbooks, this term designates both Nazi Germany and the Soviet Union. Corresponding paragraphs contain information and visual material about the co-operation between these aggressor states at the beginning of the war. Photographs from a joint German–Soviet parade in Brest are present.[18] There is an indication toward the change in Soviet propaganda rhetoric, which earlier expressed a negative attitude towards Nazi Germany. In the 2018 textbook by Vitalii Vlasov and Stanislav Kulchytskiy, a well-chosen historical source characterises this:

> From the report of the German ambassador to Berlin in Moscow, dated 6 September 1939: "The sudden turn in the policy of the Soviet Union, after many years of propaganda directed against the German aggressors, is not yet

16 Ibid., 193 [author's trans.].

17 Ibid., 196.

18 Vitalii Vlasov and Stanislav Kulchytskyi, *Istoriya Ukrayiny: Pidruchnyk dlya 10 klasu zakladiv zagalnoyi serednoyi osvity (A History of Ukraine: A Textbook for the 10th Grade of Institutions of General Secondary Education)* Kyiv: Litera LTD, 2018, 244.

> very clearly understood by the population. Statements by official agitators that Germany is no longer an aggressor are particularly dubious. The Soviet government is doing everything possible to change the population's attitude toward Germany. The press seems to have been replaced".[19]

The more recent textbooks also contain information about ethnic Ukrainians who were in the Polish Army in 1939 and participated in warfare on its side.[20]

The 2011/2012 and 2018 textbooks' narratives present the 1939–1940 Sovietisation (the politics of the transfer to the Soviet system) of western parts of the territory of present-day Ukraine in two ways. Specifically, the books point to positive aspects of this process (i.e., overcoming unemployment and Ukrainisation) and negative ones (i.e., repression and terror). The textbooks focus, however, on the negative aspects of the Sovietisation. For instance, they indicate that in the Soviet 'occupation zone' in Poland, which was two times smaller than the German 'occupation zone', the population was three to four times more repressed by June 1941..[21] The 2011 textbooks did not similarly describe the Ukrainian territories annexed by the USSR. The selection of sources for this section includes negative personal recollections. For example, one (called "From the memories of an eyewitness") states: "There were many evil faces in the city, the foul Russian language began to be heard on the streets and in the institutions more often, and simple-minded Russian matrons, officers' wives, washed apples in the toilet bowl and were in awe about how well it washed [them]".[22]

The German-Soviet War

In the older and some of the newer textbooks, the section on the German–Soviet War of 1941–1945 begins with the German attack on the Soviet Union, followed by the unsuccessful military actions on the territory of Ukraine, mobilisation (particularly the patriotism and enthusiasm of citizens who joined the army and the people's militia during the first months of the war), the evacuation of factories to the Soviet East, and so on.[23] The recent textbooks also cover these events. However, they also include new details, such as the crimes of the Communist regime, which took place after the beginning of the German invasion. They describe the scorched-earth

19 Ibid., 247 [author's trans.].

20 Oleksii Strukevych, *Istoriya Ukrayiny: Ptidruchnyk dlya 10 klasu zakladiv zagalnoyi serednoyi osvity (A History of Ukraine: A Textbook for the 10th Grade of General Secondary Education Institutions)*, Kyiv: Gramota, 2018, 179, 180.

21 Ibid., 182.

22 Olha Sorochinska and Natalia Hisem, *Istoriya Ukrayiny: Pidruchnyk dlya 10 klasu zakladiv zahalnoyi serednoyi osvity (A History of Ukraine: A Textbook for the 10th Grade of Institutions of General Secondary Education)* Ternopyl: Navchalna knyha – Bohdan, 2018, 197 [author's trans.].

23 Pometun and Hupan, *Istoriya Ukrayiny*, 2012, 17–24.

policy and the mass repressions of political prisoners, mainly in Western Ukraine. Thus, newer textbooks draw attention to the repressive nature of the mobilisation of Soviet society by the Soviet authorities to fight the Nazis. Under this falls the deliberate detonation of many buildings in the Kyiv city centre, on Khreshchatyk Street. The textbooks emphasise that this led to the destruction of more than 300 historical buildings, great casualties among residents of Kyiv, and the loss of housing.[24]

Collaboration

The textbook's authors pay considerable attention to the difficult topic of collaboration during WWII. Entire explanatory paragraphs are devoted to this phenomenon. The enumeration of reasons for collaboration is diverse: survival, careerism, and/or the desire to take revenge on the Soviet authorities and to gain Ukraine's independence with the assistance of Germany. Some textbooks provide a list of Ukrainian armed formations that fought on the German side at various stages of the war.[25] The textbooks note that for Ukraine, an unequivocal identification of 'cooperation' and 'traitor' is not acceptable. The 2018 *History of Ukraine* textbook (written by Olha Sorochinska and Natalia Hisem) asks students to answer the following questions: "What was the Soviet regime for Ukrainians on the eve of the war? Who was 'betrayed' by Ukrainians?"[26] The textbooks separately highlight the activity of self-governing bodies under the German occupation. They indicate that the government was focused on providing adequate conditions for the survival of the civilian population, and the prevention of hunger and epidemics, if the occupation authorities were not interested in these issues.[27]

The Nazi Occupation Regime and the Holocaust

Generally, both generations of textbooks present the Nazi occupation regime during the war as extremely negative. They refer to Nazis robbing and economically exploiting the occupied territories, referencing *Generalplan Ost*, 'the new order' with its unbelievable cruelty, the life of the inhabitants under the occupation, and forced labour in Germany, among other things.[28] The coverage of the Holocaust in the textbooks has evolved significantly.

24 Vlasov and Kulchytskyi, *Istoriya Ukrayiny*, 212–213.

25 Marian Mydriy and Olena Arkusha, *Istoriya: Ukrayina i svit, Pidruchnyk dlya 10 klasu zakladiv zahalnoyi serednoyi osvity*, (*History: Ukraine and the World, A Textbook for the 10th Grade of Institutions of General Secondary Education*), Kyiv: Geneza, 2018, 244–247.

26 Sorochinska and Hisem, *Istoriya Ukrayiny*, 219–220 [author's trans.].

27 Strukevych, *Istoriya Ukrayiny*, 203.

28 Pometun and Hupan, *Istoriya Ukrayiny*, 2012, 27–32; and Pometun and Hupan, *Istoriya Ukrayiny*, 2018, 210–216.

The textbooks of the early 2000s typically contain little information about the Holocaust and do not use this term. They provide data on the deaths of Jewish people at the beginning of the occupation and general data on the deaths of civilians and prisoners of the war.[29] The next-generation textbooks of 2011/2012 are more concerned with the tragedy of the Ukrainian Jewish population. These revised textbooks use the term 'Holocaust'.[30] They also add information about ghettos and the differences in the policies of mass extermination in different zones of the occupation, among other things.[31] The 2018 textbooks devote much more attention to the 'Final Solution', revealing the causes of the Holocaust and its peculiarities in different countries and zones of the occupation, and individually focus on the tragedy of the Babyn Yar massacre (indicating that the victims were not only Jews but also Soviet prisoners of war and figures of the Ukrainian nationalist movement). The books also discuss resistance to the Holocaust and the history of saving lives, particularly the work of Andrey Sheptytsky, the Metropolitan Bishop of the Ukrainian Greek Catholic Church.[32] Lastly, they pay considerable attention to the Ukrainians called the Righteous Among the Nations (the honorary title given to people who saved Jewish lives). This particularly focuses on Olena Viter, the abbess of a monastery, who cooperated with the Organisation of Ukrainian Nationalists (OUN) and was the first among Ukrainians to receive this title in 1976.[33]

The Resistance and the Ukrainian National Movement

All the textbooks I studied contain information on the resistance movement in Ukraine during the war years. The focus falls on the Soviet resistance movement, which sought to help the regular army in the restoration of Soviet power, and the Ukrainian nationalists, who aimed to use the German–Soviet War to create an independent Ukrainian state, fighting against both Bolshevism and Nazism. The Soviet resistance receives more attention in older textbooks. Alongside focusing on the Ukrainian nationalists, modern textbooks also pay more attention than older

---

29 Fedir Turchenko, Petro Panchenko, and Serhii Tymchenko, *Novitnya istoriya Ukrayiny (1939–2001): Pidruchnyk dlya 11-ho klasu serednikh pahalnoosvitnikh navchalnykh zakladiv* (*The Modern History of Ukraine (1939–2001): A Textbook for the 11th Grade of Secondary Comprehensive Educational Institutions*), Kyiv: Geneza, 2001, 21.

30 Fedir Turchenko, *Istoriya Ukrayiny: Pidruchnyk dlya 11 klasu zahalnoosvitnikh navchalnykh zakladiv* (*A History of Ukraine: A Textbook for the 11th Grade of General Educational Institutions*), Kyiv: Geneza, 2011, 31.

31 Oleksii Strukevich, Ivan Romaniuk, and Stepan Drovoziuk, *Istoriya Ukrayiny: Pidruchnyk dlya 11 klasu zahalnoosvitnikh navchalnykh zakladiv* (*A History of Ukraine: A Textbook for the 11th Grade of General Educational Institutions*), Kyiv: Gramota, 2011, 36.

32 Mydriy and Arkusha, *Istoriya*, 247–252.

33 Vlasov and Kulchytskyi, *Istoriya Ukrayiny*, 225–226.

versions to the different groups of the Polish liberation movement who were active on Ukrainian territories.

The history of the OUN and Ukrainian Insurgent Army (UPA), a Ukrainian nationalist military formation, went from being rarely covered and only in a very negative light during the Soviet era to becoming a key textbook subject. The 2011/2012 textbooks pay more attention to them. They point to the evolution of the OUN's worldview during the war, particularly to its democratisation.[34] Since 2014, the OUN's activities are presented positively, but, at the same time, some textbooks point to their denial of democracy, and their recognition of the principle of 'nationalocracy' (i.e., the power of an ethnic nation within the state).[35] Generally, the current textbooks present a fuller history of the OUN and the information is accompanied by rich illustrative material.[36]

Liberation Versus the Expulsion of the Nazi Invaders

There is a change of the titles of the sections devoted to 1943–1944 in the textbooks. It concerns themes describing the hostilities on the front at the time of the Nazi retreat from Ukrainian territory. In 'pre-Euromaidan' textbooks, the term 'liberation' is dominant. The sections are mostly called something like "The liberation of Ukraine from Nazi invaders", although the term 'expulsion' is also used.[37] These sections focus on the heroism of and tragedies befalling Soviet soldiers, who often died at the whims of the highest command – for instance, during the liberation of Kyiv, which was meant to be fast and to end before the day of the anniversary of the October Revolution. New textbooks prefer the term 'expulsion' when describing the warfare. This might intend to indicate in a more neutral way that the totalitarian Communist regime replaced the Nazi invaders on Ukrainian lands.

All the textbooks I studied also contain information on the deportation of Crimean Tatars and other Crimean nations, who were accused by the Soviet authorities of collaboration with the Nazi occupiers, to remote regions of the USSR. The 2018 textbooks pay more attention to the Crimean Tatars' deportation. They indicate that the accusations of collaboration (actual collaborators were evacuated with the Germans), the prohibition by the Red Army to live in Crimea, and other events were unjustified. They also noted that the Verkhovna Rada (Supreme Council) of Ukraine recognises the deportations as genocide.[38] Overall, the 2018 textbooks pay much more attention to the crimes of the Communist regime. Students learn about the

34 Strukevich, Romaniuk, and Drovoziuk, *Istoriya Ukrayiny*, 49–50.

35 Mydriy and Arkusha, *Istoriya*, 226.

36 Vlasov and Kulchytskyi, *Istoriya Ukrayiny*, 230–236.

37 Strukevich, Romaniuk, and Drovoziuk, *Istoriya Ukrayiny*, 51.

38 Sorochinska and Hisem, *Istoriya Ukrayiny*, 239.

mass Soviet mobilisation of young people who were in previously Nazi-occupied territory and the creation of infantry units called *chornosvitniki* (people who fight in a peasant's black overcoat), who were immediately thrown into the battle without proper training, leading to mass casualties among them.[39]

What's Next? The Post-2022 Generation of Textbooks

The full-scale Russian invasion has influenced the next generation of Ukrainian history textbooks. In August 2022, the Ministry of Education and Science confirmed changes to the school history syllabus. The official Ministry communication states that the group working on curricula updates included leading institutions of higher education, state authorities, deputies of the Verkhovna Rada, scientists, school principals, teachers, and representatives of public and nongovernmental human rights organisations and mass media. They relate that history programmes should highlight the intersecting lines from the past that help to explain current events. Part of the curricula changes aims at creating additional opportunities for analogies and comparisons.[40]

This can be seen, for example, in the following titles of educational projects and practical classes: "Models of historical memory about the Second World War and the contemporary world", "'For the great Russian people!': Russian nationalism as a dominant Stalinist ideology and propaganda during the German–Soviet War", and "Stalin's generals and the price of human life", among others. In the renewed curricula, the USSR and Nazi Germany are both called 'totalitarian empires' (this phrase is absent in the previous textbooks). There is also a reconceptualisation of certain elements of the Soviet Union's participation in the war. For example, the new curricula describe the crimes on the territory of Ukraine as committed by "totalitarian empires – the USSR and Germany".[41]

Russia's instrumentalisation of the current war is also reflected in the curricula updates. In the section devoted to the current Russo–Ukrainian War, students are

---

39 Strukevych, *Istoriya Ukrayiny*, 215.

40 Ministerstvo Osviti i Nauki Ukrainy (the Ministry of Education and Science of Ukraine), "Onovleno zmist navchalnyx program ZSO" ("The Content of Educational Programmes of the ZSO Has Been Updated"), 16 September 2022, https://mon.gov.ua/news/onovleno-zmist-navchalnikh-program-zso [accessed: 31.07.2024].

41 Ministerstvo Osviti i Nauki Ukrainy (the Ministry of Education and Science of Ukraine), *Istoriya Ukrayiny: Vsesvitnya istoiya 6–11 klas, Navchalna programa dlya zakladiv zagalnoyi serednoyi osvity* (*A History of Ukraine: World History for the 6–11th Grades, A Curriculum for Institutions of General Secondary Education*), 03 September 2022, 82, 100, https:/mon.gov.ua/storage/app/media/zagalna%20serednya/programy-5-9-klas/2022/08/15/Navchalna.programa.2022.WH.HU.6-11.pdf [accessed 31.07.2024].

invited to reflect on Russian propaganda terms, such as 'Banderivtsi' (the name of a wing of WWII–era Ukrainian nationalists used in current Russian propaganda to define Ukrainians), 'Ukrainian Nazis', or the supposed 'denazification of Ukraine', which are all labelled as tools used in the modern genocide of Ukrainians. The updated syllabus also includes the new construct 'Ruscism' (a contraction of 'Russian fascism'), which appears to counter Russian propaganda that calls Ukrainians 'fascists'.[42] It is possible that this term will be in not only Ukrainian textbooks. The Ukrainian president, Volodymyr Zelenskyy, suggested that in the future, this term will be included in history textbooks around the world.[43]

Conclusions

To sum up, Ukrainian history textbooks are an excellent marker of the state's memory politics, particularly as related to the Second World War. Internal political processes, and external influences, namely the brutal war unleashed by Russia, affect state politics in the field of history. A reflection of this can be traced in the dynamics of different generations of textbooks, which, in turn, should be considered in the context of the political realities of a given period.

Textbooks on the history of Ukraine widely cover the Second World War. Regardless of the generation of textbooks, topics such as the German–Soviet Nonaggression Pact of 1939, collaboration, the occupation regime, and the Holocaust are discussed. However, after 2014, the general understanding of the war underwent a significant change. The Soviet title of the 'Great Patriotic War' became a thing of the past. Some of the visual components, selections of quotations, and questions for students have also changed.

Primarily, the content of the textbooks has been affected by the shifts in the state's memory policy. Ukrainian history textbooks have been significantly influenced by Euromaidan, the beginning of the Russo–Ukrainian War in 2014, and the full-scale invasion of Ukraine in 2022. The politics of memory post-Euromaidan became more Ukrainian-centric and oriented towards the European model of remembrance. There was a transition from the heroisation to the commemoration of war victims, and not only those who were ethnic Ukrainians. This is opposed to the Soviet and post-Soviet models of WWII commemoration, which did not consider the crimes committed by the Communist regime during the war. Now, information about this is present in the new generations of textbooks.

42 Ibid., 100, 102.

43 Serhy Yekelchyk, "Naming the war: Russian aggression in Ukrainian official discourse and mass culture", *Canadian Slavonic Papers* 64/2–3, 2022, 232–246, here 236.

What could be found in the next generation of textbooks? The changes, according to the programme updates, should not be as numerous as those after the start of the war in 2014, but they will be significant as well. In 2022, we might see a radical reflection by Ukrainian society, authorities, and scholars on Russia's aggression. Largely, these transformations are focused on the representation of the Second World War. A common view of the past cannot be seen in Ukraine and Russia in the way it was before the full-scale war, especially prior to 2014. The extreme situation of Russia's war against Ukraine makes a common historical perception and narrative, as well as a united memory politics, impossible in the near future.

Bibliography

Fuchs, Eckhardt, and Marcus Otto, "Introduction Educational Media, Textbooks, and Postcolonial Relocations of Memory Politics in Europe", *Journal of Educational Media, Memory, and Society* 5/1, 2013, 1–13.

Instytut modernizatsiyi osvity (Institute of the Modernisation of Education), "4. Istoriia Ukrainy 11 klas" ("4. The History of Ukraine for the 11th Grade"), https://lib.imzo.gov.ua/yelektronn-vers-pdruchnikv/11-klas/4-storya-ukrani-11-klas/ [accessed: 16.07.2024].

Kasianov, Georgiy, "National Master Narrative: Vicissitudes of Method", *AREI: Journal for Central and Eastern European History and Politics* 1, 2022, 108–127.

Klymenko, Lina, "Narrating the Second World War: History Textbooks and Nation Building in Belarus, Russia, and Ukraine", *Journal of Educational Media, Memory, and Society* 8/2, 2016, 35–57.

Klymenko, Lina, "World War II in Ukrainian School History Textbooks: Mapping the Discourse of the Past", *Compare: A Journal of Comparative and International Education* 44/5, 2014, 756–777.

Ministerstvo Osviti i Nauki Ukrainy (the Ministry of Education and Science of Ukraine), "Onovleno zmist navchalnyx program ZSO" ("The Content of Educational Programmes of the ZSO Has Been Updated"), 16 September 2022, h ttps://mon.gov.ua/news/onovleno-zmist-navchalnikh-program-zso [accessed: 07.02.2023].

Ministerstvo Osviti i Nauki Ukrainy (the Ministry of Education and Science of Ukraine), *Istoriya Ukrayiny: Vsesvitnya istoiya 6–11 klas, Navchalna programa dlya zakladiv zagalnoyi serednoyi osvity* (*A History of Ukraine: World History for the 6–11th Grades, A Curriculum for Institutions of General Secondary Education*), 03 September 2022, https:/mon.gov.ua/storage/app/media/zagalna%20serednya/programy-5-9-klas/2022/08/15/Navchalna.programa.2022.WH.HU.6-11.pdf [accessed 16.07.2024].

Mydriy, Marian, and Olena Arkusha, *Istoriya: Ukrayina i svit, Pidruchnyk dlya 10 klasu zakladiv zahalnoyi serednoyi osvity*, (*History: Ukraine and the World, A Textbook for the 10th Grade of Institutions of General Secondary Education*), Kyiv: Geneza, 2018.

Pometun, Olena, and Nestor Hupan, *Istoriya Ukrayiny: Pidruchnyk dlya 10 klasu zakladiv zagalnoyi serednoyi osvity* (*A History of Ukraine: A Textbook for the 10th Grade of General Secondary Education Institutions*) Kyiv: Orion, 2018.

Pometun, Olena, and Nestor Hupan, *Istoriya Ukrayiny: Pidruchnyk dlya 11 klasu zagalnoosvitnix navchalnyx zakladiv* (*A History of Ukraine: A Textbook for the 11th Grade of Secondary Schools*), Kharkiv: Sycyya, 2012.

Popson, Nancy, "The Ukrainian History Textbook: Introducing Children to the 'Ukrainian Nation'", *Nationalities Papers: The Journal of Nationalism and Ethnicity* 29/2, 2001, 325–350.

Poroshenko, Petro, "Pro uvichnennya peremohy nad natsyzmom u Druhiy svitoviy viyni 1939–1945 rokiv" ("On the Perpetuation of the Victory over Nazism in the Second World War of 1939–1945"), Verkhova Rada Ukrainy (Ukraine's Verkhova Rada), 9 April 2015, https://zakon.rada.gov.ua/laws/show/315-19#Text [accessed 16.07.2024].

Portnov, Andrii, *Istoriyi dlya domashnogo vzhytku: Eseyi pro polsko-rosijsko-ukrayinskyj trykutnyk pamyati* (*Histories for Home Use: Essays on the Polish–Russian–Ukrainian Triangle of Memory*), Kyiv: Krytyka, 2013.

Pryshchepa, Kateryna, "Nation-building and school history lessons in Ukraine after 2014", in: Tomasz Stryjek and Joanna Konieczna-Sałamatin (eds.), *The Politics of Memory in Poland and Ukraine: From Reconciliation to De-Conciliation*, London: Routledge, 2022, 120–135.

Sorochinska, Olha, and Natalia Hisem, *Istoriya Ukrayiny: Pidruchnyk dlya 10 klasu zakladiv zahalnoyi serednoyi osvity* (*A History of Ukraine: A Textbook for the 10th Grade of Institutions of General Secondary Education*) Ternopyl: Navchalna knyha – Bohdan, 2018.

Studenna-Skrukwa, Marta, "What history? What homeland? The nationalization of history in the school education before the breakthroughs in 2014–15 and after", in: Tomasz Stryjek and Joanna Konieczna-Sałamatin (eds.), *The Politics of Memory in Poland and Ukraine: From Reconciliation to De-Conciliation*, London: Routledge, 2022, 85–103.

Strukevych, Oleksii, *Istoriya Ukrayiny: Ptidruchnyk dlya 10 klasu zakladiv zagalnoyi serednoyi osvity* (*A History of Ukraine: A Textbook for the 10th Grade of General Secondary Education Institutions*), Kyiv: Gramota, 2018.

Strukevich, Oleksii, Ivan Romaniuk, and Stepan Drovoziuk, *Istoriya Ukrayiny: Pidruchnyk dlya 11 klasu zahalnoosvitnikh navchalnykh zakladiv* (*A History of Ukraine: A Textbook for the 11th Grade of General Educational Institutions*), Kyiv: Gramota, 2011.

Törnquist-Plewa, Barbara, and Yuliya Yurchuk, "Memory politics in contemporary Ukraine: Reflections from the postcolonial perspective", *Memory Studies* 12/6, 2019, 699–720.

Turchenko, Fedir, *Istoriya Ukrayiny: Pidruchnyk dlya 11 klasu zahalnoosvitnikh navchalnykh zakladiv (A History of Ukraine: A Textbook for the 11th Grade of General Educational Institutions)*, Kyiv: Geneza, 2011.

Turchenko, Fedir, Petro Panchenko, and Serhii Tymchenko, *Novitnya istoriya Ukrayiny (1939–2001): Pidruchnyk dlya 11-ho klasu serednikh pahal'noosvitnikh navchal'nykh zakladiv (The Modern History of Ukraine (1939–2001): A Textbook for the 11th Grade of Secondary Comprehensive Educational Institutions)*, Kyiv: Geneza, 2001.

UNIAN, "Rada zaminyla u zakoni Velyku Vitchyznyanu vijnu na Drugu svitovu" ("The Rada Replaced the Great Patriotic War with the Second World War in the Law"), 14 November 2017, https://www.unian.ua/politics/2242759-rada-zaminila-u-zakoni-veliku-vitchiznyanu-viynu-na-drugu-svitovu.html [accessed 16.07.2024].

Vlasov, Vitalii, and Stanislav Kulchytskyi, *Istoriya Ukrayiny: Pidruchnyk dlya 10 klasu zakladiv zagalnoyi serednoyi osvity (A History of Ukraine: A Textbook for the 10th Grade of Institutions of General Secondary Education)* Kyiv: Litera LTD, 2018.

Yekelchyk, Serhy, "Naming the war: Russian aggression in Ukrainian official discourse and mass culture", *Canadian Slavonic Papers* 64/2–3, 2022, 232–246.

"Its Own Patriotic War"

World War II in the Official Ukrainian Discourse on the Ongoing War

Denys Shatalov

For eight decades, Ukrainian society has maintained, constructed, and transformed the memory of World War II/the Great Patriotic War (WWII/GPW).[1] In the official attitude towards the GPW/WWII, profound changes took place in 2014. They were caused by the shock of Russia's annexation of Crimea and the outbreak of war in the Donbas – as well as by the decision to distance Ukraine from Russian propaganda associated with the mythology of the GPW, a decision made more necessary by Donbas separatists' use of St. George's ribbons and red banners.[2] At the same time, the outbreak of hostilities in the Donbas in April 2014, which escalated into full-scale fighting in the summer of 2014 and winter of 2015, provoked parallels with

1 I use two definitions, and each refers to one of two models of memory about this war that are present in Ukrainian society. The GPW model can be conditionally defined as (post-)Soviet and the WWII model as nationally Ukrainian. The first focuses on events of 1941–1945 and commemorates the 'Great Victory' and the liberation deeds of the Red Army. The second emphasises the Ukrainian context of the war of 1939–1945 and its victims.

2 See Julie Fedor, Simon Lewis, and Tatiana Zhurzhenko, "Introduction: War and Memory in Russia, Ukraine, and Belarus", in: Julie Fedor, Markku Kangaspuro, Jussi Lassila, and Tatiana Zhurzhenko (eds.), *War and Memory in Russia, Ukraine and Belarus*, London: Palgrave Macmillan, 2017, 4–20; Alexandr Osipian, "Historical Myths, Enemy Images, and Regional Identity in the Donbass Insurgency (Spring 2014)", *Journal of Soviet and Post-Soviet Politics and Society* 1/1, 2015, 116–118; Alexandr Osipian, "World War II Memory Politics in Russia and Ukraine and Their Uses During the Conflict in the Donbas (Spring–Summer 2014)", in: Korine Amacher, Andrii Portnov, and Victoriia Serhienko (eds.), *Official History in Eastern Europe*, Osnabrück: Fibre, 2020, 282–288; and Dmytro Tytarenko, "'Vrah vnov vstupyl na nashu zemlyu...': Velyka Vitchyznyana / II svitova viyna v politytsi pamyati na terytoriyi samoproholoshenoyi DNR (2014–2016 rr.)" ("'The Enemy Has Again Set Foot on Our Land...': The Great Patriotic/World War II in the Memory Politics on the Territory of the Self-Proclaimed DPR (2014–2016)"), Historians.in.ua, https://www.historians.in.ua/index.php/en/istoriya-i-pamyat-vazhki-pitannya/2399-dmitro-titarenko-vrag-vnov-vstupil-na-nashu-zemlyu-velika-vitchiznyana-ii-svitova-vijna-v-polititsi-pam-yati-na-teritoriji-samoprogoloshenoji-dnr-2014-2016-rr [accessed: 31.07.2024].

the events of WWII. Ukrainian officials also embraced the rhetoric and clichés from the Soviet vision of the GPW in 2014 and 2015.[3] While the May 2014 commemoration slogan was "Never Again!", in 2015 the emphasis shifted to "We Remember. We are winning". In the public discourse, a vision of continuity was created, from the generation of WWII veterans as defenders/liberators of the Ukrainian homeland then to the contemporary Anti-Terrorist Operation fighters as successors to their cause now.[4]

At the same time, the reaction of the Ukrainian authorities, and in particular the Ukrainian Institute of National Memory (UINP), as well as civil activists, was to intentionally distance public discourse from the (post-)Soviet vision of the GPW that is accepted in Russia.[5] In its methodological materials, the UINP proposed to move away from martial displays towards emphasising the human face of war, such as the fate of Ukrainians caught in the conflict. Additionally, a move was made to break down the concept of the GPW and reframe the conflict in the broader context of WWII.[6] A visual manifestation of the change in discourse was the choice of the

---

3 Andrii Portnov, "Velikaya Otechestvennaya voyna 2014–2015" ("The Great Patriotic War of 2014–2015"), http://urokiistorii.ru/node/52475 [accessed: 31.07.2024].

4 Jochen Hellbeck and Dmytro Tytarenko, "'My pobedim, kak pobedili 70 let nazad nashi dedy i pradedy'. Ukraina: prazdnovaniye Dnya Pobedy v teni novoy voyny" ("'We Will Win as Our Grandfathers and Great-Grandfathers Won 70 Years Ago'. Ukraine: Celebrations of Victory Day in the Shadow of the New War"), *Neprikosnovennyy zapas* (*Untouchable Reserve*) 4/108, 2016, http://magazines.russ.ru/nz/2016/4/my-pobedim-kak-pobedili-70-let-nazad-nashi-dedy-i-pradedy.html [accessed: 27.02.2023]; Andriy Stets, "Memorial voyinam ATO roztashuyut na terytoriyi muzeyu Druhoyi svitovoyi viyny u Kyyevi" ("A Memorial to the ATO Soldiers Will be Placed on the Territory of the Second World War Museum in Kyiv"), *Zaxid.net*, 08 May 2017, https://zaxid.net/memorial_voyinam_ato_roztashuyut_na_teritoriyi_muzeyu_drugoyi_svitovoyi_viyni_u_kiyevi_n1425349 [accessed: 27.02.2023]; and Informatsiyne ahentstvo PRAVDA (PRAVDA Information Agency), "V muzeyi istoriyi Ukrayiny u Druhiy svitovoyi viyny vidkrylas vystavka 'Chetverte pokolinnya'" ("The Exhibition 'The Fourth Generation' Opened in the Museum of the History of Ukraine during the Second World War"), YouTube video, 3:26, 08 May 2017, https://www.youtube.com/watch?v=kgseHqpDltc [accessed: 31.07.2024].

5 On the change of discourse in legislative acts, see: Oleksandr Hrytsenko, *Dekomunizatsiya v Ukrayini yak derzhavna polityka i yak sotsiokulturne yavyshche* (*Decommunisation in Ukraine as a State Policy and as a Sociocultural Phenomenon*), Kyiv: Instytut politychnykh i etnonatsionalnykh doslidzhen im. I. F. Kurasa NAN Ukrayiny; Instytut kulturolohiyi NAM Ukrayiny, 2019, 168–169.

6 Detector Media, "Yak vysvitlyuvaty Den Peremohy. Rekomendatsiyi Instytutu natsionalnoyi pamyati" ("How to Cover Victory Day: Recommendations of the Institute of National Memory"), 05 May 2014, https://ms.detector.media/profstandarti/post/898/2014-05-05-yak-vysvitlyuvaty-den-peremogy-rekomendatsii-instytutu-natsionalnoi-pamyati/ [accessed: 31.07.2024]. Oleksandr Hrytsenko analysed in detail the discourse of the UINP and the 'decommunisation laws' in the context of WWII. See: Hrytsenko, *Dekomunizatsiya*, 134–145.

red poppy as the main symbol of commemoration, a reminder of the victims of the war. A second major change was the attempt to shift the main day of remembrance to 8 May, the Day of Remembrance and Reconciliation, thereby moving closer to European practices. However, celebrations of Victory Day on 9 May continued as well.

A new narrative and concept of how the war should be remembered were presented in the exhibition *Ukrainian World War II* by the UINP. The exhibition placed local events of the war in a global context, with the story beginning with the fate of Carpathian Ukraine in March 1939. In general, not much space was given to the combat actions themselves; instead, the focus fell on the fate of people and included topics such as the Holocaust, *Ostarbeiter*, prisoners of war, collaboration, life under occupation, punitive actions, the nationalist and Soviet resistance movements, and the Ukrainian–Polish conflict.[7]

On 24 February 2022, Ukrainians, following Russia's full-scale invasion, became participants in a new war. Already in February, numerous caricatures and comparisons of the Russian invasion forces with the troops of the Third Reich were circulating on social media. This reaction shows that for Ukrainians, the images from WWII history are a kind of mental standard: it is through comparison with them that contemporary events are presented and comprehended. Similar comparisons were made by officials at various levels. In 2022, the main slogan for 8 and 9 May was: "We defeated Nazism – we will defeat Ruscism!" Such a slogan draws explicit parallels between WWII and the ongoing war. It also echoes the 2015 slogan, "We Remember. We are winning."

In this paper, I analyse the rhetoric of Ukrainian government agencies and officials of various levels to determine how the topic of WWII is exploited in the context of the full-scale Russo–Ukrainian War. What aspects of the myth of WWII are in demand in the crisis conditions of the invasion? And what (comparative) language is used to describe the Second World War and the ongoing Russo–Ukrainian War? I aim to answer these questions using discourse analysis.

For the analysis, I selected posts from the first year of the war, from 24 February 2022 to 24 February 2023, from official Facebook pages, which in the current and recent Ukrainian reality serve as one of the means of disseminating official information. These pages represent different levels of government and military leadership. Namely, these are the pages of the President of Ukraine, Volodymyr Zelenskyy, the Commander-in-Chief of the Armed Forces of Ukraine (AFU), and the General Staff of the AFU. Meanwhile, regionally, the analysis focuses on the

---

7 Institute of National Memory (UINP), "Vystavka 'Ukrayinska Druha svitova'" ("'The Ukrainian Second World War' Exhibition"), https://uinp.gov.ua/vystavkovi-proekty/vystavka-ukrayinska-druga-svitova [accessed: 31.07.2024]. About changes in the presentation of WWII in official memory policy see also: Tadeus Olszański, "The Great Decommunisation: Ukraine's Wartime Historical Policy", *OSW Point of View* 65, September 2017, 26–40.

Dnipropetrovsk Oblast, which represents Southern Ukraine. Before the full-scale invasion, sociological research characterised the oblast as strongly emotionally connected to the historical memory of WWII. In my work, this oblast is represented by the pages of Head of the Dnipropetrovsk Oblast State Administration Valentyn Reznichenko (dismissed from office on 24 January 2023), Head of the Dnipro Oblast Council Mykola Lukashuk, and the military Operational Command (OC) "East" ("*Skhid*"), situated in Dnipro. Lastly, locally, I look at Kryvyi Rih, the second most populous city in the Dnipropetrovsk Oblast.[8] Its officials do not have their own presence on social media, apart from Oleksandr Vilkul. Vilkul was appointed head of the Military–Civilian Administration of Kryvyi Rih on 26 February 2022 and is the head of the city's Defence Council. His official Facebook page is the main source of information on the situation in Kryvyi Rih since the beginning of the war.

The President's and regional officials' pages are presented as personal, containing only names and titles. The content of all the selected pages is thematically homogeneous and designed to communicate with citizens: it features reports on current activities, newsletters, daily summaries in text or video format, posts on holidays or memorable dates, and motivational posts. Thus, the language and message of these posts are intended for the widest possible audience among Ukrainians. Vilkul's appeals to the WWII topic are of particular interest given his background: over the past couple of decades, he has been a consistent supporter of the idea of 'protecting the memory of the Victory' – that is, the post-Soviet discourse at the regional and all-Ukrainian level. In addition, his page is the only one from the selection that has some posts in Russian. Nevertheless, the posts on the analysed pages generally represent a single discourse, which allows us to perceive them as a kind of metatext. The only exception is the content from the General Staff of the AFU page, where the discourse produced by the UINP is strongly represented.

The posts related to WWII topics in the sample are mostly commemorative, written on memorial days or anniversaries connected to WWII. The table below allows us to visualise the frequency of appeals on specific dates.

8 The Facebook pages of Kryvyi Rih military units limit their posts to information about the life and activity of military departments, without references to the past. Therefore, I did not include their content in this analysis.

Figure 1: Reference to WWII by Date and Ukrainian Official

	Day of Remembrance and Reconciliation 8.05.	Victory Day 9.05.	Day of Remembrance and Sorrow 22.06.	Anniversary of the Start of WWII 1.09.	Day of Partisan Glory 22.09.	Babyn Yar Anniversary 29.09.	Day of the Liberation of Ukraine 28.10.
President of Ukraine Volodymyr Zelenskyy	+++	+	++	+		+	+
Commander-in-Chief of the AFU	+	+				+	
General Staff of the AFU	++++	+	+	+		+	+
Head of the Dnipropetrovsk Oblast State Administration Valentyn Reznichenko	+	+	+			+	+
Head of the Dnipropetrovsk Oblast Council Mykola Lukashuk	+	+				+	+
OC "East"	++++	+	+				+
Head of the Military–Civilian Administration of Kryvyi Rih Oleksandr Vilkuk	+++		+		+		+

There is also a single 'spontaneous' post without any apparent reference to current events or the WWII calendar: on 20 March 2022, the Commander-in-Chief's page presented modern Ukrainian warriors as descendants of Red Army soldiers who fought against the German invaders.[9]

Enemies Then and Now

The most common references to WWII in the posts of the selected pages refer to the image of the enemy. The activities of the modern Russian Federation are clearly identified with those of the Nazi Third Reich. Russia is presented as the reincarnation of Hitler's Germany. For example, the page of the General Staff shares, "the criminal history of Nazism did not end in 1945, but [...] continued in the modern Russian Federation".[10] Lukashuk posted a similar idea on 8 May: "Nazism has transformed into Ruscism. Putin's regime wants to destroy our nation, as the Nazis once tried to destroy us".[11] In a post he published the next day, he states that "the sign of equality between hitler and putin [lower case in the original] has long been set", and the reason for this is the repetition of Nazi acts by Russians.[12] President Zelenskyy's posts also draw similar parallels. In a speech on 8 May, he stated:

> In Ukraine, a bloody reconstruction of Nazism has been organised. Fanatical imitation of this regime. Its ideas, actions, words, and symbols. Maniacal reproduction – down to the detail – of its atrocities and "alibis" that seem to give evil a sacred purpose.[13]

9 Holovnokomanduvach ZS Ukrayiny / CinC AF of Ukraine, "Nikoly znovu... Na zhal, tse ne tak..." ("Never again... Unfortunately, that's not the case..."), Facebook post, 08 May 2022, https://www.facebook.com/watch/?v=3060183750958951 [accessed: 27.02.2023].

10 Heneralnyy shtab ZSU / General Staff of the Armed Forces of Ukraine, "Do Dnya pamyati ta prymyrennya..." ("To the Day of Remembrance and Reconciliation..."), Facebook post, 07 May 2022, https://www.facebook.com/GeneralStaff.ua/posts/pfbidoQ9isApXrZxWAGpjuoydLhF6CnZxrmADixLZJKfy3VCD93mNv2uAtVVfGeHKZPk1Ul [accessed: 27.02.2023] [author's trans.].

11 Mykola Lukashuk, "'Holovne – shchob ne bulo viyny'..." ("'The main thing is that there should be no war'..."), Facebook post, 08 May 2022, https://www.facebook.com/MVLukashuk/posts/pfbidoHt3c2wPdpv1jRF8UbG97Sh7Nzm8fyidu8EtQicWwQ3jCnhAzf57ap3CUzZd7WKCLl [accessed: 27.02.2023] [author's trans.].

12 Mykola Lukashuk, "Sohodni my vidznachayemo 77-mu richnytsyu..." ("Today we celebrate the 77th anniversary..."), Facebook post, 09 May 2022, https://www.facebook.com/MVLukashuk/posts/pfbidoSsCLn4zA1F1oxx4ggVRHSMHw1QvYLwNJwKFjyimswgRMnHFfNGud3XBUmp7KiqtAl [accessed: 31.07.2024].

13 Volodymyr Zelenskyy, "Tsohorich my kazhemo 'Nikoly znovu' inakshe..." ("This year we say 'Never again' in a different way..."), Facebook post, 08 May 2022, https://www.facebook.com/watch/?v=442165114339716 [accessed: 31.07.2024] [author's trans.]. For the text

Numerous parallels are drawn between the Nazi crimes committed during WWII throughout Europe and the atrocities committed by Russians in Ukraine today. The General Staff's page makes a similar comparison in a post dedicated to the Day of Remembrance and Reconciliation:

> Austria's annexation [is like] the attempt of the illegal temporary occupation of Crimea, the protection of German-speaking people in the Sudetenland [is like] the protection of Russian-speakers in Eastern Ukraine, the denial of the existence of Poland and the people of Israel by Hitler and German Nazism [is like] the denial of the existence of Ukraine and its people by Putin and Russian Nazism.[14]

On the anniversary of the Babyn Yar massacre, the page of the Commander-in-Chief of the AFU stated: "it is painfully difficult to talk about its repetition in Mariupol, Bucha, Irpin, Izyum and other cities".[15] Crimes were similarly compared on Zelenskyy's page on 27 October: "[Russia] organises blockades and filtration camps. And Syrets becomes Olenivka. It destroys towns and villages. And Koriukivka becomes Bucha".[16] Similarly, after the de-occupation of the Kharkiv Oblsast, Zelenskyy pointed to direct parallels regarding the occupant's actions: "Torture was a widespread practice in the occupied territory. The Nazis did it. This is what the Rus-

---

version, see: President of Ukraine, Volodymyr Zelenskyy, Official Website, "Zvernennia Prezydenta Ukrainy z nahody Dnia pamiati ta prymyrennia" ("Address of the President of Ukraine on the Occasion of the Day of Remembrance and Reconciliation"), 08 May 2022, https://www.president.gov.ua/news/zvernennya-prezidenta-ukrayini-z-nagodi-dnya-pamyati-ta-prim-74885 [accessed: 31.07.2024].

14 Heneralnyy shtab, "Do Dnya pamyati ta prymyrennya".

15 Holovnokomanduvach ZS Ukrayiny / CinC AF of Ukraine, "Sohodni mav chest poznayomytysya..." ("Today I had the honour to meet..."), Facebook post, 29 September 2022, https://www.facebook.com/CinCAFU/posts/pfbidoTYJ8S325QEhCVmuFMnHvmZUba5wNvwyzxAopDKthaFX5Hu1hQa7NSWCYa2F8ionql [accessed: 27.02.2023] [author's trans.].

16 Volodymyr Zelenskyy, "Zlo zavzhdy pochynaye odnakovo..." ("Evil always starts in the same way..."), Facebook post, 27 October 2022, https://www.facebook.com/watch/?v=574046394479712 [accessed: 31.07.2024] [author's trans.]. During the Nazi occupation, about 30,000 Soviet activists, POWs, and Jews were murdered in the Syrets concentration camp in Kyiv. In the village of Olenivka, an explosion at a prison for Ukrainian POWs on the night of 29 July 2022 killed a few dozen Ukrainian prisoners and injured more than 150. In Koryukivka, a town in the Chernihiv Oblast, occupants massacred about 7000 people of the population in 1943, while in Bucha, a suburb of Kyiv, Russian troops killed more than 400 civilians during the occupation in March 2022.

cists do".[17] In this way, 'Ruscism' is labelled a repetition of Nazism with equivalent accompanying atrocities.[18]

The identification of Russian atrocities with those of the Nazis is also seen in the narration of uploaded videos. On 9 May, the Commander-in-Chief of the AFU's page uploaded a video with English subtitles in which footage of Nazi atrocities and destruction in Europe is presented in parallel with footage of the suffering and destruction caused by the Russian invasion.[19] Alongside direct identification, it is also common practice to present the 'succession' of enemies, as the Commander-in-Chief of the AFU did on 8 May: "In 1939–1945 the enemy was the Nazis, and today it is the Ruscists – the Russian version of imperial nationalism and fascism".[20] At the same time, the Nazis remain the 'etalon' with which modern Russia is compared. For example, on 28 October, Vilkul mentioned the liberation of Ukraine "from German fascists": "We are at war with an enemy who is no less cruel. This enemy is the Russian fascist".[21]

References to WWII in posts not devoted to commemorative dates appear in the vocabulary used to describe current events. Such references include mentions of the "Kremlin Fuhrer"[22] or "the horrors of the Russian Auschwitz [in Ukrainian text used

---

17 Volodymyr Zelenskyy, "Sohodni v Izyumi Kharkivskoyi oblasti..." ("Today in Izyum in the Kharkiv Oblast..."), Facebook post, 17 September 2022, https://www.facebook.com/watch/?v=1519134511858182 [accessed: 31.07.2024] [author's trans.].

18 Volodymyr Zelenskyy, "Tak samo, yak Kyyivshchynu..." ("In the same way as in the Kyiv Oblast..."), Facebook post, 18 September 2022, https://www.facebook.com/zelenskiy.official/posts/pfbid0244YxALVV6Ga6WMT4RZUvTkxhdujyHxqcwcBrxGL99iqoaY7ACogZGcYS2w28ey38l [accessed: 31.07.2024].

19 Holovnokomanduvach ZS Ukrayiny / CinC AF of Ukraine, "Never again?...", Facebook post, 09 May 2022, https://www.facebook.com/CinCAFU/videos/526275025573107/ [accessed: 31.07.2024].

20 Heneralnyy shtab ZSU / General Staff of the Armed Forces of Ukraine, "Peremohly natsyzm – peremozhemo i rashyzm!..." ("We defeated Nazism – we will defeat Ruscism!..."), Facebook post, 08 May 2022, https://www.facebook.com/GeneralStaff.ua/posts/pfbid02fQD8geqPcFWTPYxhMiwcsCp6pvrukK2TP2asGZPKgWpmL9dTZc6Y9ibkYUXtiXVel [accessed: 31.07.2024] [author's trans.].

21 Oleksandr Vilkul, "Bryfinh nachalnyka viyskovoyi administratsiyi Kryvoho Rohu O.Vilkula 28 10 22..." ("Briefing of the Head of the Military Administration of Kryvyi Rih O.Vilkul 28 10 22..."), Facebook post, 28 October 2022, https://www.facebook.com/watch/?v=666158901742437 [accessed: 31.07.2024] [author's trans.].

22 Heneralnyy shtab ZSU / General Staff of the Armed Forces of Ukraine, "My zirvaly plany kremlivskoho fyurera!..." ("We foiled the plans of the Kremlin Führer!..."), Facebook post, 05 April 2022, https://www.facebook.com/watch/?v=553634419287322 [accessed: 31.07.2024] [author's trans.].

'Oświęcim' – D.S.]".[23] The reference to the 'Russian Auschwitz' appears on the page of the OC "East". This post exposes the hollowness of Russian promises about the humane treatment of prisoners. However, it is significant that at the same time, the OC "East" referenced the traditions of the Soviet repressive system and called Russians the "heirs to the almost century-old experience of the NKVD".[24] In this way, Nazi and Soviet crimes are combined in the same context.

One post on the page of the General Staff of the AFU was structured similarly, although it looks strange from a logical standpoint. The post discusses finding a container with metal dentures in a Russian torture chamber in the de-occupied Kharkiv Oblast.[25] It opens with a hashtagged headline: "#putin's_ruscism = #hitler's_nazism" and is accompanied by an image comparing the recent find with a container of dentures from Buchenwald found in the spring of 1945. However, the text of the post does not mention Nazis and instead states that "Russian military executioners are descendants of *Oprichniki*[26] executioners, tsarist executioners, human-hating executioners of the diabolical organs of the Soviet Union – the Cheka-OGPU, NKVD, SMERSH, KGB".[27] As we can see, in the modern Ukrainian context, the images of Nazi concentration camps and bodies like the Gestapo are less significant than the images of the Soviet repressive system.

However, it is noteworthy that although the agencies of national memory (and above all the UINP) present a narrative that shows both the Soviet and Nazi regimes as hostile to Ukraine, and present-day Russia also manifests its succession from the USSR in various forms, the exploitation of the topic of Soviet crimes during WWII (for example, the massive looting and rape by Soviet soldiers in Germany in 1945, which could be compared with Russian crimes in Ukraine) is not widespread in the analysed discourse. This can be explained by the practice of referring to WWII

---

23 Operatyvne komanduvannya "Skhid" (Operational Command "East"), "Kreml vzhe vstyh obminyaty..." ("The Kremlin has already exchanged..."), Facebook post, 29 October 2022, https://www.facebook.com/watch/?v=5853012694737823 [accessed: 31.07.2024] [author's trans.].

24 Operatyvne komanduvannya "Skhid", "Kreml vzhe vstyh obminyaty".

25 Later, it turned out that the container most likely belonged to a local dentist and was just seized by the Russians. *Khmarochos*, "Politsiya pereviryaye, chy nalezhaly zoloti zuby z kativni sela Pisky-Radkivski mistsevomu stomatolohu" ("Police Check Whether Gold Teeth From the Pisky-Radkivski Torture Chamber Belonged to a Local Dentist"), 06 October 2022, https://hmarochos.kiev.ua/2022/10/06/policziya-pereviryaye-chy-nalezhaly-zoloti-zuby-z-kativni-sela-pisky-radkivski-misczevomu-stomatologu/ [accessed: 31.07.2024].

26 *Oprichniki* were members of the bodyguard corps established by Tsar Ivan the Terrible in the 16th century.

27 Heneralnyy shtab ZSU / General Staff of the Armed Forces of Ukraine, "#putinskyy_rashyzm = #hitlerivskyy_natsyzm..." ("#putin's_ruscism = #hitler's_nazism"...), Facebook post, 05 October 2022, https://www.facebook.com/GeneralStaff.ua/posts/pfbid03XDieGmr4xdKVABD2GYJr6E3DwXvAaL6PLS9VAVLnp3e8Y8Q7GbYGiisPQLMHuMtl [accessed: 31.07.2024] [author's trans.].

mostly on former Soviet anniversaries, thereby not providing the right context for references to Soviet crimes. But on the other hand, direct or implicit contemporary self-identification with the generation of Ukrainian fighters of the Red Army (more on this below) naturally does not imply solidarity with or emphasis on the crimes of the Red Army. Thus, Soviet crimes are mentioned on other dates, such as Holodomor Remembrance Day, the Day of the Deportation of Crimean Tatars, or the Day of Remembrance of Victims of Political Repression, during which WWII is 'left out'. In the analysed selection, discussions of Soviet responsibility for these crimes and the accompanying presentation of the succession of Stalin's Soviet Union by present-day Russia appear only in the posts on the page of the General Staff of the AFU, which for the most part amount to compilations of UINP materials.

When Did That War Begin for Ukraine?

The rejection of the concept of the 'Great Patriotic War' is a central tenet of the new discourse that the UINP has promoted since 2014. WWII–era events in Ukraine are now placed in the wider framework of the history of WWII. One result of this change is that the years of significance have expanded from the traditional years of the Great Patriotic War, 1941–1945, to the wider timeframe of 1939–1945. Currently, the official date of the beginning of the Second World War in Ukraine is no longer 22 June 1941, when Nazi Germany attacked the Soviet Union, but 1 September 1939. At this point, Hitler invaded Poland; the territories of the present-day Ukrainian regions of Galicia and Volhynia, then part of the Polish state, became a battlefield.

However, in the context of the full-scale war of 2022, 1 September 1939 did not cause reflection in my analysed sources. It was mentioned on only two of the pages – that of Zelenskyy and of the General Staff. And in both cases, the posts addressed the Polish people (yet both are also in Ukrainian). In his speech, Zelenskyy compares the beginning of the war on 1 September 1939 – with the bombing of the Polish city of Wieluń – to the 24 February 2022 attack on Ukrainian cities. He also compares Nazi crimes against the Polish people to the current crimes of Russia against Ukrainians. He then says that "the morning of 1 September, the morning of 22 June, and the morning of 24 February" should not be repeated.[28] This list seems revealing: the

28 Volodymyr Zelenskyy, "1 veresnya 1939 roku..." ("1 September of the year 1939..."), Facebook post, 01 September 2022, https://www.facebook.com/watch/?v=3174257042887794 [accessed: 31.07.2024]. For the text version of the speech, see: ArmiiaInform (ArmyInformation), "Prezydent zvernuvsia do narodu Polshchi u 83-tiu richnytsiu pochatku Druhoi svitovoi viiny" ("The President Addressed the People of Poland on the 83rd Anniversary of the Beginning of World War II"), 01 September 2022, https://armyinform.com.ua/2022/09/01/prezydent-zvernuvsya-do-narodu-polshhi-u-83-tyu-richnyczyu-pochatku-drugoyi-svitovoyi-vijny/ [accessed: 31.07.2024].

'Polish' date is put on par with the two 'Ukrainian' dates, and 1 September is not presented as Ukraine's 'own' date.

The post published on 1 September on the page of the General Staff is eclectic in structure and broad in content. Discursively, it presents the aforementioned position of the UINP. It begins by expressing solidarity with the Polish Army and the Polish people, quoting the Deputy Prime Minister of the National Defence of Poland, who drew parallels between the attacks on Poland in 1939 and Ukraine in 2022. What follows is a lengthy piece based on materials developed by the UINP, which also uses fragments of the presidential speech (without indicating the source). There is a revealing supplement to his words: the text adds that, along with Wieluń, "Lviv and other Western Ukrainian cities were bombed". It then describes the participation of Ukrainians in the armies of the United Nations and presents a deconstruction of myths (prepared by the UINP) of the Soviet Russian discourses around WWII. Already the first paragraph states that "[t]he chronological framework of the 'Great Patriotic War' [...] does not correspond to the experience of the Ukrainian people during World War II".[29]

Two months earlier, the page of the General Staff presented 22 June 1941 as the day the war "between Nazi Germany and the Communist Soviet Union" began, as well as just a part of the larger war raging in Europe. The post emphasised the victims of both regimes, German and Soviet:

> The German–Soviet War demonstrated the destructive power of both totalitarian regimes. Everyone knows the crimes of the Nazis in the occupied territories of Ukraine: the Holocaust, the shooting of civilians, the creation of death camps, and the burning of villages. No less brutal were the crimes of the Stalinist regime: the executions of political prisoners in Western Ukraine in June–July 1941, the destruction of the centre of Kyiv in the fall of that year, the blowing up of the DniproHES [the Dnipro Hydroelectric Station], and then the deportation of the Crimean Tatars, the forced eviction of indigenous Ukrainians from their ethnic lands.[30]

---

29 Heneralnyy shtab ZSU / General Staff of the Armed Forces of Ukraine, "1 veresnya, Zbroyni Syly Ukrayiny solidaryzuyutsya..." ("1 September, the Armed Forces of Ukraine Stand in Solidarity..."), Facebook post, 01 September 2022, https://www.facebook.com/GeneralStaff.ua/posts/pfbidoijjcqMXCWFFkKEwTVzXAc2eBk2wgGGvqCNuUj4eENcZg8RRDyAtWD4eiDjtfEFcal [accessed: 31.07.2024] [author's trans.].

30 Heneralnyy shtab ZSU / General Staff of the Armed Forces of Ukraine, "22 chervnya – Den skorboty i vshanuvannya..." ("22 June is the Day of Mourning and Commemoration..."), Facebook post, 22 June 2022, https://www.facebook.com/GeneralStaff.ua/posts/pfbid02v88PBfWCvdyuMJm1hjwR3epqgx1GAKzJ36GghuzaVnGbjSjXvmMwz3uEaYx3gRsyl [accessed: 31.07.2024] [author's trans]. The quoted phrase was not originally written by the author of the post, it has been actively disseminated on various websites since at least 2020.

Nevertheless, rather than 1 September, it was 22 June that gave rise to historical parallels: posts on that day appeared on five out of the seven pages covered in this study. The page of the OC "East" posted a simple banner – red poppies against a background of plaques with names from soldiers' graves, and text overlay with the date's denomination: "The Day of Mourning and Commemoration of the Victims of the War in Ukraine".[31] Reznichenko recalled the Ukrainian victims of WWII and drew parallels to the present: "Missiles are flying into Ukraine again, and again we are ruthlessly destroyed".[32] This comparison refers to the identification of Russia with Nazi Germany.

Zelenskyy's page, first noting 22 June as a day to commemorate the victims of WWII, claims that events from the past are repeating themselves in the present: "On 24 February the occupiers came to our land". The post is accompanied by photos that present the destruction and suffering of the population during the ongoing war.[33] In his daily address on the same day, Zelenskyy said: "Today there is no shortage of words that what Russia did on 24 February was the same as [what] the Nazis did on 22 June".[34] Vilkul expresses a similar opinion, noting that "the two tragic dates will forever be a part of the history of our people", meaning 22 June and 24 February.[35] The page of the Commander-in-Chief of the AFU also mentions the dates of the German

31 Operatyvne komanduvannya "Skhid" (Operational Command "East"), "[Den skorboty i vshanuvannya]" ("[The Day of Mourning and Commemoration]"), Facebook post, 22 June 2022, https://www.facebook.com/EastOC/posts/pfbidoXRAVQv499dANTsoCXxgSVnnQojbuNckbWDTuJwEinh6EhFNNsd49bqTXp1a9HM1Bl [accessed: 31.07.2024].

32 Valentyn Reznichenko, "U tsey den my zhaduyemo..." ("On this day we remember..."), Facebook post, 22 June 2022, https://www.facebook.com/Valentyn.Reznichenko/posts/pfbidoWFLguUKzPnVxwBbjzYrGw6ioFFzxFAapFPEcYTUxmevuBxCRaU5cbZ8HkSPCmg3al [accessed: 31.07.2024] [author's trans.].

33 Volodymyr Zelenskyy, "Shchoroku 22 chervnya..." ("Every year on 22 June..."), Facebook post, 22 June 2022, https://www.facebook.com/zelenskiy.official/posts/pfbidoTWz9Gqbt6mNTQ4vu8Cs6j4NfNp2EAwiatMCrFGkfD9QK9b42S2DbYxhj41iAaQztl [accessed: 31.07.2024] [author's trans.].

34 Volodymyr Zelenskyy, "Vid samoho ranku prodovzhyv..." ("Since the morning, I have continued..."), Facebook post, 22 June 2022, https://www.facebook.com/watch/?v=2814332868861296 [accessed: 27.02.2023] [author's trans.]. A text version of the speech is available here: President of Ukraine, Volodymyr Zelenskyy, Official Website, "Zvilnyty nashu zemliu i pryity do peremohy – tse nasha natsionalna meta, nad realizatsiieiu yakoi maiemo pratsiuvaty shchodnia – zvernennia Prezydenta Ukrainy" ("To Liberate Our Land and Achieve Victory Is Our National Goal, Which We Must Work on Every Day – the President of Ukraine's Address"), 23 June 2022, https://www.president.gov.ua/news/zvilniti-nashu-zemlyu-i-prijti-do-peremogi-ce-nasha-nacional-76001 [accessed: 31.07.2024].

35 Oleksandr Vilkul, "Dve tragicheskiye daty..." ("Two tragic dates..."), Facebook post, 22 June 2022, https://www.facebook.com/OleksandrVilkul/posts/pfbidoHPKiMdtufXVbkMfGg3kruKNT3bRXGujfyBypENFPxNYbn7Pwur5PT5b8C9Wv9Nahl [accessed: 31.07.2024] [author's trans.].

and Russian attacks in March.[36] Drawing the same comparison on the following 9 May, Lukashuk wrote: "On 24 February, Ukraine's own Patriotic War began".[37]

Bureaucratic circumstances partially explain the 'inattention' paid to 1 September as compared to the 'popularity' of 22 June. The September date is not recorded in the official calendar, while 22 June is the official date for the Day of Mourning and Commemoration of the Victims of War in Ukraine.[38] Unsurprisingly, as an official date, it has a higher value for officials and shapes their reaction. But the content of the posts also shows that 22 June 1941 is still perceived as the day that WWII began in Ukraine.

We Will Not Give Away the Victory of Our Grandfathers

In addition to the idea of the relationship between Ukraine's enemies during WWII and now, the idea of the relationship of the defenders – that is, the heredity of the Red Army frontline soldiers to modern Ukrainian fighters – is exploited in the contemporary context. Thus, on 20 March, the page of the Commander-in-Chief of the AFU posted a video with reconstructed scenes of the Red Army's battle against the Wehrmacht, which transformed into an image of today's Ukrainian Army at war.[39] An analogous video appeared on this page on 8 May.[40] On the same day, the page of the OC "East" posted a similar video. It begins with footage from Leonid Bykov's popular Soviet war movie *Only "Old Men" Are Going into Battle* (1973). The video presents the modern Russian Army as analogous to Nazi Germany's troops, while the fighters of the Red Army are combined with the representation of the modern AFU.[41] Reznichenko's page presents the same idea in the form of a banner with the silhouettes of a Soviet soldier and a modern Ukrainian soldier against the backdrop of destruction taken from both wars and the slogan "We won then – we will win now".[42]

36 Holovnokomanduvach ZS Ukrayiny / CinC AF of Ukraine, "Viyna. Viyna nikoly ne zminyuyetsya..." ("War. War never changes..."), Facebook post, 20 March 2022, https://www.facebook.com/watch/?v=497146995321410 [accessed: 31.07.2024].

37 Lukashuk, "Sohodni my vidznachayemo 77-mu richnytsyu".

38 This is the commemorative date introduced by a decree of Ukrainian President Leonid Kuchma on 17 November 2000. Obviously, after 24 February 2022, the date's name needed to be adjusted, as now the idea of 'war in Ukraine' does not automatically refer to the events of WWII.

39 Holovnokomanduvach ZS Ukrayiny, "Viyna. Viyna nikoly ne zminyuyetsya".

40 Holovnokomanduvach ZS Ukrayiny, "Nikoly znovu... Na zhal, tse ne tak".

41 Operatyvne komanduvannya "Skhid" (Operational Command "East"), "Sohodni v Ukrayini vidznachayut..." ("Today in Ukraine is being celebrated..."), Facebook post, 08 May 2022, https://www.facebook.com/watch/?v=566804038083537 [accessed 31.07.2024].

42 Valentyn Reznichenko, "Buty ukrayintsem – tse buty vilnym..." ("To be Ukrainian means to be free..."), Facebook post, 09 May 2022, https://www.facebook.com/Valentyn.Reznichenk

It is quite telling that, although the participation of Ukrainians in other armies of the anti-Hitler coalition is mentioned,[43] this is not presented in any way.

Zelenskyy's posts also talk about the continuity of generations: "The deeds of grandfathers become the victories of grandchildren. The liberation of Ukraine from the Nazis [...] becomes a symbol: the result of our struggle will certainly be the liberation of our Ukraine!"[44] Vilkul expresses a similar idea: "Our grandfathers and great-grandfathers won. Now it is the turn of our generation to stand up for the country!"[45] On 22 February 2023, the Day of the Liberation of Kryvyi Rih from Nazi Invaders, he emphasised the same parallel: "our ancestors liberated Kryvyi Rih from the Nazi occupiers", and now "we, like our ancestors, are forced to fight, to liberate our Ukraine from another occupant".[46] Earlier, Vilkul mentioned a succession of not only soldiers but also partisans of the two wars. On September 22, Vilkul noted at a briefing:

> Today is the Day of Partisan Glory in Ukraine. For the seventh month in our native Ukraine, a full-scale war unleashed by Russia has been going on, and once again, Ukrainian partisans, just like 80 years ago, are striking fear into the enemy.[47]

It is noteworthy that there is no specification of which partisans were meant as predecessors of the present-day ones, given the existence of both nationalist and Soviet partisan formations during WWII. However, in general, this case is an interesting example of the direct incorporation of elements from the memory of the GPW into contemporary circumstances. Established by President Leonid Kuchma in 2001 "in support of the initiative of war veterans and with the aim of nationally honouring

---

o/posts/pfbidobUqU2PeyrQdCFTz98aukPeXhDjyQaZHmMEdwbFqNkfYqnZBxVHKkNVNdWzSY9qyLl [accessed 31.07.2024] [author's trans].

43 Holovnokomanduvach ZS Ukrayiny, "Nikoly znovu... Na zhal, tse ne tak".

44 Volodymyr Zelenskyy, "Zlo zavzhdy pochynaye odnakovo".

45 Oleksandr Vilkul, "Bryfinh nachalnyka viys'kovoyi administratsiyi Kryvoho Rohu O.Vilkula 28 10 22...". See also: Oleksandr Vilkul, "Rivno 78 rokiv tomu..." ("Exactly 78 years ago..."), Facebook post, 28 October 2022, https://www.facebook.com/OleksandrVilkul/posts/pfbidoUuUGMZN5RyFEypFUuHtyRRjUfqGmdX13aKNBZpm8nmDj3S4yLZBfgGKrTCxhNyJSl [accessed 31.07.2024].

46 Oleksandr Vilkul, "U tsey den 79 rokiv tomu..." ("On this day 79 years ago..."), Facebook post, 22 February 2023, https://www.facebook.com/OleksandrVilkul/posts/pfbido29Mn78nhwXyg2CWvQVRwsoWMWUuov7X8yHWkuaLosJCBtMW5981LbCkQtYpGuFTkXl [accessed 31.07.2024] [author's trans].

47 Oleksandr Vilkul, "Bryfinh nachalnyka viyskovoyi administratsiyi Kryvoho Rohu O.Vilkula 22 09 22..." ("Briefing of the Head of the Military Administration of Kryvyi Rih O.Vilkul 22 09 22..."), Facebook post, 22 September 2022, https://www.facebook.com/watch/?v=628544058975647 [accessed: 31.07.2024] [author's trans].

the feats of partisans and underground fighters during the Great Patriotic War",[48] the Day of Partisan Glory was a clear 'bow' to the leftist electorate with pro-Soviet sympathies. Since 2014, it has been almost forgotten. However, in 2022, extensive Ukrainian guerrilla activity in the Russian-occupied territories provided a new reason to resurrect this neglected holiday.

As seen from the discourse discussed above, there is a current self-identification with Ukrainian Red Army soldiers who resisted the Nazi invasion that began in 1941. It is organically combined with the identification of enemies in the ongoing and past war. In most of the analysed posts, the Second World War is perceived as 'our' war from the Soviet perspective, although this is not directly stated. At the same time, a direct correlation between modern Ukraine and the Ukrainian Soviet Socialist Republic does not follow. In the analysed discourses, Ukraine's participation in WWII is isolated from the Soviet context. For example, Lukashuk presents Ukraine as an independent participant in WWII: "The victory over Nazism was won by the anti-Hitler coalition, which included dozens of countries. Ukraine played a huge role in this victory".[49]

Lukashuk's statement that Ukrainians "are once again forced to fight for their statehood, for the nation, once again forced to confront the aggressor" indicates that their motives are the same as those of their predecessors. Almost the same words appear in Zelenskyy's speech on 9 May:

> We have never fought against anyone. We always fight for ourselves. For our freedom. For our independence. For the victory of our ancestors to be not in vain. They fought for freedom for us and won. We are fighting for our freedom, for freedom for our children, and therefore we will win.[50]

---

48 Verkhovna Rada of Ukraine, "Ukaz Prezydenta Ukrayiny 'Pro Den partyzanskoyi slavy'" ("A Decree of the President of Ukraine 'On the Day of Partisan Glory'"), 30 October 2001, https://zakon.rada.gov.ua/laws/show/1020/2001#Text [accessed: 31.07.2024] [author's trans.].

49 Lukashuk, "Sohodni my vidznachayemo 77-mu richnytsyu".

50 For an unclear reason, this address was not published on Volodymyr Zelenskyy's page, although it contains material similar to other days. Instead, it is available on other official Facebook pages, including the General Staff of the AFU. Heneralnyy shtab ZSU / General Staff of the Armed Forces of Ukraine, "Zvernennya Prezydenta Ukrayiny Volodymyra Zelenskoho..." ("Address of the President of Ukraine, Volodymyr Zelenskyy..."), Facebook post, 09 May 2022, https://www.facebook.com/watch/?v=1059693961283990 [accessed: 31.07.2024] [author's trans.]. For the text version of the speech, see: President of Ukraine, Volodymyr Zelenskyy, Official Website, "Zvernennia Prezydenta Ukrainy z nahody Dnia peremohy nad natsyzmom u Druhii svitovii viini" ("Address of the President of Ukraine on the Occasion of the Day of Victory over Nazism in World War II"), 09 May 2022, https://www.president.gov.ua/news/zvernennya-prezidenta-ukrayini-z-nagodi-dnya-peremogi-nad-na-74925 [accessed: 27.02.2022]. See also: Zelenskyy, "Tsohorich my kazhemo 'Nikoly znovu' inakshe"; and Zelenskyy, "Zlo zavzhdy pochynaye odnakovo".

The post by the Commander-in-Chief of the AFU reads similarly: "Never again? We are again fighting for freedom".[51] At the same time, in all cases, the context excludes the possibility that they are referring to the independence aspirations of the Ukrainian nationalist underground.[52]

Looking at the analysed posts, this continuity from the generation of winners in WWII also implies the inheritance of the previous generation's victory and status as winners. A common theme in officials' posts on the May commemorative dates is 'protection of the victory'. For example, Zelenskyy's address on 9 May reads:

> Today we celebrate the Day of Victory over Nazism and we will not give away a single piece of our history to anyone [...] We will not allow this victory to be annexed, we will not allow it to be appropriated.[53]

At the same time, he speaks of denying or depriving modern Russia of this status: "And very soon there will be two Victory Days in Ukraine. And someone will have none".[54] According to Zelenskyy, Russia has lost its WWII winner's status due to its actions being similar to those of Nazi Germany:

> By such actions, the Russian Federation has lost any moral right to appeal to the legacy of the victory over Nazism because by its actions it de facto repeats Nazi atrocities and desecrates the memory of the deeds of veterans and participants of the Second World War.[55]

Lukashuk's post is in the same vein:

> The Russian Federation has erased the common victory in World War II. It is trying with all its might to 'privatise' this achievement, to put only itself on a pedestal. [...] Therefore, the Russian Federation should be deprived of the status of winner in World War II, because now their country is promoting Ruscism. Our

---

51 Holovnokomanduvach ZS Ukrayiny, "Never again?".

52 I would like to note that references to the Ukrainian Insurgent Army (UPA) and the nationalist movement do not at all appear in the posts of the selected pages. The UPA was not even mentioned on 14 October, except for one (rather unexpected) exception. Only Vilkul noted in his congratulatory post that this is not only the Day of Defenders of Ukraine, the Intercession of the Mother of God, and the Day of the Cossacks, but also the Day of the UPA. Oleksandr Vilkul, "Bryfinh nachalnyka viyskovoyi administratsiyi Kryvoho Rohu O.Vilkula 14 10 22..." ("Briefing of the Head of the Military Administration of Kryvyi Rih O.Vilkul 14 10 22..."), Facebook post, 14 October 2022, https://www.facebook.com/watch/?v=443747554408624 [accessed: 31.07.2024].

53 Heneralnyy shtab ZSU, "Zvernennya Prezydenta Ukrayiny Volodymyra Zelenskoho".

54 Ibid.

55 Heneralnyy shtab ZSU, "Peremohly natsyzm – peremozhemo i rashyzm!".

> task is not to give the Russians the common achievement of millions of citizens, not to let them appropriate this victory.[56]

Meanwhile, Vilkul divides the inheritance between the two sides in this way:

> We are the heirs of the victorious warriors.
>
> And the children of those who are now coming to us 'izzaporebrika' [i.e., from Russia] and bombing peaceful Ukrainian cities will now become the heirs of the fascist occupiers. Forever.[57]

He also speaks out against Russia's "appropriation" and "distortion" of the "Great Victory".[58]

It is noteworthy that he does not specify what exactly "appropriating" the Great Victory or "depriving" Russia of its right to victory means. However, the context lets the reader infer that a possible Ukrainian refusal to present itself as the victorious party and celebrate Victory Day will mean allowing Russia to appropriate the victory. Therefore, when (rather sensationally, given his longstanding efforts to preserve the post-Soviet model of the memory of the Great Patriotic War) this year Vilkul called for the celebration of Victory Day on 8 May "together with Europe", he justified it with the need to have nothing in common with Russia. At the same time he claimed, "we have no right to allow the orcs [Russians] to steal and appropriate this great holiday for themselves", suggesting that this could occur were Ukraine to refuse to celebrate Victory Day altogether.[59]

The rhetoric of these analysed posts reveals a simple, everyday level of the perception of history as if it were a material object. Accordingly, in this way of looking

---

56 Mykola Lukashuk, "Sohodni my vidznachayemo 77-mu richnytsyu".

57 Oleksandr Vilkul, "Imenno my – nasledniki voinov-pobediteley..." ("It is we who are the heirs of the victorious warriors..."), Facebook post, 07 March 2022, https://www.facebook.com/OleksandrVilkul/posts/pfbid0NgRwWF1B2ki2UmhAHt8ETioK7Gu6HnX18HrHQ7LpCyXdSsARC4tnK4yeAGLhSbUMl [accessed: 31.07.2024] [author's trans.]. I would like to note that this post is the only one in the selection where the 'dispute over Victory' is not tied to 8–9 May. The quoted text is accompanied by a photo of the Victory Monument in Kryvyi Rih, with the Soviet soldier on the pedestal now holding a Ukrainian flag. This modification of the monument is likely to have been the information trigger for the post.

58 Oleksandr Vilkul, "Vmeste s krivorozhanami..." ("Together with Kryvyi Rih residents..."), Facebook post, 06 May 2022, https://www.facebook.com/OleksandrVilkul/posts/pfbid033zHrmDA7T9uya30E3BCkZHHpTjgweKKvpDVGLdnhPni8BpP2tE6kaQn2TUxjrhp5l [accessed: 31.07.2024] [author's trans.].

59 Ibid.

at the world, there is only one Victory Day and it can be physically stolen – in whole or in part ("a single piece"[60]).

Conclusions

In the context of the full-scale Russian invasion that began on 24 February 2022, Ukrainian officials actively use parallels with World War II in their appeals to citizens. However, these links are mostly one-sided. On the occasions of Second World War commemorative dates, connections to the present situation are made. Meanwhile, the current events are not described with references to the past war. The only exception in the latter case is war crimes: the Nazis' atrocities are used as a kind of standard for the evaluation of contemporary Russian atrocities.

Appeals to WWII notwithstanding, the vision of the past that is called up is still based on the Soviet framework. We can see this in the perception of the year 1941 as the start of the war, as well as in the presentations of a genealogy of modern defenders of Ukraine who reach back to their grandfathers, the Red Army soldiers who fought the Nazis, and the importance of the victory over Nazism as their inheritance. However, this vision does not include pro-Soviet sentiments. The Soviet context of Ukraine's participation in the events of WWII is completely ignored, while Ukrainian resistance to the Nazis is presented as an independent act, undertaken along with other allied nations. In this exploitation of the topic of WWII, there is a continuation of practices established during the period of Anti-Terrorist Operation in Eastern Ukraine (2014–2022), which was the first stage of the Russo-Ukrainian War. This analysis of the appeals to WWII history in official public communication shows us that the new narrative promoted by the UINP over the past nine years, which offers a radical break with the Soviet and post-Soviet vision of WWII, is still not fully accepted in Ukraine.

Bibliography

Amacher, Korine, Andrii Portnov, and Victoriia Serhienko (eds.), *Official History in Eastern Europe*, Osnabrück: Fibre, 2020, 282–288.

ArmiiaInform (ArmyInformation), "Prezydent zvernuvsia do narodu Polshchi u 83-tiu richnytsiu pochatku Druhoi svitovoi viiny" ("The President Addressed the People of Poland on the 83rd Anniversary of the Beginning of World War II"), 01 September 2022, https://armyinform.com.ua/2022/09/01/prezydent-zvernuvs

60 Heneralnyy shtab ZSU, "Zvernennya Prezydenta Ukrayiny Volodymyra Zelenskoho".

ya-do-narodu-polshhi-u-83-tyu-richnyczyu-pochatku-drugoyi-svitovoyi-vijny / [accessed: 16.06.2024].

Detector Media, "Yak vysvitlyuvaty Den Peremohy. Rekomendatsiyi Instytutu natsionalnoyi pamyati" ("How to Cover Victory Day: Recommendations of the Institute of National Memory"), 05 May 2014, https://ms.detector.media/profstandarti/post/898/2014-05-05-yak-vysvitlyuvaty-den-peremogy-rekomendatsii-instytutu-natsionalnoi-pamyati/ [accessed: 16.07.2024].

Fedor, Julie, Simon Lewis, and Tatiana Zhurzhenko, "Introduction: War and Memory in Russia, Ukraine, and Belarus", in: Julie Fedor, Markku Kangaspuro, Jussi Lassila, and Tatiana Zhurzhenko (eds.), *War and Memory in Russia, Ukraine and Belarus*, London: Palgrave Macmillan, 2017, 4–20.

Hellbeck, Jochen, and Dmytro Tytarenko, "'My pobedim, kak pobedili 70 let nazad nashi dedy i pradedy'. Ukraina: prazdnovaniye Dnya Pobedy v teni novoy voyny" ("'We Will Win as Our Grandfathers and Great-Grandfathers Won 70 Years Ago'. Ukraine: Celebrations of Victory Day in the Shadow of the New War"), *Neprikosnovennyy zapas (Untouchable Reserve)* 4/108, 2016, http://magazines.russ.ru/nz/2016/4/my-pobedim-kak-pobedili-70-let-nazad-nashi-dedy-i-pradedy.html [accessed: 27.02.2023].

Heneralnyy shtab ZSU / General Staff of the Armed Forces of Ukraine, "#putinskyy_rashyzm = #hitlerivskyy_natsyzm…" ("#putin's_ruscism = #hitler's_nazism"…), Facebook post, 05 October 2022, https://www.facebook.com/GeneralStaff.ua/posts/pfbid03XDieGmr4xdKVABD2GYJr6E3DwXvAaL6PLS9VAVLnp3e8Y8Q7GbYGiisPQLMHuMtl [accessed: 16.07.2024].

Heneralnyy shtab ZSU / General Staff of the Armed Forces of Ukraine, "1 veresnya, Zbroyni Syly Ukrayiny solidaryzuyutsya…" ("1 September, the Armed Forces of Ukraine Stand in Solidarity…"), Facebook post, 01 September 2022, https://www.facebook.com/GeneralStaff.ua/posts/pfbid0ijjcqMXCWFFkKEwTVzXAc2eBk2wgGGvqCNuUj4eENcZg8RRDyAtWD4eiDjtfEFcal [accessed: 16.07.2024].

Heneralnyy shtab ZSU / General Staff of the Armed Forces of Ukraine, "22 chervnya – Den skorboty i vshanuvannya…" ("22 June is the Day of Mourning and Commemoration…"), Facebook post, 22 June 2022, https://www.facebook.com/GeneralStaff.ua/posts/pfbid02v88PBfWCvdyuMJm1hjwR3epqgx1GAKzJ36GghuzaVnGbjSjXvmMwz3uEaYx3gRsyl [accessed: 27.02.2023].

Heneralnyy shtab ZSU / General Staff of the Armed Forces of Ukraine, "Do Dnya pamyati ta prymyrennya…" ("To the Day of Remembrance and Reconciliation…"), Facebook post, 07 May 2022, https://www.facebook.com/GeneralStaff.ua/posts/pfbid0Q9isApXrZxWAGpjuoydLhF6CnZxrmADixLZJKfy3VCD93mNv2uAtVVfGeHKZPk1Ul [accessed: 27.02.2023].

Heneralnyy shtab ZSU / General Staff of the Armed Forces of Ukraine, "My zirvaly plany kremlivskoho fyurera!…" ("We foiled the plans of the Kremlin Führer!…"),

Facebook post, 05 April 2022, https://www.facebook.com/watch/?v=553634419287322 [accessed: 16.07.2024].

Heneralnyy shtab ZSU / General Staff of the Armed Forces of Ukraine, "Zvernennya Prezydenta Ukrayiny Volodymyra Zelenskoho..." ("Address of the President of Ukraine, Volodymyr Zelenskyy..."), Facebook post, 09 May 2022, https://www.facebook.com/watch/?v=1059693961283990 [accessed: 16.07.2024].

Heneralnyy shtab ZSU / General Staff of the Armed Forces of Ukraine, "Peremohly natsyzm – peremozhemo i rashyzm!..." ("We defeated Nazism – we will defeat Ruscism!..."), Facebook post, 08 May 2022, https://www.facebook.com/GeneralStaff.ua/posts/pfbid02fQD8geqPcFWTPYxhMiwcsCp6pvrukK2TP2asGZPKgWpmL9dTZc6Y9ibkYUXtiXVel [accessed: 16.07.2024].

Holovnokomanduvach ZS Ukrayiny / CinC AF of Ukraine, "Never again?...", Facebook post, 09 May 2022, https://www.facebook.com/CinCAFU/videos/526275025573107/ [accessed: 16.07.2024].

Holovnokomanduvach ZS Ukrayiny / CinC AF of Ukraine, "Nikoly znovu... Na zhal, tse ne tak..." ("Never again... Unfortunately, that's not the case..."), Facebook post, 08 May 2022, https://www.facebook.com/watch/?v=3060183750958951 [accessed: 16.07.2024].

Holovnokomanduvach ZS Ukrayiny / CinC AF of Ukraine, "Sohodni mav chest poznayomytysya..." ("Today I had the honour to meet..."), Facebook post, 29 September 2022, https://www.facebook.com/CinCAFU/posts/pfbidoTYJ8S325QEhCVmuFMnHvmZUba5wNvwyzxAopDKthaFX5Hu1hQa7NSWCYa2F8ionql [accessed: 27.02.2023].

Holovnokomanduvach ZS Ukrayiny / CinC AF of Ukraine, "Viyna. Viyna nikoly ne zminyuyetsya..." ("War. War never changes..."), Facebook post, 20 March 2022, https://www.facebook.com/watch/?v=497146995321410 [accessed: 16.07.2024].

Hrytsenko, Oleksandr, *Dekomunizatsiya v Ukrayini yak derzhavna polityka i yak sotsiokulturne yavyshche* (*Decommunisation in Ukraine as a State Policy and as a Sociocultural Phenomenon*), Kyiv: Instytut politychnykh i etnonatsionalnykh doslidzhen im. I. F. Kurasa NAN Ukrayiny; Instytut kulturolohiyi NAM Ukrayiny, 2019.

Informatsiyne ahentstvo PRAVDA (PRAVDA Information Agency), "V muzeyi istoriyi Ukrayiny u Druhiy svitovoyi viyny vidkrylas vystavka 'Chetverte pokolinnya'" ("The Exhibition 'The Fourth Generation' Opened in the Museum of the History of Ukraine during the Second World War"), YouTube video, 3:26, 08 May 2017, https://www.youtube.com/watch?v=kgseHqpDltc [accessed: 16.07.2024].

Institute of National Memory (UINP), "Vystavka 'Ukrayinska Druha svitova'" ("'The Ukrainian Second World War' Exhibition"), https://uinp.gov.ua/vystavkovi-proekty/vystavka-ukrayinska-druga-svitova [accessed: 16.07.2024].

Khmarochos, "Politsiya pereviryaye, chy nalezhaly zoloti zuby z kativni sela Pisky-Radkivski mistsevomu stomatolohu" ("Police Check Whether Gold Teeth From Pisky-Radkivski Torture Chamber Belonged to a Local Dentist"), 06 October

2022, https://hmarochos.kiev.ua/2022/10/06/policziya-pereviryaye-chy-nalezhaly-zoloti-zuby-z-kativni-sela-pisky-radkivski-misczevomu-stomatologu/ [accessed: 16.07.2024].

Lukashuk, Mykola, "Sohodni my vidznachayemo 77-mu richnytsyu..." ("Today we celebrate the 77th anniversary..."), Facebook post, 09 May 2022, https://www.facebook.com/MVLukashuk/posts/pfbid0SsCLn4zA1F1oxx4ggVRHSMHw1QvYLwNJwKFjyimswgRMnHFfNGud3XBUmp7KiqtAl [accessed: 16.07.2024].

Lukashuk, Mykola, "'Holovne – shchob ne bulo viyny'..." ("'The main thing is that there should be no war'..."), Facebook post, 08 May 2022, https://www.facebook.com/MVLukashuk/posts/pfbid0Ht3c2wPdpv1jRF8UbG97Sh7Nzm8fyidu8EtQicWwQ3jCnhAzf57ap3CUzZd7WKCLl [accessed: 16.07.2024].

Olszański, Tadeus, "The Great Decommunisation: Ukraine's Wartime Historical Policy", *OSW Point of View* 65, September 2017, 26–40.

Operatyvne komanduvannya "Skhid" (Operational Command "East"), "Kreml vzhe vstyh obminyaty..." ("The Kremlin has already exchanged..."), Facebook post, 29 October 2022, https://www.facebook.com/watch/?v=5853012694737823 [accessed: 16.07.2024].

Operatyvne komanduvannya "Skhid" (Operational Command "East"), "[Den skorboty i vshanuvannya]" ("[The Day of Mourning and Commemoration]"), Facebook post, 22 June 2022, https://www.facebook.com/EastOC/posts/pfbid0XRAVQv499dANTsoCXxgSVnnQojbuNckbWDTuJwEinh6EhFNNsd49bqTXp1a9HM1Bl [accessed: 16.07.2024].

Operatyvne komanduvannya "Skhid" (Operational Command "East"), "Sohodni v Ukrayini vidznachayut..." ("Today in Ukraine is being celebrated..."), Facebook post, 08 May 2022, https://www.facebook.com/watch/?v=566804038083537 [accessed 16.07.2024].

Osipian, Alexandr, "World War II Memory Politics in Russia and Ukraine and Their Uses During the Conflict in the Donbas (Spring–Summer 2014)", in: Korine Amacher, Andrii Portnov, and Victoriia Serhienko (eds.), *Official History in Eastern Europe*, Osnabrück: Fibre, 2020, 282–288.

Osipian, Alexandr, "Historical Myths, Enemy Images, and Regional Identity in the Donbass Insurgency (Spring 2014)", *Journal of Soviet and Post-Soviet Politics and Society* 1/1, 2015, 116–118.

Portnov, Andrii, "Velikaya Otechestvennaya voyna 2014–2015" ("The Great Patriotic War of 2014–2015"), http://urokiistorii.ru/node/52475 [accessed: 27.02.2023].

President of Ukraine, Volodymyr Zelenskyy, Official Website, "Zvilnyty nashu zemliu i pryity do peremohy – tse nasha natsionalna meta, nad realizatsiieiu yakoi maiemo pratsiuvaty shchodnia – zvernennia Prezydenta Ukrainy" ("To Liberate Our Land and Achieve Victory Is Our National Goal, Which We Must Work on Every Day – the President of Ukraine's Address"), 23

June 2022, https://www.president.gov.ua/news/zvilniti-nashu-zemlyu-i-prijti-do-peremogi-ce-nasha-nacional-76001 [accessed: 16.07.2024].

President of Ukraine, Volodymyr Zelenskyy, Official Website, "Zvernennia Prezydenta Ukrainy z nahody Dnia peremohy nad natsyzmom u Druhii svitovii viini" ("Address of the President of Ukraine on the Occasion of the Day of Victory over Nazism in World War II"), 09 May 2022, https://www.president.gov.ua/news/zvernennya-prezidenta-ukrayini-z-nagodi-dnya-peremogi-nad-na-74925 [accessed: 16.07.2024].

President of Ukraine, Volodymyr Zelenskyy, Official Website, "Zvernennia Prezydenta Ukrainy z nahody Dnia pamiati ta prymyrennia" ("Address of the President of Ukraine on the Occasion of the Day of Remembrance and Reconciliation"), 08 May 2022, https://www.president.gov.ua/news/zvernennya-prezidenta-ukrayini-z-nagodi-dnya-pamyati-ta-prim-74885 [accessed: 16.07.2024].

Reznichenko, Valentyn, "U tsey den my zhaduyemo..." ("On this day we remember..."), Facebook post, 22 June 2022, https://www.facebook.com/Valentyn.Reznichenko/posts/pfbid0WFLguUKzPnVxwBbjzYrGw6i0FFzxFAapFPEcYTUxmevuBxCRaU5cbZ8HkSPCmg3al [accessed: 16.07.2024].

Reznichenko, Valentyn, "Buty ukrayintsem – tse buty vilnym..." ("To be Ukrainian means to be free..."), Facebook post, 09 May 2022, https://www.facebook.com/Valentyn.Reznichenko/posts/pfbid0bUqU2PeyrQdCFTz98aukPeXhDjyQaZHmMEdwbFqNkfYqnZBxVHKkNVNdWzSY9qyLl [accessed 16.07.2024].

Stets, Andriy, "Memorial voyinam ATO roztashuyut na terytoriyi muzeyu Druhoyi svitovoyi viyny u Kyyevi" ("A Memorial to the ATO Soldiers Will be Placed on the Territory of the Second World War Museum in Kyiv"), *Zaxid.net*, 08 May 2017, https://zaxid.net/memorial_voyinam_ato_roztashuyut_na_teritoriyi_muzeyu_drugoyi_svitovoyi_viyni_u_kiyevi_n1425349 [accessed: 16.07.2024].

Tytarenko, Dmytro, "'Vrah vnov vstupyl na nashu zemlyu...': Velyka Vitchyznyana / II svitova viyna v politytsi pamyati na terytoriyi samoproholoshenoyi DNR (2014–2016 rr.)" ("'The Enemy Has Again Set Foot on Our Land...': The Great Patriotic/World War II in the Memory Politics on the Territory of the Self-Proclaimed DPR (2014–2016)"), Historians.in.ua, https://www.historians.in.ua/index.php/en/istoriya-i-pamyat-vazhki-pitannya/2399-dmitro-titarenko-vrag-vnov-vstupil-na-nashu-zemlyu-velika-vitchiznyana-ii-svitova-vijna-v-polititsi-pam-yati-na-teritoriji-samoprogoloshenoji-dnr-2014-2016-rr [accessed: 16.07.2024].

Verkhovna Rada of Ukraine, "Ukaz Prezydenta Ukrayiny 'Pro Den partyzanskoyi slavy'" ("A Decree of the President of Ukraine 'On the Day of Partisan Glory'"), 30 October 2001, https://zakon.rada.gov.ua/laws/show/1020/2001#Text [accessed: 16.07.2024].

Vilkul, Oleksandr, "Bryfinh nachalnyka viyskovoyi administratsiyi Kryvoho Rohu O.Vilkula 28 10 22..." ("Briefing of the Head of the Military Administration of

Kryvyi Rih O.Vilkul 28 10 22…"), Facebook post, 28 October 2022, https://www.facebook.com/watch/?v=666158901742437 [accessed: 16.07.2024].

Vilkul, Oleksandr, "Rivno 78 rokiv tomu…" ("Exactly 78 years ago…"), Facebook post, 28 October 2022, https://www.facebook.com/OleksandrVilkul/posts/pfbid0UuUGMZN5RyFEypFUuHtyRRjUfqGmdX13aKNBZpm8nmDj3S4yLZBfgGKrTCxhNyJSl [accessed 16.07.2024].

Vilkul, Oleksandr, "Bryfinh nachalnyka viyskovoyi administratsiyi Kryvoho Rohu O.Vilkula 14 10 22…" ("Briefing of the Head of the Military Administration of Kryvyi Rih O.Vilkul 14 10 22…"), Facebook post, 14 October 2022, https://www.facebook.com/watch/?v=443747554408624 [accessed: 18.07.2024].

Vilkul, Oleksandr, "Bryfinh nachalnyka viyskovoyi administratsiyi Kryvoho Rohu O.Vilkula 22 09 22…" ("Briefing of the Head of the Military Administration of Kryvyi Rih O.Vilkul 22 09 22…"), Facebook post, 22 September 2022, https://www.facebook.com/watch/?v=628544058975647 [accessed: 18.07.2024].

Vilkul, Oleksandr, "Dve tragicheskiye daty…" ("Two tragic dates…"), Facebook post, 22 June 2022, https://www.facebook.com/OleksandrVilkul/posts/pfbid0HPKiMdtufXVbkMfGg3kruKNT3bRXGujfyBypENFPxNYbn7Pwur5PT5b8C9Wv9Nahl [accessed: 18.07.2024].

Vilkul, Oleksandr, "Vmeste s krivorozhanami…" ("Together with Kryvyi Rih residents…"), Facebook post, 06 May 2022, https://www.facebook.com/OleksandrVilkul/posts/pfbid033zHrmDA7T9uya30E3BCkZHHpTjgweKKvpDVGLdnhPni8BpP2tE6kaQn2TUxjrhp5l [accessed: 18.07.2024].

Vilkul, Oleksandr, "Imenno my – nasledniki voinov-pobediteley…" ("It is we who are the heirs of the victorious warriors…"), Facebook post, 07 March 2022, https://www.facebook.com/OleksandrVilkul/posts/pfbid0NgRwWF1B2ki2UmhAHt8ETioK7Gu6HnX18HrHQ7LpCyXdSsARC4tnK4yeAGLhSbUMl [accessed: 18.07.2024].

Zelenskyy, Volodymyr, "Zlo zavzhdy pochynaye odnakovo…" ("Evil always starts in the same way…"), Facebook post, 27 October 2022, https://www.facebook.com/watch/?v=574046394479712 [accessed: 18.07.2024].

Zelenskyy, Volodymyr, "Tak samo, yak Kyyivshchynu…" ("In the same way as in the Kyiv Oblast…"), Facebook post, 18 September 2022, https://www.facebook.com/zelenskiy.official/posts/pfbid0244YxALVV6Ga6WMT4RZUvTkxhdujyHxqcwcBrxGL99iqoaY7ACogZGcYS2w28ey38l [accessed: 27.02.2023].

Zelenskyy, Volodymyr, "Sohodni v Izyumi Kharkivskoyi oblasti…" ("Today in Izyum in the Kharkiv Oblast…"), Facebook post, 17 September 2022, https://www.facebook.com/watch/?v=1519134511858182 [accessed: 18.07.2024].

Zelenskyy, Volodymyr, "1 veresnya 1939 roku…" ("1 September of the year 1939…"), Facebook post, 01 September 2022, https://www.facebook.com/watch/?v=3174257042887794 [accessed: 18.07.2024].

Zelenskyy, Volodymyr, "Shchoroku 22 chervnya..." ("Every year on 22 June..."), Facebook post, 22 June 2022, https://www.facebook.com/zelenskiy.official/posts/pfbid0TWz9Gqbt6mNTQ4vu8Cs6j4NfNp2EAwiatMCrFGkfD9QK9b42S2DbYxhj41iAaQztl [accessed: 27.02.2023].

Zelenskyy, Volodymyr, "Vid samoho ranku prodovzhyv..." ("Since the morning, I have continued..."), Facebook post, 22 June 2022, https://www.facebook.com/watch/?v=2814332868861296 [accessed: 18.07.2024].

Zelenskyy, Volodymyr, "Tsohorich my kazhemo 'Nikoly znovu' inakshe..." ("This year we say 'Never again' in a different way..."), Facebook post, 08 May 2022, https://www.facebook.com/watch/?v=442165114339716 [accessed: 18.07.2024].

"My War" as a Means of Preserving the Individual and Collective Memories of Ukrainians During the Russian Invasion of 2022

Olha Polishchuk

Tragic events marked European society in the 20th century. Revolutions took place throughout almost all of Europe, along with the First and Second World Wars. After the Second World War, which claimed millions of lives and left much of Europe in ruins, Europeans vowed to make every effort to ensure that war would never happen again. But at the beginning of the 21st century, new armed conflicts in Yugoslavia, Afghanistan, and Iraq shook humanity. In 2014, the Russian Federation annexed Crimea, and an armed confrontation between Russia and Ukraine began, localised in the eastern part of Ukraine, bordering Russia. On 2 March 2022, the UN General Assembly adopted the resolution "Aggression against Ukraine", which condemned the Russian Federation's invasion of Ukraine and demanded that the Russian Federation immediately withdraw its troops from Ukraine, hoping to resolve the conflict politically. However, unfortunately, it was not possible to avoid a full-scale invasion of Ukraine, the largest country in Europe, by Russian troops. The horrors of the 20th century arrived in the 21st century with a new force: the Russo–Ukrainian War.

This war has been going on for centuries,[1] but it escalated on 24 February 2022. For all Ukrainians, that morning began with the roar of Russian planes and explosions in their hometowns. At that moment, the reality of Ukrainian society split into a 'before' and an 'after'. Beyond the basic preservation of life in the face of military aggression, this war raises several other issues important to humanity: a global food shortage, which is leading to famine in several countries; irreversible environmental damage; the moral degradation of humanity; and mass terrorism, among other things. As Ronald Eyerman, Alexander Jeffrey, and Elizabeth Butler Bresse noted, "[i]nevitably, mass individual suffering will produce a process of collective trauma, much less a mitigating social narrative to restore social fragmentation".[2]

1 Andrii Bulvinskyi, *Ukrainsko-rosiiska viina 1658–1659 (The Ukrainian–Russian War of 1658–1659)*, dissertation abstract, Kyiv: Taras Shevchenko Kyiv University, 1998, 19.

2 Ronald Eyerman, Alexander Jeffrey, and Elizabeth Butler Bresse, *Narrating Trauma: On the Impact of Collective Suffering*, 2011, 20.

However, this war is terrible not only for Ukraine and for Ukrainians but also for Europe. Today, Ukraine is a shield that protects all European countries.[3] If this shield falls, the security of Europe will collapse as well. The Ukrainian people are paying too high a price not only for their freedom, independence, and their democratic vector of development, but also for defending the democratic values of Europe and the whole world.

In 2014, the Russo–Ukrainian War became hybrid. Battles were fought not only in the physical spaces of the country, but primarily in the information space. Accordingly, the tactics for confronting a modern hybrid war must be different than those for 'traditional' warfare. Digital technologies make it possible to document and share the truth about events directly from the ground. History is no longer written only by scholars in academic institutions. It is also written by ordinary people, direct participants in tragic events.

People worldwide have been learning about the Russian Army's war crimes and the experience of Russian aggression on the territory of Ukraine through the media – without being in the combat zone or in the range of Russian missiles. For the world to hear the truth about the Russo–Ukrainian War, the Ukrainian Ministry of Culture and Information Policy created the platform My War.[4] This project is designed to provide "an opportunity for every Ukrainian who witnessed the brutal war of the Russian Federation against Ukraine, against democracy, against freedom, and against humanity, to describe their history".[5]

These personal stories are modern literature. Natalia Dovganych notes that literature is "a factor in the formation and transfer of memory about the past, both personal and collective".[6] Since 2013, new literary studies have appeared on the collective trauma of Ukrainians. Particularly important have been the works of Tamara Hundorova, Olena Suchy, Vadym Vasylenko, Hrystyna Rutar, Marta Somyk, and Vi-

3 For more, see: Raisa Ivanchenko, *Ukraina – skhidnyi shchyt Yevropy: Uroky istorii i suchasnist (Ukraine – The Eastern Shield of Europe: Lessons of History and Modernity)*, Kyiv: Dnipro, 2022.

4 My War, https://mywar.mkip.gov.ua/, [accessed: 30.01.2023]. Currently, only the mobile version of the platform works.

5 Ibid.

6 Nataliia Dovganych, "Pamiat, travma, i literatura: Sproby representatsii ta interpretatsii" ("Memory, Trauma, and Literature: Attempts at Representation and Interpretation"), *Ukrainske literaturoznavstvo (Ukrainian Literature Studies)*, 2020, 51–59, here 51 [author's trans.].

taliy Ohienko.[7] Looking at this scholarship can help to better understand the current collective trauma of Ukrainians caused by Russian aggression in 2022.

Today, the first published works of art, which highlight the tragic events of the full-scale Russian invasion, are beginning to appear. The individual poems of Eastern Ukrainian poet-volunteers, such as Serhiy Zhadan, Lyuba Yakymchuk, Natalka Marynchak, and others, can be found on social media networks.[8] This literature is only now being written, and it will take time for the world to see it. However, the platform My War is already recording and publishing the stories of direct eyewitnesses of the war. As I see it, these stories are nonfiction literature. This is important for understanding these tragic events.

Stories preserving the war's memory are my research object. This article aims to analyse these personal stories of eyewitnesses of the Russo–Ukrainian War and to identify signs of collective trauma caused by the military aggression of the Russian Federation against Ukraine. This research is significant because the experience of a collective trauma of a society in the 20th century showed that it is necessary not only for doctors or psychologists to respond to these problems, but also for scientists, journalists, politicians, and civil society in general. After all, I know from my

---

7 For specific works by these authors, see: Tamara Hundorova, *Tranzytna Kultura: Symptomy poskolonialnoi travmy, Statti ta esei* (*Transit Culture: Symptoms of Postcolonial Trauma, Articles and Essays*), Kyiv: Grani-T, 2013; Olena Suchy, "Problema kolektyvnoi travmy v ukrainskomu sotsiumi ta poshuk stratehii ii opanuvania" ("The Problem of Collective Trauma in Ukrainian Society and the Search for Strategies to Overcome It"), *Naukovi zapysky* (*Scientific Notes*) 74/6, 2014, 18–32; Vadym Vasylenko, "Zbyraiuchy ulamky dosvidu: Teoretyschna (re)kontseprualizatsiia travmy" ("Gathering Fragments of Experience: A Theoretical (Re)conceptualisation of Trauma"), *Slovo i chas* (*Word and Time*) 11, 2018, 109–122; Hrystyna Rutar, "Travmovana chy mifologichna pamiat? (na materiali romanu 'Tango smerti' Yuriia Vynnychuka)" ("Traumatised or Mythologised Memory? (Based on the Novel *Tango of Death* by Yury Vinnychuk)"), *Modern problems of linguistics and literary studies* 23, 2018, 294–298; Marta Somyk, "Bumerang pamiati: pro stydki i strashni spohady v ukrainskii literature" ("Boomerang of Memory: About Styles and Terrible Memories in Ukrainian Literature"), *Ukraino-polska mediaplatforma* (*U.P.M.P*) (*Ukrainian–Polish Media Platform*), 06 February 2018, https://upmp.news/ua-in-ukraine/bumerang-pam-yati-pro-stidki-i-strashni-spogadi-v-ukrayinskij-literaturi/ [accessed: 31.07.2024]; and Vitaliy Ohienko, "Posttravmatychnyi stresovyi syndrom i kolektyvna travma v osobystyh naratyvah svidkiv Holodomoru" ("Post-Traumatic Stress Syndrome and Collective Trauma in Personal Narratives of Holodomor Witnesses), *Ukraina Moderna* (*Modern Ukraine*), 06 April 2018, https://uamoderna.com/md/ogienko-holodomor-trauma [accessed: 31.07.2024].

8 Works by these authors can be found on their respective Facebook pages or profiles: Serhiy Zhadan, official Facebook page, https://www.facebook.com/serhiy.zhadan [accessed: 20.01.2023]; Liubov Yakymchuk, Facebook profile, https://www.facebook.com/iakymchuk [accessed: 31.07.2024]; and Natalka Marynchak, Facebook profile, https://www.facebook.com/vetra.smi [accessed: 31.07.2024].

own experience that understanding and acknowledging the presence of psychological trauma, both individual and collective, is an important step towards overcoming it.

My research methodology uses a cultural-historical method, through which I analyse personal stories as documents testifying to the military aggression of the Russian Federation against Ukraine. I apply a hermeneutic method when individual stories are ambiguous. On the one hand, these materials are documentations and reflect the circumstances and facts of reality. On the other hand, these stories are also literary works. Lastly, I use a phenomenological approach to reveal the existential significance of individuals' concerns, assessments, and attitudes.

I analysed the stories of 100 people posted on the My War platform. Overall, as of 31 December 2022, there are 3,691 stories on this platform. The stories are mainly written in Ukrainian and Russian, and sometimes, though rarely, in English. The platform has an automatic translation function, converting the texts into one of 75 languages. Therefore, people from all parts of the world can read the stories of ordinary Ukrainians. In this way, everyone who wants to know the truth about this war, can.

My study's timeframe covers stories written during the first six months of the war, running until the end of August 2022. People of different ages wrote these stories, ranging from 15 to 65 years old. A trauma experienced in the not-so-distant past hurts people and needs to be 'told' in the present tense. Hundorova emphasises that a traumatic past cannot be distanced from the present: "People who do not get rid of the trauma of the past will not be able to fully exist in the present, and accordingly in the future. Therefore, it is very important to 'work out' the memory".[9] The leading researcher in trauma theory, Cathy Caruth, also stresses the need to understand the essence of trauma. "Trauma seems to be much more than a pathology, or the simple illness of a wounded psyche", she writes, "it is always the story of a wound that cries out, that addresses us in the attempt to tell us of a reality or truth that is not otherwise available".[10] Investigating the trauma of Ukrainians, Hundorova states that "trauma is a constant and unconscious fear, caused by explicit or implicit factors when the mechanisms of psychological protection simply do not work".[11] Accordingly, a traumatic experience often remains in a person's memories.

9 Hundorova, *Tranzytna Kultura*, 16 [author's trans.].

10 Cathy Caruth, *Unclaimed Experience: Trauma, Narrative, and History*, Baltimore: John Hopkins University Press, 1996, 4. For more classic studies on the theory of memory and trauma, see: Arthur G. Neal, *National Trauma and Collective Memory: Major Events in the American Century*, Armonk: M.E. Sharpe, 1998; and Joshua Pederson, "Speak, Trauma: Toward a Revised Understanding of Literary Trauma Theory", *Narrative* 22/3, 2014, 333–353.

11 Hundorova, *Tranzytna Kultura*, 14–15.

In her work *Cultural Memory and Western Civilization*, Aleida Assmann, a scholar of English and literary studies, writes that "memories arise only when the experience to which they relate is completed and has gone into the past".[12] On the My War platform, people jot down their memories of the terrible events that they have experienced. Often, contributors explain why they write their stories on this platform: it is to not forget the events of the Russian military invasion of Ukraine, to remember the treachery and cruelty of the enemy, and to pass this memory on to future generations. Sometimes, contributors write their stories a few days after the experience. But more often, they do so after several weeks.

On the platform, ordinary people share their stories, personal experiences, and fears of the Russian aggression against Ukraine; they describe their powerlessness and, sometimes, feelings of madness stemming from hopelessness. In most cases, these are reflections on past events. But these reflections demonstrate how they affect the present. These individual, narrativised experiences become direct evidence of the crimes of Russian military aggression. The My War platform is a means of preserving individual and collective memories. As evidence, the texts surpass being purely literary material. This falls in line with theories by Ukrainian literary critic Vasylenko, who writes that

> testimony texts are rarely included in traditional narrative forms and canons – this is not always and not only literature, but the territory of writing aimed not so much at the reconstruction of "physiological tissue" as at "restoring the presence of a trace", repressed by language, i.e., witnessing the ethical, psychological, and physiological consequences of the traumatic experience of the body and memory.[13]

Many of the stories begin in a similar way: on the morning of 24 February 2022, people peacefully slept when they heard the first explosions in their hometowns. Dasha Yurchenko (I give the names of the contributors as they appear on the My War platform) from Bucha (in the Kyiv Oblast) writes: "February 24. Bucha, I wake up at 6 in the morning without an alarm clock, I go to the shower and in a half-asleep state I hear two very loud explosions in a row".[14] Similarly, Inessa Pustovalova, from Kharkiv, writes "05.12 in the morning. Explosions", and Anastasia Zapeka, from Chernihiv, begins, "[i]n one moment, all my terrible dreams became reality

---

12 Aleida Assmann, *Prostory spohadu. Formy ta transformatsii kulturnoi transformatsii (Cultural Memory and Western Civilization)*, trans. K. Dmytrenko, L. Doronicheva, and O. Yudin. Kyiv: Nika Centre, 2012, 20 [author's trans.].

13 Vasylenko, "Zbyraiuchy ulamky dosvidu", 110 [author's trans.].

14 Dasha Yurchenko, My War, https://mywar.mkip.gov.ua/user/madness.dy [accessed: 11.01.2023].

when I woke up on Thursday morning at 6:40 to the blood-curdling wail of sirens and two powerful rockets".[15]

Stories of people not yet personally experiencing Russian aggression but learning about it through messages or calls from friends and relatives are the second most frequently recurring narrative. "On February 24 at 5:25 an unexpected call from Odesa from my brother Andriy 'The war has begun! Cities are being bombed!'" writes Yeliena Trutnieva from Hostomel.[16] "Around five in the morning, my sleep was interrupted by a phone call from the father of my children. 'World, wake up, the war has begun', and a few minutes later I heard explosions!" posts Svetlana from Kharkiv.[17] Mariia Murashko, from Kyiv, contributes that "The morning started suddenly! Around five-thirty in the morning, my mother called and said that Boryspil was being bombed!"[18]

In all the stories, the date of 24 February 2022 is a key moment. For most, it is a point of bifurcation, when the usual reality, the established picture of the world, is divided into a 'before' and an 'after'. Such a division of reality became an acute stress for all of Ukrainian society. These traumatic memories left an imprint on the psyche of both adults and children.

In many stories, there are memories of a time before the full-scale Russian invasion, yet this is still a time when there were already many warnings in information spaces about the possibility of it. People remember that they did not believe these warnings. For instance, Yulia from Kharkiv writes:

> We discussed a possible attack with family and friends and thought with a smile: "No, he (fascist Putin) has enough sense not to attack a peaceful country", "What kind of attack can we talk about in the 21st century", "This old [Putin] will not commit yes, because then his country will go to the bottom" [...] We thought so on February 23, on the eve of the start of the war...[19]

Similarly, Serhii Huzenko from Kherson remembers thinking: "It's just ridiculous, it can't happen! Who in the 21st century could be so insane as to unleash a full-scale

---

15 Inessa Pustovalova, My War, https://mywar.mkip.gov.ua/user/inessa_pustovalova [accessed: 10.01.2023]; and Anastasia Zapeka, My War, https://mywar.mkip.gov.ua/user/anastasiya_zapeka [accessed: 10.01.2023].

16 Yeliena Trutnieva, My War, https://mywar.mkip.gov.ua/user/elena_trutneva [accessed: 10.01.2023].

17 Svetlana, My War, https://mywar.mkip.gov.ua/user/Svetlyachok [accessed: 10.01.2023].

18 Mariia Murashko, My War, https://mywar.mkip.gov.ua/user/mariya_sokolovskaya [accessed: 10.01.2023].

19 Yulia, My War, https://mywar.mkip.gov.ua/user/yuliya_shypko [accessed: 10.01.2023].

war in the center of Europe?"[20] The rejection of even the thought of this kind of threat to people's lives meant that when this reality arrived, many people refused to accept it.

The whole world saw the shocking footage of Bucha. The people who stayed in this city during the Russian occupation, and who return to these events through their memories, also do not accept that this reality took place. To distance themselves from deep trauma, they try to displace the memory of the events, assuring themselves that it was, for instance, a dream. Dasha Yurchenko recalls living under occupation in Bucha as follows:

> And then begins a dream, long as eternity, which will never leave the memory again [...] The words 'fear' and 'panic' will not describe what we feel when the whole house shakes from the first tank shot on Vokzalna, a street 5 minutes from your house. The explosions become more frequent and louder, and you run to the basement in a panic, not thinking about anything else. In the cold and darkness, your body stops obeying you, and the explosions are so loud that, out of ignorance, you are already 100% sure that there are no houses above.[21]

Analysing the stories from the first month of the war, it is possible to distinguish categories in their authors' memories. Anger, a hatred of the enemy, and fear feature most prominently. Olena from Ovruch writes, "[a]nd every day you live in fear... Tension, despair, and tears are already the norm".[22] Inna Tokarieva from Mykolaiv, a city that was not shelled for only about 20 days in the first six months of the war, admits: "I have never hated before in my life. I was angry – yes, I was offended – yes. And now I HATE it. Openly and unequivocally". Further on, she adds, "THE TITANIUM SHIELD OF HATE. People. People are simply enchanting. It seems that the entire city has been covered with a single impenetrable shield of titanic Hate".[23] Andrii Lisovyi from Kyiv similarly expresses that "[t]his is unforgivable. I hate everyone who dares to set foot on our land and I despise everyone who, having the opportunity to learn the truth, chooses the path of a slave without going out into the streets".[24]

Frequently, it is not customary to talk openly about hatred in society; this is a taboo. But here, on the platform, people capitalise the word and use it as an association. As a result of trauma, people break the taboo by exposing their emotions.

---

20 Serhii Huzenko, My War, https://mywar.mkip.gov.ua/user/sergei_guzenko [accessed: 10.01.2023].

21 Yurchenko, My War.

22 Olena, My War, https://mywar.mkip.gov.ua/user/Olena [accessed: 10.01.2023].

23 Inna Tokarieva, My War, https://mywar.mkip.gov.ua/user/inna_tokarjeva [accessed: 10.01.2023].

24 Andrii Lisovyi, My War, https://mywar.mkip.gov.ua/user/andrii_lisovyi [accessed: 10.01.2023].

This emotion is directed against the enemy, the 'Other'. In this way, the contributors try to distance themselves from their emotions or redirect them towards the enemy. At the same time, they do not openly mention the horrors of war. Often the contributors use words such as "fear", "horror", "death", "basement", "broken", and "burned", among others.[25] Rather than depicting the horrors of the war in detail, they describe their emotions. This demonstrates their self-isolation and the presence of their trauma, which are painful to write about. Therefore, here we can see the contributors' attempts to bypass traumatic memories or redirect their anger and rage at the enemy. Assmann points out that silencing trauma is a "purposeful strategy", through which people think they protect themselves from traumatic experiences.[26]

In the material I analysed on the platform, it was possible to single out a stage when the contributors began to understand their new reality. Here, I distinguished two opposing strategies: an acceptance of the thought of imminent death and/or the desire to die so as not to see everything; and a surge of energy and a desire to do something. Those adopting the first strategy, as seen in the stories on My War, delay evacuating to safer places and fantasise of a quick death, without suffering. Alyona Mazurenko, from Kyiv, writes:

> Tonight I already came to terms with death when my house was shaking when planes flew so low one after another [...] Somehow it got cold. Siren. Explosion, cry, death. Now the day can be described as follows. I look at the photo, and I hear about death... sorrow has come. But now there are no tears because the horror has passed, emptiness and wild coldness remain in the soul. I am afraid that I can no longer cry. I am afraid that the news of death is not shocking...[27]

When people accept reality as one in which death cannot be avoided, they are often in a state of anxiety that has not yet left them. On the My War platform, anxiety is often expressed in descriptions of heart palpitations, sudden waking in the night, dreams of the horrors of war, the inability to sleep, the anticipation of coming under fire, the phantom sounds of roaring aeroplanes, and air raid sirens.

In the second strategy, people try to leave dangerous places or, despite fear or panic attacks, actively help the military and those who need it. "We started actively volunteering", writes Maria Murashko. "Dad went to dig trenches, mom baked bread for our defenders, and they donated canned goods, some clothes, blankets, and mattresses to receive refugees", she continues.[28] Inessa Pustovalova states that "[p]eople

---

25 My War, https://mywar.mkip.gov.ua/.

26 Assmann, *Prostory spohadu*, 296.

27 Alyona Mazurenko, My War, https://mywar.mkip.gov.ua/user/mo_sparkle [accessed: 10.01.2023].

28 Murashko, My War.

are very inspiring: I coordinate financial assistance, we collect things for the army, civilians [...] seven nervous breakdowns and panic attacks are behind me. There are no more tears. And now I don't feel anything at all. I loaded myself with matters related to helping the country".[29] Svetlana expresses that "Something must be done! And it began. I registered on the official website as a volunteer. To accept a child with a family [...] The assistance of the State Emergency Service, in sorting out debris. Searching for people somewhere in the social network. This is how my battle began".[30] Or, similarly, Iryna Zlatieva from Dnipro recalls that

> In two hours, they collected four cars of food, drinks, things [...] A large amount of money was then used to buy medicine and things. And it went on...day after day... Purchasing, searching drugstores, volunteer centers, checkpoints, pest control, hospitals... At school, everyone was actively weaving camouflage nets...[31]

Most of the people who describe such stories chose a path of struggle. The reasons for choosing this seem obvious. There is a desire to be not just an observer, to not hope that someone else will help or protect you, but to change something yourself. Broadly, this collective awareness of the need to act, to rise in response to an external threat, accelerated the formation of the Ukrainian nation and accumulated nation-building processes. The war influenced many people's views of themselves as belonging to the Ukrainian nation. Sociological surveys, politicians, historians, and journalists also indicate this.[32]

---

29 Pustovalova, My War.

30 Svetlana, My War.

31 Iryna Zlatieva, My War, https://mywar.mkip.gov.ua/user/zlata_zlateva [accessed: 31.07.2024].

32 See: National Institute for Strategic Studies (NISS), "Iak viina zminyla suspilny svidomist ukraintsiv: sotsiolohichni doslidzhennia" ("How the War Changed the Public Consciousness of Ukrainians: Sociological Studies"), 09 November 2022, https://niss.gov.ua/news/komentari-ekspertiv/yak-viyna-zminyla-suspilnu-svidomist-ukrayintsiv-sotsiolohichni [accessed: 28.01.2023]; Dmytro Syniak, "'Tsia viina prizvela do formuvannia ukrainskoi natsii i zrobyla nas sylnishimi...' Prozpovidaiut holovy hromad" ("'This War Led to the Formation of the Ukrainian Nation and Made Us Stronger...' Community Leaders Say"), *Detsentralizatsiia (Decentralisation)*, 07 March 2022, https://decentralization.gov.ua/news/14620 [accessed: 31.07.2024]; Vitaliy Mykhailovskii, "Narodzheni viinoiu. Iak uprodovzh stolit zbroini konflity formuvali ukrainsku natsiiu" ("Born of War: How Armed Conflicts Shaped the Ukrainian Nation over Centuries"), *Ukrainsyi Tyzhden* (*Ukrainian Weekly*), 09 January 2023, https://tyzhden.ua/narodzheni-vijnoiu-iak-uprodovzh-stolit-zbrojni-konflikty-formuvaly-ukrainsku-natsiiu/ [accessed: 28.01.2023]; and Oleksandr Reznik, "Kolektyvna identychnist za umov viiny: vid kompleksu menshovartosti do natsii peremozhtsiv" ("Collective Identity under Conditions of War: From an Inferiority Complex to a Nation of Winners"), Ilko Kucheriv Democratic Initiatives Foundation, 24

On the platform, people began to measure reality through the categories of 'self' and 'other'. In their testimonies, the category 'self' or 'us' is defined by words and phrases such as "our", "dear", "relatives", and "our kitties".[33] The word 'own' is always associated with national and state attributes, such as the Ukrainian flag, the colours blue and yellow, the chevrons of the Ukrainian military, and other similar symbols. The contributors depict the category of 'stranger' with words such as "those", "inhumans", "enemies", "invaders", or "orcs", among others. [34] To denote the flag of the Russian Federation, Ukrainians choose derogatory expressions such as "tricolour", "aquafresh", [35] and "Russian rag".[36]

The My War platform is nonfiction literature, which preserves the individual memory of Ukrainians during the Russo–Ukrainian War. Narrativised through media, the personal memories of Ukrainians acquire the characteristics of collective memory. This is facilitated by the wide spatial scope of the memories (i.e., all the regions of Ukraine are covered), and the fact that not only direct participants and witnesses share their experiences on the platform. Some contributors bring to life the experiences of others by sharing their stories, creating indirect expressions of collective memory.

The individual stories posted on the My War platform allow Ukrainians to understand their involvement in historical events. And most importantly, they help citizens understand that they are not alone with these traumatic experiences. This understanding helps strengthen the unity of the nation. One of the consequences of this war is a stronger sense of national identity than ever before.

The My War platform is a vital tool for documenting and preserving memories of the Russo-Ukrainian War, facilitating the sharing of personal narratives to address psychological trauma. This task is of paramount importance in contemporary society, as memory shapes the ideological constructs that define a nation's cultural and historical consciousness. The Russian Federation's continued military aggression against Ukraine has caused a fundamental shift in Ukrainian identity, emphasising the importance of preserving and comprehending these memories.

The platform My War catalogues these memories and contributes to a nuanced comprehension of the Russo-Ukrainian War. These shared memories not only aid individual healing but also facilitate a greater understanding of the conflict. Eyewitness accounts provide an impartial viewpoint of the events, revealing the motives

---

July 2022, https://dif.org.ua/en/article/kolektivna-identichnist-za-umov-viyni-vid-kompleksu-menshovartosti-do-natsii-peremozhtsiv [accessed: 31.07.2024].

33 My War, https://mywar.mkip.gov.ua/.

34 Ibid.

35 Aquafresh is the name of a toothpaste that has the same colours (red, blue, and white) as the flag of the Russian Federation.

36 My War, https://mywar.mkip.gov.ua/.

behind Russia's military incursion and anticipating possible consequences for European society and global security. The narratives showcased on My War serve as a counter to the partial accounts perpetuated by the Russian media, offering an alternative and more credible perspective.

After conducting a thorough examination of the stories showcased on the platform, it is clear that the Ukrainian experience has been affected by a communal trauma due to military aggression. The trauma presents itself through multiple signs, including shock, disbelief of reality, acute awareness of impending death, intense emotions of animosity, and the division of the world into 'self' and 'other'. These categories highlight the significant psychological influence of the conflict on both individuals and the collective psyche of the Ukrainian population.

Ultimately, the My War platform acts not only as a storehouse for personal accounts but also advances comprehension of the psychological costs incurred by the Russo–Ukrainian War. Documenting and analysing these memories provide valuable insights not only into individual experiences of trauma, but also into the wider societal and geopolitical implications of the conflict. This scholarly approach promotes a nuanced understanding of the war's consequences, facilitating the development of strategies to address and alleviate the collective trauma experienced by the Ukrainian population.

Bibliography

Assmann, Aleida, Prostory spohadu. *Formy ta transformatsii kulturnoi transformatsii (Cultural Memory and Western Civilization)*, trans. K. Dmytrenko, L. Doronicheva, and O. Yudin. Kyiv: Nika Center, 2012.

Bulvinskyi, Andrii, *Ukrainsko-rosiiska viina 1658–1659 (The Ukrainian–Russian War of 1658–1659)*, dissertation abstract, Kyiv: Taras Shevchenko Kyiv University, 1998.

Caruth, Cathy, *Unclaimed Experience: Trauma, Narrative, and History*, Baltimore: John Hopkins University Press, 1996.

Dovganych, Nataliia, "Pamiat, travma, i literatura: Sproby representatsii ta interpretatsii" ("Memory, Trauma, and Literature: Attempts at Representation and Interpretation"), *Ukrainske literaturoznavstvo (Ukrainian Literature Studies)*, 2020, 51–59.

Eyerman, Ronald, Alexander Jeffrey, and Elizabeth Butler Bresse, *Narrating Trauma: On the Impact of Collective Suffering*, London and New York: Routledge, 2011.

Hundorova, Tamara, *Tranzytna Kultura: Symptomy poskolonialnoi travmy, Statti ta esei (Transit Culture: Symptoms of Postcolonial Trauma, Articles and Essays)*, Kyiv: Grani-T, 2013.

Huzenko, Serhii, My War, https://mywar.mkip.gov.ua/user/sergei_guzenko [accessed: 10.01.2023].

Ivanchenko, Raisa, Ukraina – skhidnyi shchyt Yevropy: Uroky istorii i suchasnist (Ukraine – The Eastern Shield of Europe: Lessons of History and Modernity), Kyiv: Dnipro, 2022.

Lisovyi, Andrii, My War, https://mywar.mkip.gov.ua/user/andrii_lisovyi [accessed: 10.01.2023].

Marynchak, Natalka, Facebook profile, https://www.facebook.com/vetra.smi [accessed: 18.07.2024].

Mazurenko, Alyona, My War, https://mywar.mkip.gov.ua/user/mo_sparkle [accessed: 10.01.2023].

Murashko, Mariia, My War, https://mywar.mkip.gov.ua/user/mariya_sokolovskaya [accessed: 10.01.2023].

My War, https://mywar.mkip.gov.ua/, [accessed: 30.01.2023].

Mykhailovskii, Vitaliy, "Narodzheni viinoiu. Iak uprodovzh stolit zbroini konflity formuvali ukrainsku natsiiu" ("Born of War: How Armed Conflicts Shaped the Ukrainian Nation over Centuries"), *Ukrainsyi Tyzhden (Ukrainian Weekly)*, 09 January 2023, https://tyzhden.ua/narodzheni-vijnoiu-iak-uprodovzh-stolit-zbrojni-konflikty-formuvaly-ukrainsku-natsiiu/ [accessed: 18.07.2024].

National Institute for Strategic Studies (NISS), "Iak viina zminyla suspilny svidomist ukraintsiv: sotsiolohichni doslidzhennia" ("How the War Changed the Public Consciousness of Ukrainians: Sociological Studies"), 09 November 2022, https://niss.gov.ua/news/komentari-ekspertiv/yak-viyna-zminyla-suspilnu-svidomist-ukrayintsiv-sotsiolohichni [accessed: 18.07.2024].

Neal, Arthur G., *National Trauma and Collective Memory: Major Events in the American Century*, Armonk: M.E. Sharpe, 1998.

Ohienko, Vitaliy, "Posttravmatychnyi stresovyi syndrom i kolektyvna travma v osobystyh naratyvah svidkiv Holodomoru" ("Post-Traumatic Stress Syndrome and Collective Trauma in Personal Narratives of Holodomor Witnesses), *Ukraina Moderna (Modern Ukraine)*, 06 April 2018, https://uamoderna.com/md/ogienko-holodomor-trauma [accessed: 18.07.2024].

Olena, My War, https://mywar.mkip.gov.ua/user/Olena [accessed: 10.01.2023].

Pederson, Joshua, "Speak, Trauma: Toward a Revised Understanding of Literary Trauma Theory", *Narrative* 22/3, 2014, 333–353.

Pustovalova, Inessa, My War, https://mywar.mkip.gov.ua/user/inessa_pustovalova [accessed: 10.01.2023].

Reznik, Oleksandr, "Kolektyvna identychnist za umov viiny: vid kompleksu menshovartosti do natsii peremozhtsiv" ("Collective Identity under Conditions of War: From an Inferiority Complex to a Nation of Winners"), Ilko Kucheriv Democratic Initiatives Foundation, 24 July 2022, https://dif.org.ua/en/article/kolektivna-identichnist-za-umov-viyni-vid-kompleksu-menshovartosti-do-natsii-peremozhtsiv [accessed: 18.07.2024].

Rutar, Hrystyna, "Travmovana chy mifologichna pamiat? (na materiali romanu 'Tango smerti' Yuriia Vynnychuka)" ("Traumatised or Mythologised Memory? (Based on the Novel Tango of Death by Yury Vinnychuk)"), *Modern problems of linguistics and literary studies* 23, 2018, 294–298.

Somyk, Marta, "Bumerang pamiati: pro stydki i strashni spohady v ukrainskii literature" ("Boomerang of Memory: About Styles and Terrible Memories in Ukrainian Literature"), *Ukraino-polska mediaplatforma (U.P.M.P) (Ukrainian–Polish Media Platform)*, 06 February 2018, https://upmp.news/ua-in-ukraine/bumerang-pam-yati-pro-stidki-i-strashni-spogadi-v-ukrayinskij-literaturi/ [accessed: 18.17.2024].

Suchy, Olena, "Problema kolektyvnoi travmy v ukrainskomu sotsiumi ta poshuk stratehii ii opanuvania" ("The Problem of Collective Trauma in Ukrainian Society and the Search for Strategies to Overcome It"), *Naukovi zapysky (Scientific Notes)* 74/6, 2014, 18–32.

Syniak, Dmytro, "'Tsia viina prizvela do formuvannia ukrainskoi natsii i zrobyla nas sylnishimi...' Prozpovidaiut holovy hromad" ("'This War Led to the Formation of the Ukrainian Nation and Made Us Stronger...' Community Leaders Say"), *Detsentralizatsiia (Decentralisation)*, 07 March 2022, https://decentralization.gov.ua/news/14620 [accessed: 28.01.2023].

Svetlana, My War, https://mywar.mkip.gov.ua/user/Svetlyachok [accessed: 10.01.2023].

Tokarieva, Inna, My War, https://mywar.mkip.gov.ua/user/inna_tokarjeva [accessed: 10.01.2023].

Trutnieva, Yeliena, My War, https://mywar.mkip.gov.ua/user/elena_trutneva [accessed: 10.01.2023].

Vasylenko, Vadym, "Zbyraiuchy ulamky dosvidu: Teoretyschna (re)kontseprualizatsiia travmy" ("Gathering Fragments of Experience: A Theoretical (Re)conceptualisation of Trauma"), *Slovo i chas (Word and Time)* 11, 2018, 109–122.

Yakymchuk, Liubov, Facebook profile, https://www.facebook.com/iakymchuk [accessed: 18.07.2024].

Yulia, My War, https://mywar.mkip.gov.ua/user/yuliya_shypko [accessed: 10.01.2023].

Yurchenko, Dasha, My War, https://mywar.mkip.gov.ua/user/madness.dy [accessed: 11.01.2023].

Zapeka, Anastasia, My War, https://mywar.mkip.gov.ua/user/anastasiya_zapeka [accessed: 10.01.2023].

Zhadan, Serhiy, official Facebook page, https://www.facebook.com/serhiy.zhadan [accessed: 18.07.2024].

Zlatieva, Iryna, My War, https://mywar.mkip.gov.ua/user/zlata_zlateva [accessed: 10.01.2023].

The Tonality of the Archives of the Memories of Forcibly Displaced Ukrainians

Olha Haidamachuk

> "We say to the memory – stay with us,
> don't leave us alone…"
> Serhiy Zhadan, *Voroshylovgrad*[1]

In the current Russo–Ukrainian War, Ukraine fights not only for its territorial integrity and independence but also for the memory, culture, language, faith, and history of all the peoples whose identity Russian propaganda tries to erase. The imperial discourse of this same propaganda also inspired some Western intellectuals to talk about the 'Nowhere Nation', 'Nasty Ukraine', the 'Cleft Country', and the 'Unwanted Stepchild of Soviet Perestroika', among other names for Ukraine.[2] The placement of Ukraine within the mental map of Western Europeans, was, however, also facilitated by the tonality of Ukrainian existential resistance to Russian aggression, the roots of which go deep into the past.[3]

We know about historical events thanks to preserved records held in private and public archives and libraries. The influence of archives on processes of generating cultural memory can hardly be overestimated, since, in the words of Thomas Osborne, "the archive is a means of generating ethical and epistemological credibility".[4] As Ray Edmondson points out, the power of archives rests on this credibility: "archivists, like librarians, museologists and other collecting professionals, exercise a particular kind of power over the survival, accessibility and interpretation of the

1 Serhiy Zhadan, *Voroshylovgrad*, Kharkiv: Folio, 2010, 216 [author's trans.].

2 Mykola Riabchuk, "Mapping a 'Nowhere Nation' | Ukraine! Unmuted", Cultural Strategy Institute, https://isc.lviv.ua/en/ryabchuk-ukrzriz/ [accessed: 31.07.2024]. This essay articulates some of the focal points of the Russian imperial narrative in order to deconstruct this narrative.

3 For the linguistic aspect of this confrontation, see: Michael S. Flier and Andrea Graziosi, "The Battle for Ukrainian: An Introduction", *Harvard Ukrainian Studies* 35/1–4, 2017/18, 11–30.

4 Thomas Osborne, "The ordinariness of the archive", *History of the Human Sciences* 12/2, May 1999, 51, https://doi.org/10.1177/09526959922120243.

world's cultural memory".[5] On the one hand, the growth of archives increases and complicates their influence on human interaction with reality. The traditional functions of the archive, including "to ensure rights, to provide historical sources, to participate in administration and to disseminate culture", argues Lajos Körmendy, have changed.[6] According to him, the new philosophy of archiving focuses on the following: "popularisation, transparency, openness, market approach, media culture and information-centricity".[7] On the other hand, lost records or unrecorded events[8] cannot influence the shaping of the vision of the past for future generations. Such pasts can also be controlled through the prohibition of access to recorded and preserved documents, books, artefacts, and other material.

The archive as a metaphor for collective memory makes us think not only about the authenticity of the events themselves but also about the authenticity of the archival memory of them. Lara Cox points to this double problem in her comments on Jacques Derrida's *Archive Fever*.[9] Additionally, she singles out trends such as anarchising (i.e., destroying the order of memories), which, according to Derrida, threatens stable, exclusive memory.

In the case of daily publications (which also have their own archives), it is obvious that not all everyday events attract coverage in the press. Moreover, the media coverage of events at times significantly depends on an editorial perspective or on state policy. Therefore, when reading about the seemingly same events (e.g., the beginning of full-scale Russian aggression towards Ukraine) in different news sources (e.g., in domestic or foreign ones), it is possible to get the impression that they discuss different events (e.g., in terms of the scales or evaluations of the events, etc.).[10]

5 Ray Edmonson, *Audiovisual Archiving: Philosophy and Principles*, report, Paris: UNESCO, 2004, 1, https://www.fiafnet.org/images/tinyUpload/E-Resources/Official-Documents/Philosophy-of-Audiovisual-Archiving_UNESCO.pdf [accessed: 08.12.2023].

6 Lajos Körmendy, "Changes in archives' philosophy and functions at the turn of the 20th/21st centuries", *Archival Science* 7, 2007, 167–177, here 167, https://doi.org/10.1007/s10502-007-9052-8.

7 Ibid.

8 In this case, primary sources are supposed to be not the events themselves, but their documented description.

9 Lara Cox, "Reaching for Archive Fever: A Tall Tale about Queer 'Made in France'", *Paragraph* 39/3, 319–334, https://www.jstor.org/stable/26418651. Cox responds to: Jacques Derrida, "Archive Fever: A Freudian Impression", trans. Eric Prenowitz, *Diacritics* 25/2, 1995, 9–63, https://www.jstor.org/stable/465144.

10 I discuss this further in the following texts: Olha Haidamachuk, "The 'Emergency Grab Bag' of Memory, or the Tonalities of News Headlines About the War in Ukraine – Part One", *TRAFO – Blog for Transregional Research*, 21 March 2023, https://trafo.hypotheses.org/45765; and Olha Haidamachuk, "The 'Emergency Grab Bag' of Memory, or the Tonalities of News Headlines About the War in Ukraine – Part Two", *TRAFO – Blog for Transregional Research*, 29 June 2023, https://trafo.hypotheses.org/47670.

This is important to consider because the Russian Federation behaves as aggressively on the information field as it does on the ground, distorting facts and reality,[11] and thereby trying to impose its own interpretation. And if, indeed, "[l]ife increasingly becomes lived in the shadow of the archive", as Mike Featherstone suggests, then the significance of archives is obvious.[12] Guided by the belief that history is written by the victors, Russian policy tries to justify its crimes to posterity in advance, setting itself up to approach the past only as a 'history' of its own victories. And it is for this reason that, in the occupied territories, Russians burn Ukrainian books,[13] thus

---

11 Mykola Riabchuk writes, for instance, about the "distorted perception of reality, harmful for Kyiv, beneficial for Moscow" and, ultimately, the threat of genocide. Riabchuk, "Mapping a 'Nowhere Nation'".

12 Mike Featherstone, "Archive", *Theory, Culture & Society* 23/2–3, 2006, 591–596, here 591.

13 In the occupied territories, Russians burn books about Ukrainian history and the Holodomor and even Ukrainian fairy tales, among other publications. This is regularly reported by Ukrainian mass media. See, for example: *Televiziinoi sluzhby novyn (TSN)* (*Television news service*), "Rosiiski okupanty spaliuiut ukrainsku literaturu na tymchasovo nepidkontrolnykh Ukraini tepytopiiahk – HUR" ("Russian Occupants Burn Ukrainian Literature in the Temporarily Uncontrolled Territories of Ukraine – the Defence Intelligence of Ukraine"), 24 March 2022, https://tsn.ua/ato/rosiyski-okupanti-spalyuyut-ukrayinsku-literaturu-na-timchasovo-nepidkontrolnih-ukrayini-teritoriyah-gur-2018890.html [accessed 31.07.2024]; Andrii Kushchenko, "Rosiiski okupanty spaliuiut ukrainski knyhy, u tomu chysli pidruchnyky z istorii" ("Russian Occupiers Destroyed Ukrainian Books, Including History Textbooks", *Patriot Donbasu* (*Patriot of the Donbas*) 22 May 2022, https://donpatriot.news/article/rosiyski-okupanti-spalyuyut-ukrayinski-knigi-u-tomu-chisli-pidruchniki-z-istoriyi [accessed: 08.12.2023]; *Vholos* (*Aloud*), "'Orky i dykuny': Larysa Nitsoi pro rosiian, iaki spaliuiut ukrainski knyzhky na okupovanykh terytoriiakh" ("'Orcs and Savages': Larysa Nitsoi about Russians Burning Ukrainian Books in the Occupied Territories"), 26 July 2022, https://vgolos.ua/news/okupanti-znishchuyut-ukrayinski-knigi-tomu-shcho-same-v-nih----nasha-identichnist.-i-ce-trivaie-vzhe-sotni-rokiv----pismennicya-larisa-nicoy_1425095.html [accessed 31.07.2024]; Markiian Klymkovetskyi, "Na Kharkivshchyni okupanty znyshchuiut ukrainski knyzhky, vkliuchno z dytiachymy kazkamy" ("In the Kharkiv Oblast, Occupiers Destroy Ukrainian Books, Including Children's Fairy Tales"), *hromadske*, 25 July 2022, https://hromadske.ua/posts/na-harkivshini-okupanti-znishuyut-ukrayinski-knizhki-vklyuchno-z-dityachimi-kazkami [accessed 31.07.2024]; Serhii Ziatiev, "'Literaturna' viina rashystiv, abo Pro shcho zaboroneno chytaty na tymchasovo okupovanykh terytoriiakh" ("The 'Literary' War of the Rashists, or, What is Forbidden to Read in the Temporarily Occupied Territories"), *ArmiialNFORM* (*ArmyINFORM*), 07 September 2022, https://armyinform.com.ua/2022/09/07/literaturna-vijna-rashystiv-abo-pro-shho-zaboroneno-chytaty-na-tymchasovo-okupovanyh-terytoriyah/ [accessed 08.12.2023]; *Espreso*, "Na okupovanykh terytoriiakh rosiiany spaliuiut knyzhky z ukrainskoi literatury, – Henshtab ZSU" ("Russians Burn Books of Ukrainian Literature in Occupied Territories – the General Staff of the Armed Forces of Ukraine"), 19 October 2022, https://espreso.tv/na-okupovanikh-teritoriyakh-rosiyani-spalyuyut-knizhki-z-ukrainskoi-literaturi-genshtab-zsu [accessed 31.07.2024]; and *Nezalezhne televiziine ahentstvo (NTA)* (*Independent Television Agency*), "Na Kharkivshchyni kolaborant skladav spysky ukrainskykh knyzhok dlia znyshchennia" ("In the Kharkiv Oblast,

claiming a monopoly on memory spaces and leaving no room for the possibility of an alternative. Accordingly, from the point of view of common sense, it is extremely important to instead have archives comprised of various data, documents, and testimonies about events, allowing for comprehensive studies of them in the future.

Do people still remember the German author Heinrich Heine's prophecy? In 1821, in *Almansor: A Tragedy* (*Almanso: Eine Tragödie*), the author wrote, "[t]here, where one burns books, one will in the end also burn people".[14] In the centre of Berlin, at Bebelplatz, the site of the 10 May 1933 Nazi book burnings, the monument of the Empty Library stands as a warning. Is its message still eloquently clear for humanity? How many more books connected to Ukrainian national memory should be burnt – as has also already occurred to Tatar, Moldavian, and Georgian books – recalling this prophecy? The impunity of evil only strengthens it and opens the way to new frontiers. Delay in punishing evil locally leads to the need to defend against evil globally. Human memory already contains this knowledge and Heine's prophecy reminds us of this experience.

Temporal distancing from a given event intensifies the 'anarchising' forces that Cox and Derrida wrote about, because the witnesses of the event disappear forever, taking with them unrecorded memories that could have, under the influence of time or lived experience, transformed into living archives. With digital technology, archiving possibilities have increased dramatically, but at the same time, so has the vulnerability of archives. How reliable are guarantees of protection, preservation, and access to data considering that it is easy to erase an electronic archive, without even the need to burn something? David Beer draws attention to another challenge in his reflections on mass media, asking, if social networks are an archive, how can we use them in a conversation about the life they record?[15] In this process, the dy-

---

a Collaborator Compiled Lists of Ukrainian Books to Be Destroyed"), 23 December 2022, https://www.nta.ua/na-harkivshhyni-kolaborant-skladav-spysky-ukrayinskyh-knyzhok-dlya-znyshhennya/ [accessed 31.07.2024].

14 "Dort, wo man Bücher verbrennt, verbrennt man auch am Ende Menschen" In: Heinrich Heine, *Almansor*, Digitale Bibliothek, p. 8, http://www.digbib.org/Heinrich_Heine_1797/Almansor_.pdf [accessed 31.07.2024].

15 David Beer, "Archive Fever revisited: Algorithmic archons and the ordering of social media", in: Leah Lievrouw and Brian Loader (eds.), *Routledge Handbook of Digital Media and Communication*, London: Routledge, 2020, 99–111, here 100.

namics of the archive,[16] its connection to the 'archon'[17] (for Derrida meaning those who commanded or 'the documents' guardians'[18]), and the etymological connection of both words to the ancient Greek '*arkhē*'[19] (simultaneously meaning 'commencement' and 'commandment') are emphasised. In the word *arkhē*, Derrida finds a definitional opposition between the natural and the legal and relates the latter directly to the authority of the powerful (either humans or gods).[20] I consider it necessary to also pay attention to the fact that commandments/laws are dominated by persuasive and imperative intonations. Accordingly, Beer approaches the 'archive' through a tonal range, offering to read it as a platform from which both prescripts/orders and announcements/pronouncements can be made.[21]

Archival data provides a toolbox for the accumulation of memory and, at the same time, makes prescriptions. Therefore, it is, in fact, a source of authority. Beer's approach is reminiscent of Michel Foucault's "dictation of the archive" and of the archive as a source of the formation and transformation of memory according to

---

16 Derrida uses the word 'archon' in his reflections on the new situation of speech, which seems to have to give up its 'archon' status in favour of writing. I believe that Derrida, with the help of the metaphorical 'archon', focuses our attention on nonobvious powerful forces. We should keep this in mind for things like the fact that the magazine *Archont*, published since 2017 in the Russian Federation, contains sections like "Current Geopolitics", "National Security", "Political Technologies", and "The National Question", among others. In his book *Archive Fever*, Derrida explains why it is worth to pay more attention to the archon, stating, particularly, that "[t]he archons are first of all the documents' guardians. They do not only ensure the physical security of what is deposited and of the substrate. They are also accorded the hermeneutic right and competence. They have the power to interpret the archives. Entrusted to such archons, these documents in effect state the law: they recall the law and call on or impose the law. To be guarded thus, in the jurisdiction of this *stating the law*, they needed at once a guardian and a localization. Even in their guardianship or their hermeneutic tradition, the archives could neither do without substrate nor without residence". Derrida, "Archive Fever", 10, stress in the original.

17 Derrida writes: "The meaning of 'archive,' its only meaning, comes to it from the Greek *arkheion*: initially a house, a domicile, an address, the residence of the superior magistrates, the archons, those who commanded". Derrida, "Archive Fever", 9.

18 "The archons are first of all the documents' guardians. They do not only ensure the physical security of what is deposited and of the substrate. They are also accorded the hermeneutic right and competence. They have the power to interpret the archives." Derrida, "Archive Fever", 10.

19 Specifically, Derrida wrote: "*Arkhē*, we recall, names at once the *commencement* and the *commandment*. This name apparently coordinates two principles in one: the principle according to nature or history, *there* where things *commence* – physical, historical, or ontological principle – but also the principle according to the law, *there* where men and gods *command*, *there* where authority, social order are exercised, *in this place* from which *order* is given – nomological principle". Derrida "Archive Fever", 9, stress in the original.

20 Ibid.

21 Beer, "Archive Fever revisited", 100.

Featherstone.[22] Featherstone also points to the blurring of boundaries: "[i]ncreasingly the boundaries between the archive and everyday life become blurred through digital recording and storage technologies".[23] To this, we can also add the 'decolonial mission' of archives. Siseko Kumalo, for instance, hopes that the authoritative power of such a mission can allow for substantively engaging ontologies of Indigeneity together with archives.[24]

I believe that all these conditions also apply to both collective and individual memory. Beyond this, it is important to highlight the tonal background of archiving. This is made up of the elements that are fixed in the process of archiving, controlled through preservation, and produced during familiarisation with archival data, all occurring after the archived events. Against the background of these changing tonalities (which have different attitudes and evaluations), the contents of the archive can be perceived differently,[25] ultimately affecting their status. For example, these contents can be open or closed (e.g., secret vs. public, or privately vs. publicly accessible), have different scales of value or importance, contain diverse periods of storage, and vary in terms of what they disclose or erase, among other things. Such considerations allow us to better understand the effects of war on archival processes.

How Do War and Displacement Reshape the Tonalities of Memory?

War throws a person off balance, traumatises them, destroys their confidence in the future, overturns their worldview, and tests the depth of their convictions and the strength of their relationships. War is a complete disorientation, an undermining of values, and a powerful challenge to ecology, humanity, consciousness, and all lifeforms. War can suddenly cast a person from their everyday life into complete disarray, thereby not only challenging the survival strategies applicable to life during peace, but also shaking the foundations of individual and collective memory. The

---

22 Beer, "Archive Fever revisited", 100. For the other two works, see: Michel Foucault, *The Archaeology of Knowledge and the Discourse on Language*, trans. A. M. Sheridan Smith, New York: Pantheon Books, 1972; and Featherstone, "Archive".

23 Featherstone, "Archive", 591.

24 Siseko H. Kumalo, "Resurrecting the Black Archive through the decolonisation of philosophy in South Africa", *Third World Thematics: A TWQ Journal* 5/1–2, 2020, 19–36, https://doi.org/10.1080/23802014.2020.1798276.

25 Olena Moroz investigates the correlation of textual tonality and emotional experiences during reading. Olena Moroz, "Tonalnist iak tekstova kategoriia: ontologichnyi aspekt" ("Tonality as a Textual Category: The Ontological Aspect"), *Nova Filologiia (New Philology)* 43, 2011, 94–99, here 94, http://nbuv.gov.ua/UJRN/Novfil_2011_43_18.

shock of war not only causes a reflexive revision of memories, but, in the key of disturbing tonalities, it can provoke the deconstruction of memory through a decolonisation of its intonations once the muteness caused by the shock is overcome.[26]

In my research, I consider the memories of Ukrainians who were forced to leave their homes and go abroad due to the full-scale invasion.[27] I seek to discover which tonal foundations of memory they rely on in their present, and which foundations, conversely, risk their immediate detonation. I suggest that the latter disturbing tonalities are capable of both evoking reflections on a collective past and prompting the revision of individual memories. This (re)articulation of the collective and individual past, under the influence of unrelenting anxiety, can, in turn, provoke intonational changes in the deconstruction of memory as an effort to 'rewrite it without mistakes'. Despite their focus on the past through reflection and deconstruction, both processes aim at the future and at the hope for a 'peaceful future' determined by the 'security' of the memory of the past. I consider the decolonisation of intonations to be the deepest layer of such security. That is, in this case, a conscious rejection of exposed false tonalities imposed by Russian discourse. Accordingly, I analyse the memories of forcibly displaced Ukrainians in precisely this triple key, set against the background of general anxiety. Specifically, I first look at reflexive revisions; second, I consider the provocation of the deconstruction of memory; and, third, I discuss the decolonisation of intonations.

The Reflective Revision of Memory

In a reflective revision of their memories of the day before 24 February 2022, some of the Ukrainians I interviewed, who were forced to escape the war abroad and found themselves in Berlin, indicated a premonition of anxiety or an intuitive feeling of a tense atmosphere: "we're already somewhere in the 20s [of February], but somehow

---

26 For instance, the contemporary Ukrainian philosophers Volodymyr Yermolenko and Vakhtang Kebuladze, in a conversation about the 'struggle against muteness', chose tones that range between 'laughing at the enemy' and 'love for one's own.' Kult: Podcast, "Kultura u viini: borotba z nimotoiu, smikh nad vorohom, liubov do svoikh. Pamiati Oleksandra Roitburda" ("Culture during War: Fighting Muteness, Laughing at the Enemy, Loving Your Own. In Memory of Oleksandr Roitburd"), YouTube video, 23 January 2023, 56:40, https://www.youtube.com/watch?v=GYyu9m8slrM [accessed 31.07.2024].

27 I conducted a qualitative study based on oral interviews with 13 Ukrainians from October to December 2022. The participants were 11 women and two men. Their ages ranged from 20 to 70 and they originated from the following Ukrainian oblasts: the Cherkasy Oblast, the Donetsk Oblast, the Lviv Oblast, the Kharkiv Oblast, the Kherson Oblast, the Kyiv Oblast, the Poltava Oblast, and the Sumy Oblast. I asked the questions in Ukrainian, but they were free to answer in Ukrainian or in Russian. One woman from the Kharkiv Oblast answered exclusively in Russian and one man from the Kyiv Oblast answered most of the questions in Russian.

[...] we're even at work: we already talk about concerts, but this anxiety hangs in the air... you seem to talk about concerts, but the anxiety hangs" (Ukrainian woman, 20s, Lviv Oblast). This occurred both in the west and the east of Ukraine:

> It was on that night of the 24th that I didn't sleep. I didn't even go to sleep. I was preparing for my usual things. I was preparing for lessons. But something strange held me back. I don't know how to explain it, but at 5 o'clock in the morning, as soon as I went to bed, immediately, within two minutes, I heard explosions. It was like there was some kind of energy in the air, so I couldn't sleep that night (Ukrainian woman, 40s, Kharkiv).

Neither the feelings of anxiety or tension nor the memories of these feelings result in deeper reflections in my interlocuters, regardless of whether the memories revolve around a 'we-then' or 'me-then'.

Some felt anxiety but, with hesitation, tried to distance themselves from it with 'rational' arguments. Through this hesitation, notes of panic are audible between the intuitive sense of a threat and the rational resistance to it:

> There was a lot of information, it was written on the internet that a full-scale war is possible ... it seems that on the 16th of February... [t]here was some such information, but this information was denied. Nothing started. And then we ... think: "But this ... is somehow 'another piece of nonsense'". Let's say this. Well, this is fake, I think, somehow... But on the 16th, I heard something like that information. And somehow, I was ... a little unwell. I thought something like: "What should I do? Suddenly it starts – what is it? Where are they going? Where to turn? To whom to run?" (Ukrainian man, 20s, Kherson Oblast).

It seems that these memories still cause confusing feelings, thoughts, and existential questions without answers.

However, people who were immersed in work and everyday life and preoccupied with their own affairs do not recall having had reasons for anxiety at all, thus admitting a certain conscious or unconscious insensitivity or indifference to public moods: "I didn't feel any danger at all" (Ukrainian woman, 30s, Kharkiv Oblast). Or, as someone else states, "[h]ow was I doing? I woke up in the morning, worked at one job, in the evening at another job. And after all that I had some fun [...] and we didn't watch the news. Didn't watch..." (Ukrainian woman, 20s, Poltava Oblast). Maximally focusing one's attention and efforts on set goals and thereby immersing oneself in one's microcosm is a valuable skill during times of peace. However, during war, the lack of an established connection with the macrocosm increases mental vulnerability: "I don't even remember exactly anymore, because it was a whole day of panic and inexplicable emotions" (Ukrainian woman, 30s, Kharkiv Oblast). Reflection is complicated by the scale of emotions, which, like a wall of sound, hides memories.

Of course, on the morning of 24 February 2022, everyone was shocked without exception: both those who were already anxious and those who were caught by surprise. Some refused to believe in the reality of the disaster, experiencing something like a collapse of time caused by the noise of the explosions:

> Despite the fact that both my family and I were morally prepared, there was a feeling of unreality to what was happening. Unrealities! I personally had the feeling that time had moved to the Second World War, because the sounds were exactly the same as they were back then. The first shelling was heavy artillery. The GRAD [self-propelled multiple rocket launcher] came later (Ukrainian woman, 60s, Kharkiv Oblast).

Such temporal collapses generate a layering of memory, a phenomenon described by Norman Saadi Nikro: "[T]he more distant the past becomes, the more layered are the modalities and forms of mediations by which past events resonate into the present, and become significant for the present".[28] The sounds heard or the shock waves felt by the explosions will be etched in the memory of many Ukrainians, at least from the morning of 24 February 2022.

However, for some, visuality dominates their memories from the start; they experienced similar disorders to those above, but in the form of a spatial collapse or dissociation: "It was... you know... I'll say, like in a movie, like a movie was supposedly being recorded – I felt like this at that moment" (Ukrainian woman, 40s, Kharkiv). Some experienced a spatial collapse as an alienation from space. In these cases, 'reality' appeared both as inadequate and as an experience of the 'afterlife' (or of the 'other side' of life), with a deep horror of nonexistence at its core:

> We are all smart, educated, classy people here – and this kind of violence against us is simply unacceptable! And these poor mothers with children, with those bags – it's just terrible! It's like you look at them and... And as soon as you cross the border, they give you some food or tea there, and you're like: "Wow, now you're a homeless person". Like, I'll say it like this: "That's it! In Ukraine, I was, well, at least someone, but here I am a homeless person". And I had this thought: "Well, that's it, life is over..." (Ukrainian woman, 20s, Lviv Oblast).

Similarly, someone else from Eastern Ukraine said: "it seemed to me that I was probably not in this world, or that I had died, or something like that. There was this kind of stress that I thought that everything, life, was over" (Ukrainian woman, 40s, Sumy

---

28 Norman Saadi Nikro, "Middle East and North Africa", in: Yifat Gutman and Jenny Wüstenberg (eds.), *The Routledge Handbook of Memory Activism*, New York: Routledge, 2023, 318–324, here 319.

Oblast/Kharkiv). In these examples, there is a certain echo in the memories, repetitions with stresses of varying intensity, as seen in the recurrence of "unreality [...] Unrealities!", "like in a movie, like a movie", and "homeless [...] homeless". Some repetitions can also be traced only at the semantic level, through synonymous phrases: "not in this world [...] I had died [...] life, is over". These repetitions seem to be a symptom of the pulsating obsession of anxious thoughts.

However, even those who dared to accept that war was bound to happen were not ready for it when it came. It was a shocking and painful insight:

> Although I had an opinion about that, that such an attack on the part of Russia is quite possible and rather likely, I postponed packing my emergency grab bag, although I planned it. I postponed it. I didn't want to believe it. I thought about it, but I didn't want to believe it... All the signs suggested the fact that it would happen, this war, although I still didn't want to believe it. The accumulation of troops near the borders of Ukraine, the policy – sharply anti-Ukrainian – pursued by our northern neighbour. The policy aimed at fostering a hatred towards Ukrainians – all this led me to think that they are preparing for this war, they are preparing for an invasion (Ukrainian woman, 60s, Kharkiv Oblast).

In this statement are several instances of the rhythmic repetitions of disturbing thoughts: "postponed [...] postponed", "I didn't want to believe [...] I didn't want to believe [...] I still didn't want to believe", and "they are preparing for this war, they are preparing for an invasion". Accordingly, seven to nine months after the mentioned events, the pain experienced is still acute and it is just as difficult to believe in what has already happened.

Russia's full-scale invasion of Ukraine was an even greater shock to those who refused to believe it and rejected any warnings as unfit for this time in history and the state of contemporary humanity. For instance, one respondent from Western Ukraine stated:

> My mother said a week or two earlier that this is possible. I started to laugh, I said: "What are you talking about? In general, this cannot be! ... What ... well, how could it even be imagined...? What does "full-scale" mean? What? As in the Second World War, will some army go? But this is unreal! (Ukrainian woman, 20s, Lviv Oblast).

Similarly, a respondent from the east recalled: "I didn't believe that this could happen. I didn't believe that Russia could attack" (Ukrainian woman, 40s, Sumy Oblast/Kharkiv). Originating from the centre of the country, another respondent stated:

> I knew, I knew from the mass media, but, again, never in my mind, I could not have guessed that one day it would still start. Everyone read, saw – including

> me – and watched the news, and heard a lot of information, even from Western media, but to accept the idea that this could really happen, I, for example, could never imagine... I could not... at that time imagine in my mind that such a thing could really happen in the 21st century (Ukrainian woman, 40s, Cherkasy Oblast).

Lastly, an interlocutor from the capital shared, "I didn't think this would happen, but when Russian helicopters first flew over our house on the morning of February 24th, followed by our Ukrainian fighter jets, I understood that it would be very serious" (Ukrainian man, 60s, Kyiv).

These Ukrainians' revisions of their memories about their traumatic experience are characterised by an alarming tone. While younger people (in their 20s and 30s) withstood the pressure of this anxiety through outward calm, many people with more life experience (in their 40s, 60s, and 70s) teared up or strained their voices. In this self-revision, the individual memory archives of life during peace generate resistance (even after the fact) to the awareness of a threat that has become reality. Instead, these memory archives hold deep historical knowledge that covers this experience and its resonances with the present.

The Provocation of the Deconstruction of Memory

Dissonances caused by the perception of reality as 'unrealistic' can bring reflection to the point of the deconstruction of memories. I was interested in what the respondents focus on in their memories and why. What is the (in)adequate assessment of a dangerous situation based on? This deconstruction seems to be vitally necessary. If in a tonal 'picture of the world' the known intonations suddenly do not work – that is, they do not provide a sense of support – then it is impossible to rely on them to build a strategy for the future. The provoked deconstruction of memory is not only a revision of the accents once placed on customary tonalities, but sometimes a shift in tonalities altogether. The resistance to accepting the horror that has become reality permeates these memories, provoking their deconstruction:

> I understand – this is something that should not happen and should not happen to anyone, because children should not see it, we should not experience it. There [during the war], I am more than a 20-year-old, I have to think there... I don't know... about something other than [what a 20-year-old thinks about], and about things like some UAVs [unmanned aerial vehicles] here, some Javelins there. Why do I need to know this? Why do I need to know how to make a Molotov cocktail? Well, this is not normal a priori. Why should children hear explosions? Even those in Lviv, those anywhere. They should not hear these bad words – well, even those, about the "Russian warship..." – this should not happen. That's

> all, it just wasn't meant to be. And this is not normal (Ukrainian woman, 20s, Lviv Oblast).

The insistence on erasing something from memory as an anomaly ("should not happen [...] should not happen [...] should not happen") as well as the desire to return to the past, idealised in retrospect, indicate implicit tones of rebellion and despair simultaneously. Another respondent states:

> I've analysed a lot here in these eight months and I'm actually telling my child about it now, I'll tell everyone that we should, having a peaceful life, appreciate what we really have. After all, I remember at my work I was not satisfied with a lot of things, although now analysing, turning my mind back, I had a good life. I didn't have to anger God, as they say. I had a good life and I really want to return to it. I really want to go back – to that past life that I had (Ukrainian woman, 40s, Cherkasy Oblast).

Both anger at the present and a shift to a positive tone towards the past, stemming from despair about the sense of a lost future, can accumulate in anarchising impulses in the archives of individual memory.

Those who packed their 'emergency grab bags' in advance or too quickly (recommendations to pack such a bag were heard everywhere two weeks before the start of the full-scale invasion) later admitted that some of the things turned out to be unnecessary:

> My emergency grab bag was, as I now think, not entirely successful. I put medicine [in] there, some key things necessary for children, there were things like socks, I don't know ... tights. Then, for some reason, I stuck candles in there. I still think – why candles? Then there are matches, toilet paper... and some food: some kind of cookies, some dry porridge (Ukrainian woman, 30s, Kharkiv Oblast).

This packing of 'unnecessary' items is connected to not only panicked confusion and unconsciously acquired assumptions,[29] but also to a revision of one's value system and a reassessment of the values themselves:

29 The Ukrainian Ministry of Education and Science published recommendations for what to put in the emergency grab bag. The list of recommended things does indeed include matches and candles, but no clothes. Ministry of Education and Science of Ukraine, "Tryvozhna valiza" ("Emergency Grab Bag"), https://mon.gov.ua/storage/app/media/civilniy-zahist/2022/03.02/Rekom.vmist.tryvozhnoyi.valizy.03.02.pdf [accessed 31.07.2024].

> The importance of material things in this life has greatly weakened for me. I can't say that it doesn't matter to me. It matters. After all, as long as a person lives, they need a roof over their head, food, drink, and clothing. It cannot help but interest a person, all this, but it's a globally reinterpreted meaning of the material. It is [now] secondary, tertiary, tenth [in the order of importance] in our life (Ukrainian woman, 60s, Kharkiv Oblast).

Often, the interviewees mention documents – that is, one's personal archive – and things required for self-identification – or artefacts of one's own history – among their truly valuable possessions. They recognise the items directly related to their personal memories as valuable. However, family heirlooms (e.g., photographs, souvenirs, gifts, and hand-made items such as a mother's embroidery, a grandmother's rushnyks, or children's drawings, etc.), books, and collections (e.g., of stamps or postcards) rarely find a place in the 'emergency grab bag': "I am very sorry about the photos. Well, I didn't even think that everything would be like this... So much... Still, I thought: well, maybe it won't last long" (Ukrainian woman, 70s, Donetsk Oblast/Kharkiv Oblast). During catastrophic moments, most people do not think about eternity or the distant future. Extreme conditions force them to focus on the current moment or a couple of weeks at most.

Splitting the life of every Ukrainian into a 'before' and an 'after',[30] the full-scale invasion stressed the quality of the lost former life. Most of the respondents reflect on their life 'before' in a positive tone:

> I was happy then in my own way. At that time ... everything was fine with me ... Considering that I lived off my own money, I didn't have a super well-paying profession and I didn't work very much ... but I went to the gym, went to the beautician, bought things for myself. Everything was fine with me, that's why... I lived well (Ukrainian woman, 20s, Lviv Oblast).

Or, as someone else states, "I felt very good, because this question [of feeling good] is very closely related to self-realisation for me. I feel happy when I can work, earn [money], and cover all my needs" (Ukrainian woman, 30s, Kharkiv Oblast). These positive views show their desire to return to Ukraine as soon as it becomes safe to live there.[31]

---

30 For example: "Life really split into a before and an after" (Ukrainian woman, 20s, Poltava Oblast).

31 See also: "I think this is the effect of lost opportunities. It's like the effect of lost freedoms, yes. If you have rights and you don't use them, that's fine. As soon as your right is taken away, you must have it [...]. Freedom, when you have it, you don't appreciate it. If your home, your home, your country are taken away, you start to appreciate it" (Ukrainian woman, 20s, Poltava Oblast).

However, for some, the experience of living abroad changed their perception of 'before', revealing lost opportunities in hindsight: "I think that then it seemed to us that we were happy ... I think that we were content with little, and this was enough for us, and we didn't think that it could be better" (Ukrainian woman, 40s, Kharkiv).

The intonations of the past shift, if not into a negative range, then into a neutral one, as some of the respondents question the authenticity of the happiness they remember. On the one hand, the tone of doubt in such cases, as Derrida suggested, not only provokes anarchising trends, but also threatens a stable memory. In this case, there are no rebellion, no despair, and no anger, just as there is no fear of the future. Instead, enthusiasm sounds clearly. Therefore, on the other hand, this same doubt opens the respondents' eyes to unexpectedly acquired opportunities. And, if at the core of a positive (or even an idealised) assessment of one's past is the desire to return to Ukraine, then doubts can fuel the desire to stay in Germany to create a life of a different quality in the here and now, and not in an uncertain future.

The Decolonisation of Intonations of Memory

This revolutionary update of memories actualises the fight against false tones for some Ukrainians. As I discuss above, the 'decolonial mission' is embedded in the archives themselves. Individual memory archives are no exception. In some cases, shock, reflection, and deconstruction result in the decolonisation of intonations (in fact, due to their detonation). That is, they lead to a rejection of the myths that feed these intonations and to a change of accents. For example, the tonality of the word 'brother' transformed noticeably[32] – it has become irritating to the Ukrainian ear. At the heart of this detonation is the desire to get rid of an obsessive false brotherhood, insidiously used by the enemy to lull the vigilance of Ukrainians. Similarly, the phrase 'born in the Soviet Union' also becomes irritating:

> [W]hen we [...] issued my foreign passport [...] the Germans translated that it [my birthplace] was the Soviet Union. It hurt me so much (laughs). Although I was actually born in the USSR, it affected me. I think: well, what is the Soviet Union? If I am a Ukrainian [...] [f]or me, Ukraine is my native country. Although [it was] part of the Soviet Union. Was there a Ukraine in the USSR too? – Ukraine! I never considered myself as "born in the Soviet Union". Like my [...] cousin, [...] whose

32 The Ukrainian Institute of National Memory, together with the Ministry of Culture and Information Policy, created an infographic to debunk the myth of 'fraternal' nations. The infographic is based on the history of the relationship between Ukrainians and Russians. Ukrainian Institute of National Memory, "Why Ukrainians And Russians Are Not Fraternal Nations (infographics)", https://uinp.gov.ua/informaciyni-materialy/rosiysko-ukrayinska-viyna-istorychnyy-kontekst/why-ukrainians-and-russians-are-not-fraternal-nations-infographics [accessed: 31.07.2024].

> mother is Ukrainian, he was born in Moldova, in Chisinau. [...] He currently lives in Moscow. When we started texting, he wrote to me: "...what happened to you there? You are being bombed there – that's what [is happening], right?" I said: "Yes... it's true." And he: "Well, [it's] nothing, be patient!" The words "be patient" – and then I immediately stopped writing to him. After a while, he writes to me: "You have horror over there. Just horror! What is 'grandpa' [Putin] doing!". He writes a message – and immediately deletes it. That is, he is afraid. I say: "But God forbid what he [Putin] does. Just horror! [...] Well ... you are Ukrainian! [...] You used to come to your grandmother's house, to your grandfather's house, in Ukraine, every summer. [...] Well, you know what Ukraine is. Your mother is buried here, your father is buried here in Ukraine". And he tells me: "I was born in the Soviet Union". [...] I think: "Oh, damn you! In the Soviet Union!" (laughs). For me, this is how important it is... [and] all the more so right now! Well, I was not born in the Soviet Union, I was born on Ukrainian land in Ukraine (Ukrainian woman, 40s, Sumy Oblast/Kharkiv Oblast).

The essence of this misunderstanding is that Ukrainians (even when Ukraine was a part of the Soviet Union) thought of themselves as Ukrainians, while those outside of Ukraine perceived and sometimes still perceive Ukrainians as '(post-)Soviet people' (or, as I note at the beginning of the essay, the country is seen as the 'Nowhere Nation').

For the Ukrainian ear, an important shift in tonality also occurred with the word 'nationalist'. For centuries, Ukrainians were taught to be ashamed of their identity and provincialism was imposed on them through oppressions, prohibitions, restrictions, repressions, famines, genocide, and linguicide.[33] With the new generation of Ukrainians, who were born and grew up in an independent Ukraine, there is a positive shift in self-identification, particularly in some categories. They move away from an inferiority complex and an identity conflict towards a healthy nationalism:

> [W]e really need to learn from the Germans, because they are very careful about all these things... They take care of it [culture] on a very national level, on all these holidays... [T]hey have, they constantly celebrate some personalities [writers, composers, artists, etc.]. They know about them, they are constantly talking about them. We don't have that, because... you're some kind of nationalist if you want to talk about this. But this is how everyone lives, and it is normal for everyone, but it was somehow not ok for us. And that's unusual (Ukrainian woman, 20s, Lviv Oblast).

---

33 For a brief introduction to this linguicide, see: Euromaidan Press staff, "A short guide to the linguicide of the Ukrainian language | Infographics", 22 February 2017, https://euromaidanpress.com/2017/02/22/a-short-guide-to-the-linguicide-of-the-ukrainian-language-infographics/ [accessed: 31.07.2024].

This resonates with the observations of the contemporary Ukrainian writer Andrii Lyubka, who states that "the acceptance of Ukrainianness as an attribute of a political nation is an ongoing process".[34] It is encouraging to hear such views from young people: "I feel great strength. It is a great strength that I am Ukrainian" (Ukrainian woman, 20s, Kharkiv).

Conclusions

My study considers the tonality of the memory archives of Ukrainians who were forced to put their whole lives in 'emergency grab bags'[35] by Russia's full-scale war, leave everything behind, and go abroad. It aims at discovering the (un)stable tonal foundations of their memory archives and potential risks of detonation. If an alarming tonality can provoke reflections on collective and individual memory, prompt a revision of individual memory, and cause decolonisation on both levels of memory, I found that being used to life during peace also increases resistance to an awareness of real threats. Archives of memory, enriched with historical knowledge, can cause a layering of memory, superimposing different historical events on the present and comparing them with their resonances with the present. Even if this historical baggage contributes to an adequate assessment of a threat, and perhaps shortens the decision-making time, it does, however, not overcome the psychological resistance to believing in a terrible future, even when it has already become the present.

I observed some failures in memory through dissonances connected to both time and space. For the most part, Ukrainians, more than half a year after their displacement, tend to live in a tonally positive past and (impossibly) desire to return to it, because lost opportunities dominate over their acquired opportunities. In some cases, however, Ukrainians show readiness to leave the past behind and start moving towards the future in the here and now, thereby changing their priorities. While almost all the respondents demonstrate reflexive revisions of their memories, as well as provocations of the deconstruction of them, the decolonisation of the intonations of memories only exists in isolated cases. First, this decolonisation appears in the (indignantly ironic) detonation of Soviet identity in favour of Ukrainian self-identification, and second, in the (surprising) detonation of an imposed 'inferiority' and 'provincialism' in favour of a healthy national pride. Whether these processes

34 Pershyi (The First), "Andrii Liubka: 'Pryiniattia ukrainskosti yak atrybutu politychnoi natsii – protses, yakyi tryvaie'" ("Andriy Lyubka: 'Acceptance of Ukrainianness as an Attribute of a Political Nation is an Ongoing Process'"), YouTube video, 12 March 2023, 25:38, https://www.youtube.com/watch?v=ViEQ4hspiho [accessed: 31.07.2024].

35 For example: "I was surprised when my life, when I came here, fit into one suitcase. Well… although no, I'm lying, it didn't fit. There are many things left [behind]…" (Ukrainian woman, 20s, Poltava Oblast).

of the decolonisation of intonations will spread among Ukrainians in Ukraine and beyond is an open question. This is especially the case as it relates to the broader issue of the decolonisation of other memory intonations, and particularly those of Europeans about 'good' Russians.

Bibliography

Beer, David, "Archive Fever revisited: Algorithmic archons and the ordering of social media", in: Leah Lievrouw and Brian Loader (eds.), *Routledge Handbook of Digital Media and Communication*, London: Routledge, 2020, 99–111.

Cox, Lara, "Reaching for Archive Fever: A Tall Tale about Queer 'Made in France'", *Paragraph* 39/3, 319–334, https://www.jstor.org/stable/26418651.

Derrida, Jacques, "Archive Fever: A Freudian Impression", trans. Eric Prenowitz, *Diacritics* 25/2, 1995, 9–63, https://www.jstor.org/stable/465144.

Edmonson, Ray, *Audiovisual Archiving: Philosophy and Principles*, report, Paris: UNESCO, 2004, https://www.fiafnet.org/images/tinyUpload/E-Resources/Official-Documents/Philosophy-of-Audiovisual-Archiving_UNESCO.pdf [accessed: 08.12.2023].

Espreso, "Na okupovanykh terytoriiakh rosiiany spaliuiut knyzhky z ukrainskoi literatury, – Henshtab ZSU" ("Russians Burn Books of Ukrainian Literature in Occupied Territories – the General Staff of the Armed Forces of Ukraine"), 19 October 2022, https://espreso.tv/na-okupovanikh-teritoriyakh-rosiyani-spalyuyut-knizhki-z-ukrainskoi-literaturi-genshtab-zsu [accessed 18.07.2024].

Euromaidan Press staff, "A short guide to the linguicide of the Ukrainian language | Infographics", 22 February 2017, https://euromaidanpress.com/2017/02/22/a-short-guide-to-the-linguicide-of-the-ukrainian-language-infographics/ [accessed: 18.07.2024].

Featherstone, Mike, "Archive", *Theory, Culture & Society* 23/2–3, May 2006, 591–596.

Flier, Michael S., and Andrea Graziosi, "The Battle for Ukrainian: An Introduction", *Harvard Ukrainian Studies* 35/1–4, 2017/18, 11–30.

Foucault, Michel, *The Archaeology of Knowledge and the Discourse on Language*, trans. A. M. Sheridan Smith, New York: Pantheon Books, 1972.

Haidamachuk, Olha, "The 'Emergency Grab Bag' of Memory, or the Tonalities of News Headlines About the War in Ukraine – Part Two", *TRAFO – Blog for Transregional Research*, 29 June 2023, https://trafo.hypotheses.org/47670.

Haidamachuk, Olha, "The 'Emergency Grab Bag' of Memory, or the Tonalities of News Headlines About the War in Ukraine – Part One", *TRAFO – Blog for Transregional Research*, 21 March 2023, https://trafo.hypotheses.org/45765.

Heine, Heinrich, *Almansor*. Digitale Bibliothek. 41. http://www.digbib.org/Heinrich_Heine_1797/Almansor_.pdf [accessed 18.07.2024].

Kumalo, Siseko H., "Resurrecting the Black Archive through the decolonisation of philosophy in South Africa", *Third World Thematics: A TWQ Journal* 5/1–2, 2020, 19–36, https://doi.org/10.1080/23802014.2020.1798276.

Klymkovetskyi, Markiian, "Na Kharkivshchyni okupanty znyshchuiut ukrainski knyzhky, vkliuchno z dytiachymy kazkamy" ("In the Kharkiv Oblast, Occupiers Destroy Ukrainian Books, Including Children's Fairy Tales"), *hromadske*, 25 July 2022, https://hromadske.ua/posts/na-harkivshini-okupanti-znishuyut-ukrayinski-knizhki-vklyuchno-z-dityachimi-kazkami [accessed 18.07.2024].

Körmendy, Lajos, "Changes in archives' philosophy and functions at the turn of the 20th/21st centuries", *Archival Science* 7, 2007, 167–177, https://doi.org/10.1007/s10502-007-9052-8.

Kult: Podcast, "Kultura u viini: borotba z nimotoiu, smikh nad vorohom, liubov do svoikh. Pamiati Oleksandra Roitburda" ("Culture during War: Fighting Muteness, Laughing at the Enemy, Loving Your Own. In Memory of Oleksandr Roitburd"), YouTube video, 23 January 2023, 56:40, https://www.youtube.com/watch?v=GYyu9m8sIrM [accessed: 18.07.2024].

Kushchenko, Andrii, "Rosiiski okupanty spaliuiut ukrainski knyhy, u tomu chysli pidruchnyky z istorii" ("Russian Occupiers Destroyed Ukrainian Books, Including History Textbooks", *Patriot Donbasu* (*Patriot of the Donbas*) 22 May 2022, https://donpatriot.news/article/rosiyski-okupanti-spalyuyut-ukrayinski-knigi-u-tomu-chisli-pidruchniki-z-istoriyi [accessed: 18.07.2024].

Ministry of Education and Science of Ukraine, "Tryvozhna valiza" ("Emergency Grab Bag"), https://mon.gov.ua/storage/app/media/civilniy-zahist/2022/03.02/Rekom.vmist.tryvozhnoyi.valizy.03.02.pdf [accessed 18.07.2024].

Moroz, Olena, "Tonalnist iak tekstova kategoriia: ontologichnyi aspekt" ("Tonality as a Textual Category: The Ontological Aspect"), *Nova Filologiia* (*New Philology*) 43, 2011, 94–99, http://nbuv.gov.ua/UJRN/Novfil_2011_43_18.

Nikro, Norman Saadi, "Middle East and North Africa", in: Yifat Gutman and Jenny Wüstenberg (eds.), *The Routledge Handbook of Memory Activism*, New York: Routledge, 2023, 318–324.

Nezalezhne televiziine ahentstvo (NTA) (Independent Television Agency), "Na Kharkivshchyni kolaborant skladav spysky ukrainskykh knyzhok dlia znyshchennia" ("In the Kharkiv Oblast, a Collaborator Compiled Lists of Ukrainian Books to Be Destroyed"), 23 December 2022, https://www.nta.ua/na-harkivshhyni-kolaborant-skladav-spysky-ukrayinskyh-knyzhok-dlya-znyshhennya/ [accessed 18.07.2024].

Osborne, Thomas, "The ordinariness of the archive", *History of the Human Sciences* 12/2, May 1999, 51–64, https://doi.org/10.1177/09526959922120243.

Pershyi (The First), "Andrii Liubka: 'Pryiniattia ukrainskosti yak atrybutu politychnoi natsii – protses, yakyi tryvaie'" ("Andriy Lyubka: 'Acceptance of Ukrainianness as an Attribute of a Political Nation is an Ongoing Process'"), YouTube video, 12

March 2023, 25:38, https://www.youtube.com/watch?v=ViEQ4hspiho [accessed: 18.07.2024].

Riabchuk, Mykola, "Mapping a 'Nowhere Nation' | Ukraine! Unmuted", Cultural Strategy Institute, https://isc.lviv.ua/en/ryabchuk-ukrzriz [accessed: 18.07.2024].

Televiziinoi sluzhby novyn (TSN) (Television news service), "Rosiiski okupanty spaliuiut ukrainsku literaturu na tymchasovo nepidkontrolnykh Ukraini tepytopiiahk – HUR" ("Russian Occupants Burn Ukrainian Literature in the Temporarily Uncontrolled Territories of Ukraine – the Defence Intelligence of Ukraine"), 24 March 2022, https://tsn.ua/ato/rosiyski-okupanti-spalyuyut-ukrayinsku-literaturu-na-timchasovo-nepidkontrolnih-ukrayini-teritoriyah-gur-2018890.html [accessed 18.07.2024].

Ukrainian Institute of National Memory, "Why Ukrainians And Russians Are Not Fraternal Nations (infographics)", https://uinp.gov.ua/informaciyni-materialy/rosiysko-ukrayinska-viyna-istorychnyy-kontekst/why-ukrainians-and-russians-are-not-fraternal-nations-infographics [accessed: 18.07.2024].

Vholos (Aloud), "'Orky i dykuny': Larysa Nitsoi pro rosiian, iaki spaliuiut ukrainski knyzhky na okupovanykh terytoriiakh" ("'Orcs and Savages': Larysa Nitsoi about Russians Burning Ukrainian Books in the Occupied Territories"), 26 July 2022, https://vgolos.ua/news/okupanti-znishchuyut-ukrayinski-knigi-tomu-shcho-same-v-nih----nasha-identichnist.-i-ce-trivaie-vzhe-sotni-rokiv----pismennicya-larisa-nicoy_1425095.html [accessed 18.07.2024].

Zhadan, Serhiy, *Voroshylovgrad*, Kharkiv: Folio, 2010.

Ziatiev, Serhii, "'Literaturna' viina rashystiv, abo Pro shcho zaboroneno chytaty na tymchasovo okupovanykh terytoriiakh" ("The 'Literary' War of the Rashists, or, What is Forbidden to Read in the Temporarily Occupied Territories"), *ArmiiaINFORM* (*ArmyINFORM*), 07 September 2022, https://armyinform.com.ua/2022/09/07/literaturna-vijna-rashystiv-abo-pro-shho-zaboroneno-chytaty-na-tymchasovo-okupovanyh-terytoriyah/ [accessed 23.07.2024].

Representations

The Power of Maps and Geographic Imagery in Digital Communication

Narrating Russia's War in Ukraine

Alina Mozolevska

Since 24 February 2022, internet users have been bombarded daily by thousands of war-related images, videos, and news coming from Ukraine via different digital media that are not only displaying all the complexity of the war's developments on the battlefield, but also narrating the wartime reality of many Ukrainians. For more than eight months (at the time of writing this text), we have seen the borders of Ukraine violated. Every day, the frontline shifts with the heavy marks of Russian aggression. Explosions mapped on the Ukrainian geo-body spill out into thousands of stories of heroism, resistance, displacement, and violence. Each of these stories has echoes in the world's hybrid media space, touching people far beyond Ukraine and making them 'live' the war through the screens of their devices. The current Russo–Ukrainian War can be undoubtedly called the most documented war in history because of the "digital tsunami of media content" that is generated on a daily basis.[1] This war is also extremely visual; it is experienced and perceived through the prism of the multiplicity of visual data posted and recirculated online. What, then, is the role of visuals in Russia's current invasion of Ukraine? What information and messages do they convey? In this essay, I focus on maps and their multiple interpretations in digital media. I aim at unpacking the main functions of these visuals. To do so, I created a dataset of more than 300 maps and iconographic images collected from international, Ukrainian, and Russian digital media (e.g., official media, X (formerly Twitter), Facebook, and VKontakte).

Contemporary technologies determine not only how wars are conducted but also how they are communicated. Russia's war in Ukraine is also an information war, which goes beyond the battlefield and individual experiences and is broadcasted through old and new media and processed (live) by millions. The war has become

1 Andrew Hoskins and Pavel Shchelin, "The War Feed: Digital War in Plain Sight", *American Behavioral Scientist* 67/3, 2023, 449–463, https://doi.org/10.1177/00027642221144848, here 452.

content that flows across every platform simultaneously.[2] Using this opportunity to speak to the world and to be heard, Ukrainians document the invasion in detail, share their war experiences, write war diaries, and show the destruction caused by Russian aggression. They broadcast their fights from the frontlines and express their grief. In this shared space of war documentation, the brutal reality unfolds with multiple personal interpretations of wartime experiences. Indeed, this "first TikTok war"[3] or "first social media war"[4] has many innovative means of informing and narrating the experiences that reshape the understanding of who Ukrainians are, what they fight for, and what Ukraine is.

At the same time, social media platforms amplify mis- and disinformation about the Russian invasion of Ukraine, propagating alternative narratives and fake news.[5] The flows of disinformation and anti-Ukrainian propaganda circulate Russia's vision of the geopolitical future of Ukraine, denying its agency and right to independence. Masking its true motives under the slogans of 'liberation' and 'denazification', Russia aims to resurrect the former borders of the USSR, spread its aggressive imperialism beyond its own borders, and erase Ukraine from the world map. These massive disinformation campaigns make the crucial challenges of the digital media landscape visible, exposing what Johannes Buchheim and Gilade Abirihe call "a growing epistemic divide running through liberal democracies: a situation in which substantial portions of the population believe in alternative realities on a broad range of factual issues".[6] Exploiting the existing tensions in different regions of the world, these alternative realities and fake news create divisions and draw new mental borders in the attempt to weaken the collective response of Ukraine's allies.

The above-mentioned complexity of the unfolding war narratives in contemporary digital spaces explains the urgent need to study the mechanisms of communicating and propagating the discourses of war through visual means. It is worth

2 Kyle Chayka, "Watching the World's 'First TikTok War'", The New Yorker, 03 March 2022, https://www.newyorker.com/culture/infinite-scroll/watching-the-worlds-first-tiktok-war [accessed: 31.07.2024].

3 Thomas L. Friedman, "We Have Never Been Here Before", *The New York Times*, 25 February 2022, https://www.nytimes.com/2022/02/25/opinion/putin-russia-ukraine.html [accessed: 31.07.2024].

4 Dan Ciuriak, "Social Media Warfare Is Being Invented in Ukraine", *Centre for International Governance Innovation*, 15 June 2022, https://www.cigionline.org/articles/social-media-warfare-is-being-invented-in-ukraine/ [accessed: 31.07.2024].

5 Paul Kari and agencies, "Russian disinformation surged on social media after invasion of Ukraine, Meta reports", *The Guardian*, 07 April 2022, https://www.theguardian.com/world/2022/apr/07/propaganda-social-media-surge-invasion-ukraine-meta-reports [accessed: 31.07.2024].

6 Johannes Buchheim and Abirihe Gilad, "War in Ukraine, Fake News, and the Digital Epistemic Divide", *Verfassungsblog (Constitution Blog)*, 12 May 2022, https://verfassungsblog.de/the-war-in-ukraine-fake-news-and-the-digital-epistemic-divide/ [accessed: 31.07.2024].

noting that the visual discourse of the Russo–Ukrainian War has not yet been considered in detail, although there exists some research on the use of cartoons, memes, and other types of visuals in the period between 2014 and 2022.[7] The developments of visual participatory culture during Russia's current full-scale invasion and the role of this culture as a means of resistance and resilience garnered significant media attention,[8] but the role of maps and geographic imagery specifically has not yet been studied by journalists or academics. For this reason, this essay studies these visuals and their symbolic meanings and functions in media communication. Throughout the text, I discuss examples from Ukrainian and Russian digital popular culture as well as maps used by state media.

What Do Maps Tell Us about the Russo-Ukrainian War?

Borders, reflecting the manifold consequences of the war, become spaces of violence. For some, they symbolise the demarcation of newly acquired territories, and for others, they become symbols of resistance and freedom. Indeed, maps play a crucial role in the visual representation of the war's developments, but they not only map boundaries and separation lines. They can also intensify people's sense of nationhood, identity, and belonging, as well as serve as popular mobilisers. From the constructivist perspective, maps represent powerful symbols that can visually not only materialise the territorial dimensions of a state, but also symbolise the nation.

---

7 Bradley E. Wiggins, "Crimea River: Directionality in Memes from the Russia–Ukraine Conflict", *International Journal of Communication* 10, 2016, 451–485; Myloka Makhortykh and Juan Manuel González Aguilar, "Memory, politics and emotions: internet memes and protests in Venezuela and Ukraine", *Continuum* 34/3, 2020, 342–362; Mykola Makhortykh and Maryna Sydorova, "Social media and visual framing of the conflict in Eastern Ukraine", *Media, War & Conflict* 10/3, 2017, 359–381, https://doi.org/10.1177/1750635217702539; Anastasia Denisova, "Russian Resistance and Propaganda through Memes in the 2010s", in: Anastasia Denisova, *Internet Memes and Society: Social, Cultural, and Political Contexts*, London: Routledge, 2019, 154–185; and Valentyna Ushchyna, "From conflict of discourses to military conflict: multimodality of identity construction in Russo–Ukrainian war discourse", *East European Journal of Psycholinguistics* 9/2, 2022, 130–143, https://doi.org/10.29038/eejpl.2022.9.2.ush.

8 Daryna Antoniuk, "Making sense of Ukrainian war memes: From watermelons to Saint Javelin", *Kyiv Independent*, 29 November 2022, https://kyivindependent.com/national/making-sense-of-ukrainian-memes-from-watermelons-to-saint-javelin [accessed: 31.07.2024]; Ilan Manor, "Do memes matter for the Russia–Ukraine War?", *Medium*, 13 July 2022, https://medium.com/international-affairs-blog/do-memes-matter-for-the-russia-ukraine-war-c86887b5b7f5 [accessed: 31.07.2024]; and Aja Romano, "Reckoning with the war meme in wartime: Is it ever okay to meme at a war?", *Vox*, 25 February 2022, https://www.vox.com/culture/2022/2/25/22950655/ukrainian-invasion-memes-political-cartoons-controversy [accessed: 31.07.2024].

According to Benedict Anderson, nations as 'imagined communities' are tightly connected to the spatial shape of their territory. In modern times, maps can be used as one of the pillars of building and maintaining nation-states and as skilful tools for visually associating the nation with its territory on an international scale.[9] Currently, in the age of digital media, the power of the map as a representational tool is not limited to the national community itself: maps and iconographic images that are repeatedly reproduced in media can be used as means of meaning-making and as tools of transferring national narratives to wider international audiences.

After the full-scale invasion, the geographical contours of Ukraine, previously unknown to most of the global population, suddenly monopolised the headlines of leading world media and flooded social media platforms like Facebook, X, and Instagram. Prior to the invasion, Ukraine had been an Eastern European country that was not 'European' enough to be integrated into the larger European family, yet also not so distant and unfamiliar to be interesting – a country that always resided in the shadow of its 'older brother' Russia. Yet, following 24 February 2022, it became the centre of global media attention. In this media environment, maps not only transfer factual information but also act as symbols. Alexander J. Kent and Peter Vujakovic suggest that maps offer "selective representations that preserve and promote some features while suppressing or obliterating others".[10] Maps vividly mark digital epistemic divides, consolidating different visions of the Russian aggression. While official military maps[11] track daily changes on the battlefield during the Russian invasion of Ukraine, hundreds of other maps are uploaded, shared, and circulated by internet users and the press through social and traditional media. Some maps are attempts to accurately depict the situation in Ukraine and provide additional information about the country, while others justify the Russian 'liberation' of its 'historical Russian lands'.

From the beginning of the full-scale aggression, world media used the maps not only to update about the war but also to place the country in a larger global context,

9 Anderson Benedict, *Imagined Communities: Reflections on the Origin and Spread of Nationalism*, London: Verso, 1991, 174–179.

10 Alexander J. Kent and Peter Vujakovic, "Maps and identity", in: Alexander J. Kent and Peter Vujakovic (eds.), *The Routledge Handbook of Mapping and Cartography*, New York: Routledge, 2018, 413–426, here 415.

11 See, for example, the maps of the Ministry of Defence of the United Kingdom, the interactive maps of Russia's invasion of Ukraine by the Institute of Study of War, and the maps of the war in Ukraine from DeepStateMAP, which have been published/updated daily and recirculated by Ukrainian and international media: Ministry of Defence 🇬🇧 (@DefenceHQ), https://twitter.com/DefenceHQ, X page, [accessed: 31.07.2024]; Institute for the Study of War, "Interactive Map: Russian's Invasion of Ukraine", https://www.understandingwar.org/interactive-map-russias-invasion-ukraine [accessed: 31.07.2024]; and DeepStateMAP, https://deepstatemap.live/en#6/47.828/25.005 [accessed: 31.07.2024].

to show why Ukraine is important to Europe, and to tell the story of an invasion that reverberates all over the world.[12] Unlike military maps that often focus only on Ukrainian territory and the development of the war,[13] these maps try to teach international audiences to think and talk about Ukraine as an integral part of the European or even global landscape.[14] They show not only the geography and size of Ukraine but also provide information about its history, politics, and languages. In this case, maps are used not as a neutral representation of the territory, but as social constructs[15] that convey important messages, integrating the Ukrainian geobody into the mental map of the European continent and making it a part of a larger imaginary. They are also important in giving Ukraine agency and subjectivity and in showing the international community that EU political actors should not ignore this large European state.

Ukrainian government organisations and nongovernmental organisations (NGOs) have also released several map projects intended to make global audiences see Russian aggression not only as a Ukrainian war, but also as a war against Europe and global democratic values. These maps manifested the cruelty of Russia and the heroism of Ukrainian people, were largely shared on social media (e.g., X and Facebook), and provoked vivid discussions among internet users. For example, in July 2022, the independent analytical platform *VoxUkraine* published a map of occupied Ukrainian territory together with a series of maps of France, Germany, Italy, Hungary, and other EU countries that illustrate the scale of the invasion (e.g., Figure 2). They use orange to mark territories occupied by Russian troops and to transfer these contours onto the maps of other countries. These maps reflect the general tendencies of military maps of the Russian invasion by using red or orange – colours associated with violence – to mark occupied territories and blue to show de-occupation.

---

12 Sara Chodosh et al., "How to Think About Ukraine, in Maps and Charts", *The New York Times*, 25 February 2022, https://www.nytimes.com/interactive/2022/02/25/opinion/russia-ukraine-invasion-maps.html [accessed: 31.07.2024].

13 This statement can be illustrated by the military map of the Russian invasion by the UK Ministry of Defence, which is often used by Ukrainian social media information channels: Ministry of Defence 🇬🇧 (@DefenceHQ), "The illegal and unprovoked invasion...", X post, 15 May 2022, https://twitter.com/DefenceHQ/status/1525767592316747776 [accessed: 31.07.2024].

14 The map used in the article of Sara Chodosh et al., "How to Think About Ukraine, in Maps and Charts" (*The New York Times*, 25 February 2022, https://www.nytimes.com/interactive/2022/02/25/opinion/russia-ukraine-invasion-maps.html [accessed: 31.07.2024]), for example, places the geographical countours of Ukraine on a map of Europe to illustrate the spatial dimensions of the country.

15 Jeremy W. Crampton, "Maps as social constructions: power, communication and visualization", *Progress in Human Geography* 25/2, 2001, 235–252, here 240.

Figure 2: Image from VoxUkraine Eng, "Russia occupied 125 000 km2 of Ukraine's territory..."

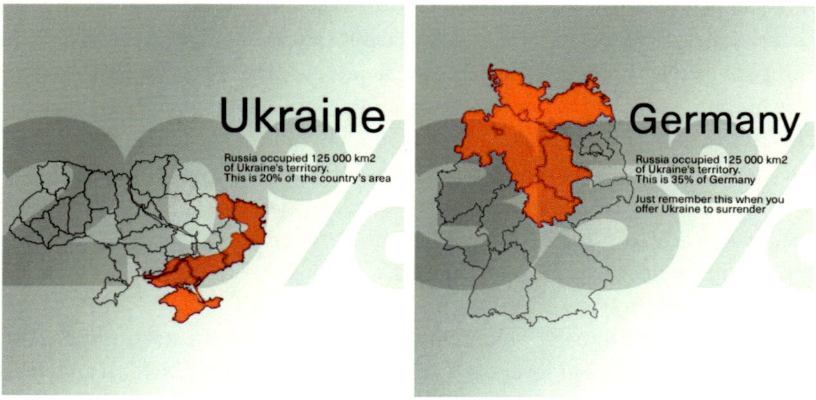

VoxUkraineEng, Facebook post, 01 June 2022, https://m.facebook.com/voxukraine/posts/3185241458401847/ [accessed: 24.07.2024].

The Ministry of Defence of Ukraine posted another series of maps on X in July 2022 to visualise the length of the frontline of the Russo–Ukrainian War. By placing the frontline in the middle of Europe, on the US–Mexican border, or in Japan, the authors wanted to demonstrate the scale of the resistance of Ukrainians, who, with a frontline of more than 2,000 kilometres, stand "between Freedom and tyranny".[16] The Ministry of Defence claimed that now more than a million Ukrainians hold the line, "protecting Europe from the Russian horde"[17] (Figure 3). The German magazine *Katapult*, for example, also used similar geographical visualisations of Ukrainian resistance (Figure 4).

These maps make the Ukrainian experience more recognisable, bringing it closer to a European or Western geographical landscape. This spatial recontextualisation of wartime experiences of the occupation and resistance, and their placement into a geographical space familiar to media users from the referenced parts of the world, could lead them to think about further threats of the Russian invasion and its scale. These maps not only reshape and refine the image of Ukraine but also change the perception of the 'Other', the aggressor, by making the consequences of the war more visible.

16 Defense of Ukraine (@DefenceU), "The front line of more than 2,000 km...", X post, 13 July 2022, https://twitter.com/defenceu/status/1547324237895110657 [accessed: 24.07.2024].

17 Ibid.

Figure 3: . Image from Defense of Ukraine, "The front line of more than 2,000 km..."

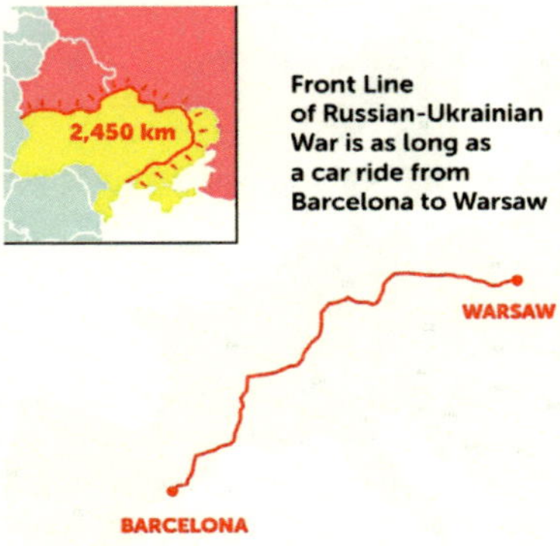

Defense of Ukraine (@DefenceU), "The front line of more than 2,000 km...", X post, 13 July 2022, https://twitter.com/defenceu/status/1547324237895110657 [accessed: 23.07.2024].

Figure 4: Image from KATAPULT Magazin, "Davon werden an 1.105 Kilometern aktive..."

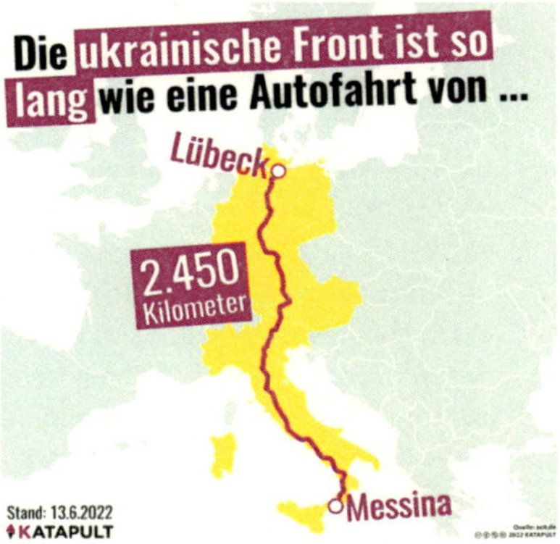

KATAPULT Magazin (@Katapultmagazin), "Davon werden an 1.105 Kilometern aktive...", X post, 14 June 2022, https://twitter.com/Katapultmagazin/status/1536691735514038275 [accessed: 23.07.2024].

Another politics of representation through maps and mapping exists in the Russian media space. Official Russian media used different mechanisms of territorial representation to justify the Russian invasion after 2014. The intentional use of mapmaking started years before the beginning of the full-scale invasion, when spatial relationships between Russia and Ukraine were redefined and the narrative of the nonexistence of Ukraine was instrumentalised to normalise the occupation of Crimea. The official media used maps as tools of imperialism; they explained the 'correct' visions of the historical development of Ukraine and deconstructed its territorial integrity. For example, Russian official news media repeatedly circulated a map of Ukraine where different parts of the country were marked by different colours. This map indicates the dates and historical personalities who "offered" these territories to Ukraine.[18] It was used to propagate the narrative that Ukraine is an artificial state composed of disparate territories that historically belonged to Russia and were only incorporated into Ukraine through the actions of Russian tsars or Soviet government representatives.[19]

18 Roman Golovanov, "Ukraina sostoit iz podarkov russkikh tsarey i sovetskikh gensekov" ("Ukraine Consists of the Gifts from Russian Tsars and Soviet General Secretaries"), Komsomolskaya Pravda (Komsomol Truth), 18 May 2017, https://www.kp.ru/daily/26680.3/3702227 [accessed: 31.07.2024].

19 For more examples, see: Natalya Pupkova, "Territorialnyy pazl Dlya Ukrainy on slozhilsya blagodarya 'okkupantam' – rossiyskim tsaryam I bolshevikam" ("The Territorial Puz-

The same narrative was reproduced on Russian social media. Pro-Kremlin groups on VKontakte and Facebook, as well as individual users, posted and shared in comments maps that misrepresented Ukrainian historical development.[20]

zle: For Ukraine, It Was Formed Thanks to the 'Occupiers' – the Russian Tsars and Bolsheviks"), *Krymskaya Pravda* (*Crimean Truth*), 10 July 2014, https://c-pravda.ru/news/2014-07-10/territorialnyjj-pazl [accessed: 23.07.2024]; Yuriy Baranchik, "Ukraina: byt ili ne byt?" ("Ukraine: To Be or Not to Be?"), *regnum*, 08 January 2017, https://regnum.ru/news/polit/2224728.html [accessed: 23.07.2024]; Aleksandr Gorokhov, "A ne 'dekommunizirovat' li nam territoriyu Ukrainy?" ("Should We 'Decommunise' the Territory of Ukraine?"), *Novoross*, 2019, https://www.novoross.info/politiks/55184-a-ne-dekommunizirovat-li-nam-territoriyu-ukrainy-mnenie.html [accessed: 23.07.2024]; Kirill Somov, "Ukraina na tret sostoit iz rossiyskikh 'podarkov'" ("Ukraine is One-Third Comprised of Russian 'Gifts'"), *Federalcity.ru*, 19 March 2021, https://federalcity.ru/10283-ukraina-na-tret-sostoit-iz-rossijskih-podarkov-jekspert.html [accessed: 23.07.2024]; *Sevastopol.su*, "V GD predlozhili vernut' Rossii pol-Ukrainy posle slov ob 'okkupatsii'" ("In the State Duma, They Proposed to Return Half of Ukraine to Russia after Talk about 'Occupation'"), 08 January 2018, https://sevastopol.su/news/v-gd-predlozhili-vernut-rossii-pol-ukrainy-posle-slov-ob-okkupacii [accessed: 23.07.2024]; Maria Lisitsyna, "Rossiya 24 pokazala kartu s 'territoriyami-podarkami' Ukraine" ("Russia 24 Showed a Map with 'Gift Territories' to Ukraine"), *RBC*, 23 February 2022, https://www.rbc.ru/politics/23/02/2022/6216280c9a794717da17a93d [accessed: 23.07.2024]; Alexander Samsonov, "Pohoronit antiruskiy proyekt 'Ukraina'" ("Bury the Anti-Russian Project 'Ukraine'"), *Voennoe Obozrenie* (*Military Review*), 2022, https://topwar.ru/192827-pohoronit-antirusskij-proekt-ukraina.html [accessed: 23.03.2023]; Elena Bylkina, "VGTRK pokazal kartu Ukrainy s territoriyami, podarennymi tsaryami i gensekami" ("VGTRK Showed a Map of Ukraine with Territories Gifted by Tsars and Secretaries-General"), *Pravda* (*Truth*), 23 February 2022, https://www.pravda.ru/news/society/1685414-ukraina/ [accessed: 23.07.2024]; Daria Dmitrova, "Telekanal 'Rossiya 24' sostavil kartu podarennikh Ukraine territoriy" ("TV Channel 'Russia 24' Compiled a Map of Territories Gifted to Ukraine"), *Gazeta.ru* (*Newspaper.ru*), 23 February 2022, https://www.gazeta.ru/social/news/2022/02/23/17334445.shtml?updated [accessed: 23.07.2024].

20 For example, such publications and comments can be found in the pro-Kremlim VKontakte groups like Chto Tam U Khryuklov? (ChTUKh) (What's Up with the Oinkers?) or Zapadenets News. See: Chto Tam U Khryuklov? (ChTUKh) (What's Up with the Oinkers?), VKontakte page, https://vk.com/chto_tam_u [accessed: 23.07.2024]; and Zapadenets News, VKontakte page, https://vk.com/zapadeneznews [accessed: 14.03.2024]. A series of publications, *Ukraine does not exist*, are also available on VKontakte through the page Stalinskii Polk – Sovinformbyuro (Stalin's Regiment – the Soviet Information Bureau): Stalinskii Polk – Sovinformbyuro (Stalin's Regiment – the Soviet Information Bureau), VKontakte page, https://vk.com/sovinformburo [accessed: 23.07.2024]. Moreover, the image *Gifts for Ukraine from Russian Tsars* has more than four million likes on the patriotic platform Prezidentpress.ru, which incited a wide spread of this visual: Prezidentpress.ru, https://prezidentpress.ru/news/2816-ukraina-podarki-russkih-carey.html [accessed:14.03.2024]. Individual users also post similar maps to their personal pages. See, for example: Alexander Ulyanov, "esli USSR vykhodit iz sostava..." ("if the Ukrainian SSR leaves..."), VKontakte post, 01 April 2022, https://vk.com/wall249749579_8993 [accessed: 14.03.2024].

Other maps reconstructed the geographical contours of Russia, joining to it the annexed territories of the Crimean Peninsula and representing the 'new' space of the Russian Federation. The marking of Crimea as Ukrainian or Russian on international maps and the use of typical geographical representations of the two states (with or without Crimean Peninsula) remained a sensitive topic for more than eight years and became one of the emblems of the epistemic divide. While Ukrainian government and official media recirculated the slogan 'Crimea is Ukraine'[21] and desperately fought for the visual recognition of its geographical integrity, Russian officials claimed to have the right to mark Crimea as a part of their territory. The ambiguous mapping and the clashing media narratives provoked a series of scandals that reflected one or another spatial vision of the Russo–Ukrainian War that started in 2014.[22] Similar strategies of the integration of Ukrainian regions into Russian topography appeared after the fraudulent referendums on occupied Ukrainian territories in September 2022.[23] Even though the 'new' map of Russia has not yet been officially issued, it is broadly circulated in news media to mark political decisions and confirm the 'successes' of the Russian troops in the 'special military operation'. Again in this case, mapping does not serve to represent internationally recognised borders, but to reaffirm the political decisions and imperial ambitions of Russian officials. Thus, maps reproducing Russian aggression function as propaganda, a construction that recreates space following the demands and ambitions of people in power.

These documentary or pseudo-documentary forms of content often overlap in new media with artistic and symbolic representations of the two nation-states that create new visual narratives of the war or metaphorically reproduce existing narratives. Rebeca Pop notes that as the war develops and the narrative of the aggression

---

21 This slogan was first introduced in 2015 and used by the Ukrainian Ministry of Culture and Information Policy and the Ukrainian Ministry of Foreign Affairs in numerous information campaigns. For more, see: Zhytomyrska oblasna derzhavna administratsiia (Zhytomyr Oblast State Administration), "V Ukraini startuvala komunikatsiina kampaniia 'Krym – tse Ukraina'" ("Communication Campaign 'Crimea is Ukraine' Launched in Ukraine"), 01 March 2016, https://oda.zht.gov.ua/news/v-ukrayini-startuvala-komunikatsijna-k/ [accessed: 23.07.2024]; and *Radio Svoboda* (*Radio Freedom*), "MZS Ukrainy bude monitoryty, yak poznachaiut Krym na kartakh svitu" ("Ukraine's Foreign Ministry Will Monitor How Crimea Is Marked on World Maps"), 02 December 2015, https://www.radiosvoboda.org/a/27402854.html [accessed: 23.07.2024].

22 *The Moscow Times*, "Crimean Map Scandals: Choice Between Offending Russia or Ukraine", 29 July 2016, https://www.themoscowtimes.com/2016/07/29/map-scandals-topography-after-annexations-a54796 [accessed: 23.07.2024].

23 For example, Russian official media outlets published a new map of Russia which incorporates the occupied Ukrainian territories: Polina Devyatova, "Novaya karta Rossii. Infografika" ("New Map of Russia: Infographics"), *Argumenty i Fakty (Arguments and Facts)*, 28 September 2022, https://aif.ru/politics/russia/novaya_karta_rossii_infografika [accessed: 14.12.2022].

becomes more complex, new maps appear to tell a multifaceted story of the invasion.[24] Maps themselves not only represent places physically but become conceptual containers filled with new meanings, both for those who live inside and outside the borders of Ukraine. These geographic representations of Ukraine and Russia are intimately integrated into the visual mediascape of the two countries, constructing opposite visions of war experiences.

Geographical Imagery and a New Spatial Reality

In today's digital media, geographical outlines of Ukraine and Russia are highly recurring symbols. Hundreds of images circulate on social media, combined with other symbolic representations of the countries, such as the colours of their flags (yellow and blue for Ukraine and red, white, and blue for Russia), national emblems (the trident for Ukraine and the two-headed eagle for Russia), or other symbols (e.g., sunflowers for Ukraine and a bear for Russia). These emblematic images not only stand for the respective geographical spaces but, in some cases, might also act as symbolic representations of the countries' populations. Similarly, they convey messages that have deep conceptual, cultural, and epistemological meanings for their nations, helping to support and construct national narratives. In the case of Ukraine, visual narratives widely shared by internet users on social media through groups and private profiles incorporate iconographic geographic images to tell the story of Ukrainian resistance and fighting. Meanwhile, for the Russian regime, the recurring visual narratives serve to affirm Russian imperialism.

From the very first days of the Russian aggression, images inspired by the geographic contours of Ukraine, including artistic and popular ones, flooded Ukrainian media spaces. They served to tell the story of the invasion and the violation of the borders of Ukraine, or were used to express and share collective emotions. Simple visuals conveyed complex information and helped not only to relate to the grief and sorrow of Ukrainians but also had the potential to join people around a common goal and form a narrative of victory and heroism. Often, these images function as metaphors that convey the fight against the invader and portray the nation heroically. In these cases, the geographical representations of Ukraine are combined with images of Ukrainian soldiers. The representations of Ukrainian combatants can be incorporated into the geographical contours of the country or they can stand between the Ukrainian geo-body and the aggression of the enemy. For instance, the artwork of Oleksiy Bondarenko depicts a Ukrainian soldier "holding the sky" in order

24 Rebeca Pop, "Similar Stories, Different Maps – A Visual Narrative of the War in Ukraine", *Everviz*, 10 May 2022, https://www.everviz.com/blog/similar-stories-different-maps-a-visual-narrative-of-the-war-in-ukraine/ [accessed: 23.07.2024].

to protect Ukrainian lands (see Figure 5). Often, the cartographic imagery is combined with the visualisation of ordinary Ukrainian people and Ukrainian national symbols to reinforce a sense of unity and national belonging. This can be illustrated by the work of Alyona Zhuk, where the map of Ukraine is composed of a multitude of faces of ordinary people of different ages and professions united by the common goal to defeat the enemy (see Figure 6). Some works personify the Ukrainian geo-body to illustrate the active participation of different parts of Ukrainian society in the country's war efforts.[25] These images often carry slogans such as "no to war", "stand with Ukraine", or "I am Ukraine/Ukrainian", as well as the word "freedom". The images convey the existential position of many Ukrainians, for whom this war turned into a battle for the survival of their nation. Lastly, the images' messages are easily recognisable for those seeing them beyond the borders of Ukraine, suggesting that they mean to mobilise people from all over the world.

Carrying important national symbols, these images tend to express significant messages for Ukrainians and intensify their feelings of national belonging. The clearest example of this are maps that combine words with similar spellings but opposing meanings: "Бійся – бийся" ("*Biisia – byisia*", "Be afraid – fight") or "Війна – Вільна" ("*Viina – Vilna*", "War – Freedom").[26] These conflicting concepts placed in a single iconographic image aim to reflect the contradictory reality of many Ukrainians and help to mobilise the population in their fight for freedom. Other common phrases include, "Home", "I love Ukraine", "Ukraine – my home", and "Ukraine my zone of comfort". These express affection and love towards the homeland and also tend to reinforce a sense of belonging.

The unity of the nation is particularly important in the visualisation of Ukrainian resistance and is also expressed by the combination of the spatial contours of the country and the common phrase "Як ти?" ("*Yak ty*?", "How are you?"). In the digital space of social media, there are several anonymous works in this style. Another common motif incorporates real stories of resistance or common difficulties that

---

25 For example, an illustration by Nikita Titov posted on Facebook depicts the collective body of Ukraine as a courageous and fearless creature ready to fight the aggressor. This illustration was also used by official outlets to showcase how Ukrainian artists visualise the resistance and resilience of Ukrainians in the face of war. For more details, see: Iryna Petrenko, "Kakym byl 2022 god: retrpspectiva v illustratsyyah Grekhova, Maydukova, Titova, Drachkovskoy" ("How was the year 2022?: retrospective in illustrations by Grekhov, Maidukov, Titov, Drachkovskaya"), *Liga.net*, 28 December 2022, https://life.liga.net/ru/rozvagy/cards/kakim-byl-2022-god-retrospektiva-v-illyustratsiyah-grekova-maydukova-titova-drachkovskoy [accessed: 14.07.2024].

26 For example, the artwork of Natali Hall combines the geographic contours of Ukraine, the colours of the national flag and the slogan "Війна – Вільна", insisting on the importance of freedom for the Ukrainian nation: Natali Hall, "Ukraine will always be free!", 30 March 2022, https://www.artstation.com/artwork/aGB4Kk [accessed: 14.07.2024].

Ukrainians have experienced daily during the last 10 months (e.g., power cuts or massive drone attacks). For example, the story of the unbreakable kitchen cupboard in one of the destroyed houses in the village of Borodianka inspired a widely shared image of Ukraine.[27] These maps of Ukraine, combined with simple symbols or slogans of unbreakable resistance, aim to convey the collective feelings of Ukrainians and to mobilise the nation, providing hope for the future.

Figure 5: Image from Oleksiy Bondarenko, "Hold the Sky"

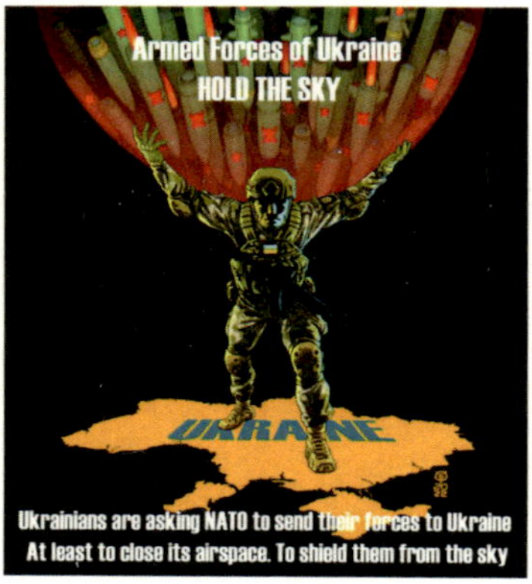

Image from Oleksiy Bondarenko, "Oleksiy Bondarenko – Donate To Artist", ArtDopomoga, https://artdopomoga.com/oleksiy-bondarenko/ [accessed: 14.12.2022].

Figure 6: Image from Alyona Zhuk, "Razom peremozhemo..." ("We'll do it together...")

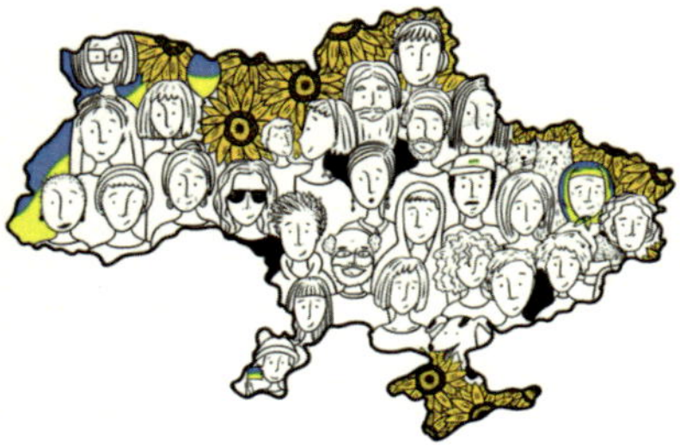

Image from Alyona Zhuk (@zhuk_alyona), "Razom peremozhemo..." ("We'll do it together..."), Instagram post, 20 April 2022, https://www.instagram.com/p/CckoEhBN6Pq/ [accessed: 14.12.2022].

Moreover, the mapmaking also helps to express emotions, negative and positive, and to share them with other members of the community. The images present the pain of loss and the traumatic experience of the violation of Ukraine's borders through red, the colour of blood and one associated with aggression, as well as symbols like scars, bandages, or adhesive plasters that indicate collective trauma. For example, an illustration by Anna Foralberg visualises the war trauma of Ukrainians through the combination of the individual body of a human being and the collective

27 Kyiv24.news, "'Ty yak? Trymayus!' Kukhonna shafa, yaka vtsilila pislia znyshchennia budynku u Brodyantsi, stala symvolom vytrymky Ukrayiny" ("'How Are You? Holding On!': The Kitchen Cabinet That Survived the Destruction of a House in Borodianka Has Become a Symbol of Ukraine's Resilience"), 09 April 2022, https://kyiv.media/news/ty-yak-trymayus-kuhonna-shafa-yaka-vczilila-pislya-znyshhennya-budynku-u-borodyanczi-stala-symvolom-vytrymky-ukrayiny [accessed: 23.07.2024].

body of the country, reflecting the deep trauma inflicted by the conflict and symbolising how the pain of war permeates both personal and collective identities (see Figure 7). Artem Gusev's artwork depicts Ukraine's war trauma using the image of the bleeding collective body of Ukraine while highlighting the healing effect of popular mobilisation and consolidation in the face of danger (see Figure 8). Positive emotions such as love, affection, and belonging to the homeland are expressed with floral motives or depictions such as a heart incorporated into the contours of Ukraine.[28]

These representations of the geo-body are directly associated with the physical body of Ukrainians, as they openly stand for the suffering of many people or the intensification of a sense of belonging and an affirmation of national unity and sovereignty.

Figure 7: Image from Anna Foralberg, "V dome mnoho sveta..." ("There's a lot of light in the house...")

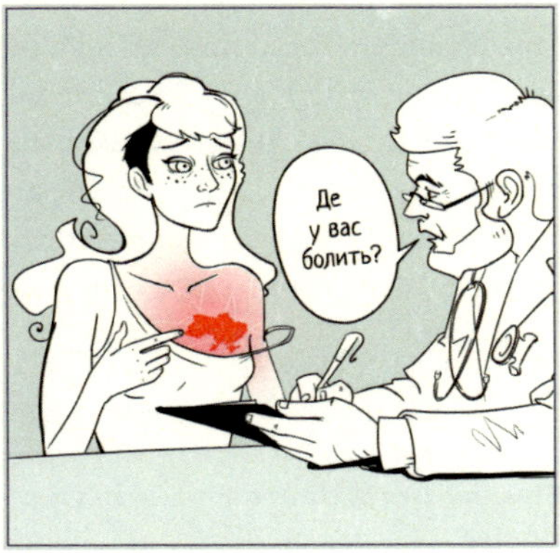

Anna Foralberg (@foralberg_art), "V dome mnoho sveta..." ("There's a lot of light in the house..."), Instagram post, 27 March 2022, https://www.instagram.com/p/CbnoYNQNffi/ [accessed: 14.12.2022].

Figure 8: Image from Artem Gusev, "9 udariv po Poltavshchyni..." ("9 strikes on Poltava Oblast")

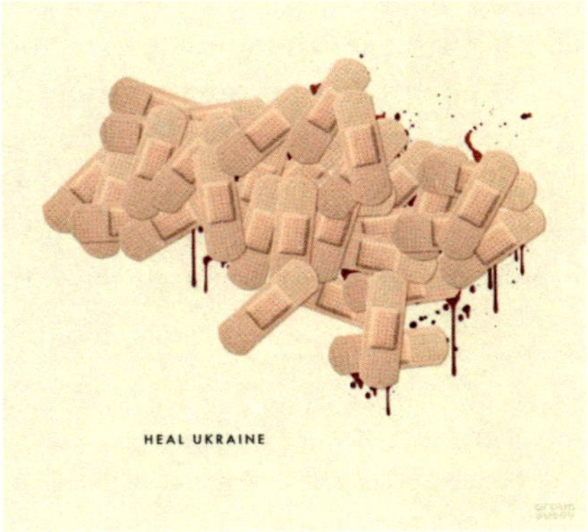

Artem Gusev (@gusev_art), "9 udariv po Poltavshchyni..." ("9 strikes on Poltava Oblast"), Instagram post, 25 April 2022, https://www.instagram.com/p/Ccw9XnjNJCw/ [accessed: 31.07.2024].

28 For example, an image posted on Instagram in March 2022 created by Oleksandra Olishevska portrays a young girl who is holding tightly to the collective body of Ukraine. A painted heart at the centre of Ukraine's body symbolises the deep emotional connection between the land and its people. Later, this artwork was shared by the official page of Ukraine on Facebook: Ukraine.ua, "Hold you tight and will never give you to anybody. Our one and only Ukraine", Facebook post, 24 March 2022, https://www.facebook.com/photo/?fbid=336827915142831&set=a.237166015109022 [accessed: 28.02.2023].

Despite the variety of the messages and ideas expressed through the maps, the spatial integrity of Ukraine is present in all the analysed images, with Crimea and the Donbas included within its borders. The wholeness and unity of the nation and its territory are the most important parameters in the spatial expressions of Ukrainian artists.

In Russian digital discourse on social media, geographical imagery about Ukraine reproduces the main narratives of Russian state propaganda. Ukraine is always shown as an object: it is not given agency, and its territory is violated, manipulated, or used as a tool.[29] In many visual representations, Russia is presented as a saviour, an older brother ready to help, while the US and NATO are depicted as enemies who want to invade Ukraine or take advantage of it.[30] The images portray relationships of superiority and inferiority through the representation of Ukraine as weak, helpless, and always threatened by external dangers. They also often depict Ukrainian geography as a stage or arena for the 'political games' of superpowers and lack any of the affective components present in Ukrainian digital discourse.

This visual discourse reaffirms Russian imperialism and strives to incorporate new territories into the collective visions of Russia. Since 2014, Ukraine has been depicted without Crimea in Russian official media and on social media, and after the beginning of the full-scale invasion, new practices of ordering reality appeared, especially in social networks like VKontakte and pro-Kremlin Telegram channels. Paralleling official propaganda, 'new' or 'improved' maps of Russia and Ukraine are created and widely circulated on social media.[31] They map the newly occupied territories in the colours of the Russian flag. Interestingly, some of these maps move be-

29 For example, a cartoon created by Aleksandr Troitsky depicts Ukraine as a bullet, labelled NATO, loaded into a weapon. This visual metaphor not only deprives Ukraine of its agency but also propagates the narrative that Ukraine is a tool used by NATO to advance its geopolitical interests against the Russian Federation. See: Zlobodnevnye Karikatury, "Odna iz oboimy – Aleksandr Troitsky" ("One from the clip – Aleksandr Troitsky"), Telegram post, 10 October 2022, https://t.me/caricaturaru/1097 [accessed: 31.07.2024].

30 For example, an image depicting the US and NATO as monstrous creatures devouring Ukraine while a human hand in the colours of the Russian flag (blue, red, and white) reaches out to protect or save the country is often used on Russian social media to visually frame the Russo-Ukrainian War. See: Nonamenews, "Otobrazhenye realnoi sytuatsyy na Ukrayne ("Reflection of the real situation in Ukraine"), Pikabu.ru post, 14 March 2022, https://pikabu.ru/story/otobrazhenie_realnoy_situatsii_na_ukraine_8924195 [accessed: 31.07.2024].

31 For instance, the telegram channel "Povernutye na Z voyne" ("Crazy about Z war") that has more than seven hundred thousand subscribers posted an image of the 'correct' map of Ukraine, where the occupied Ukrainian territories were marked with the colours of the Russian flag, openly indicating their belonging to the Russian Federation. See: Povernutye na Z voyne (Crazy about Z war), "Pravilnaya karta" ("The correct map"), Telegram post, 30 September 2022, https://t.me/voenacher/30076 [accessed: 31.07.2024].

yond Ukraine and spread to the European continent.[32] These maps reflect Russian *pobedobesie*[33] and slogans that propagandists used since the beginning of the full-scale invasion,[34] revealing Russian imperial aspirations. These images show that in the spatial imaginary of the artists and those who share the images, Russian borders are not firm and can be modified according to political needs.

Conclusions

Maps are powerful tools for re- and deconstructing, communicating, and sharing spatial imagery and collective identities. This article revealed that the Russian aggression against Ukraine provoked the emergence of (counter-) mapping practices that propagate different visions of geographical spaces and serve to support or co-construct the existing narratives of war. In the case of the Russian regime, the modified maps of Russia that include the annexed Ukrainian territories are used to justify aggression against a sovereign state and the realisation of the special military operation. In the case of Ukraine and its Western allies, the visualisation of the spatial integrity of Ukrainian territory represents the support and reaffirmation of Ukrainian sovereignty and independence. Ukrainian popular cultural productions inspired by the geographic contours of the state considered in this text represent an attempt to assert the collective identity and spatial wholeness of the nation-state. They are also combined with other images and symbols of war and aim to consolidate and share collective experiences and emotions triggered by the war. Meanwhile, in the Russian digital social media space, maps reaffirm a Russian vision of the historical developments of Ukraine and its role in today's political arena and strive to propagate Russia's imperial narratives.

---

32 For example, the image of a map of the Russian-backed self-proclaimed Donetsk and Luhansk People's Republics that incorporated European countries using red contours was widely shared on Russian social media. This map visually extended the influence of these territories across Europe, symbolically asserting Russian power and geopolitical dominance. See: Tyurbab, "Strategicheskaya_Karta_Genshtaba_Rossii" ("Strategic map of the Russian General Staff"), Pikabu.ru post, 25 February 2022, https://pikabu.ru/story/strategicheskaya_karta_genshtaba_rossii_8867983 [accessed: 31.07.2024].

33 *Pobedobesie* is a pejorative term used to describe the Victory Cult in the Russian Federation.

34 For instance, the maps are combined with slogans that support continuing the 'special military operation', such as "Go till La Manche" or "Go till Berlin". See: Olesia Bida, "Pryishli zvilnyaty vid natsikiv. Shcho na rosiyskomu telebachenni govoriat pro viynu z Ukrayinoyu" ("They Came to Liberate from the Nazis: What Russian Television Says about the War with Ukraine"), *Hromadske*, 2022, https://hromadske.ua/posts/prijshli-zvilnyati-vid-nacikiv-sho-na-rosijskomu-telebachenni-govoryat-pro-vijnu-z-ukrayinoyu [accessed: 23.07.2024].

Bibliography

Baranchik, Yuriy, "Ukraina: byt ili ne byt?" ("Ukraine: To Be or Not to Be?"), *Regnum*, 08 January 2017, https://regnum.ru/news/polit/2224728.html [accessed: 23.07.2024].

Benedict, Anderson, *Imagined Communities: Reflections on the Origin and Spread of Nationalism*, London: Verso, 1991.

Bida, Olesia, "Pryishli zvilnyaty vid natsikiv. Shcho na rosiyskomu telebachenni govoriat pro viynu z Ukrayinoyu" ("They Came to Liberate from the Nazis: What Russian Television Says about the War with Ukraine"), *Hromadske*, 2022, https://hromadske.ua/posts/prijshli-zvilnyati-vid-nacikiv-sho-na-rosijs komu-telebachenni-govoryat-pro-vijnu-z-ukrayinoyu [accessed: 23.07.2024].

Buchheim, Johannes, and Abirihe Gilad, "War in Ukraine, Fake News, and the Digital Epistemic Divide", *Verfassungsblog* (*Constitution Blog*), 12 May 2022, https: //verfassungsblog.de/the-war-in-ukraine-fake-news-and-the-digital-epistem ic-divide/ [accessed: 23.07.2024].

Bylkina, Elena, "VGTRK pokazal kartu Ukrainy s territoriyami, podarennymi tsaryami I gensekami" ("VGTRK Showed a Map of Ukraine with Territories Gifted by Tsars and Secretaries-General"), *Pravda* (*Truth*), 23 February 2022, ht tps://www.pravda.ru/news/society/1685414-ukraina/ [accessed: 23.07.2024].

Chayka, Kyle, "Watching the World's 'First TikTok War'", *The New Yorker*, 03 March 2022, https://www.newyorker.com/culture/infinite-scroll/watching-the-world s-first-tiktok-war [accessed: 23.07.2024].

Chodosh, Sara, et al., "How to Think About Ukraine, in Maps and Charts", *The New York Times*, 25 February 2022, https://www.nytimes.com/interactive/2022/02/2 5/opinion/russia-ukraine-invasion-maps.html [accessed: 23.07.2024].

Chto Tam U Khryuklov? (ChTUKh) (What's Up with the Oinkers?), VKontakte page, https://vk.com/chto_tam_u [accessed: 23.07.2024].

Ciuriak, Dan, "Social Media Warfare Is Being Invented in Ukraine", *Centre for International Governance Innovation*, 15 June 2022, https://www.cigionline.org/articles /social-media-warfare-is-being-invented-in-ukraine/ [accessed: 23.07.2024].

Crampton, Jeremy W., "Maps as social constructions: power, communication and visualization", *Progress in Human Geography* 25/2, 2001, 235–252.

DeepStateMAP, https://deepstatemap.live/en#6/47.828/25.005 [accessed: 23.07. 2024].

Defense of Ukraine (@DefenceU), "The front line of more than 2,000 km…", Twitter post, 13 July 2022, https://twitter.com/defenceu/status/1547324237895110657 [accessed: 24.07.2024].

Denisova, Anastasia, "Russian Resistance and Propaganda through Memes in the 2010s", in: Anastasia Denisova, *Internet Memes and Society: Social, Cultural, and Political Contexts*, London: Routledge, 2019, 154–185.

Dmitrova, Daria, "Telekanal 'Rossiya 24' sostavil kartu podarennikh Ukraine territoriy" ("TV Channel 'Russia 24' Compiled a Map of Territories Gifted to Ukraine"), *Gazeta.ru* (*Newspaper.ru*), 23 February 2022, https://www.gazeta.ru/social/news/2022/02/23/17334445.shtml?updated [accessed: 24.07.2024].

Friedman, Thomas L., "We Have Never Been Here Before", *The New York Times*, 25 February 2022, https://www.nytimes.com/2022/02/25/opinion/putin-russia-ukraine.html [accessed: 23.07.2024].

Gorokhov, Aleksandr, "A ne 'dekommunizirovat' li nam territoriyu Ukrainy?" ("Should We 'Decommunise' the Territory of Ukraine?"), *Novoross*, 2019, https://www.novoross.info/politiks/55184-a-ne-dekommunizirovat-li-nam-territoriyu-ukrainy-mnenie.html [accessed: 23.03.2023].

Hoskins, Andrew, and Pavel Shchelin, "The War Feed: Digital War in Plain Sight", *American Behavioral Scientist* 67/3, 2023, 449–463, https://doi.org/10.1177/00027642221144848.

Institute for the Study of War, "Interactive Map: Russian's Invasion of Ukraine", https://www.understandingwar.org/interactive-map-russias-invasion-ukraine [accessed: 25.02.2024].

Kari, Paul, and agencies, "Russian disinformation surged on social media after invasion of Ukraine, Meta reports", *The Guardian*, 07 April 2022, https://www.theguardian.com/world/2022/apr/07/propaganda-social-media-surge-invasion-ukraine-meta-reports [accessed: 23.07.2024].

Kent, Alexander J., and Peter Vujakovic, "Maps and identity", in: Alexander J. Kent and Peter Vujakovic (eds.), *The Routledge Handbook of Mapping and Cartography*, New York: Routledge, 2018, 413–426.

Kyiv24.news, "'Ty yak? Trymayus!' Kukhonna shafa, yaka vtsilila pislia znyshchennia budynku u Brodyantsi, stala symvolom vytrymky Ukrayiny" ("'How Are You? Holding On!': The Kitchen Cabinet That Survived the Destruction of a House in Borodianka Has Become a Symbol of Ukraine's Resilience"), 09 April 2022, https://kyiv.media/news/ty-yak-trymayus-kuhonna-shafa-yaka-vczilila-pislya-znyshhennya-budynku-u-borodyanczi-stala-symvolom-vytrymky-ukrayiny [accessed: 23.07.2024].

Lisitsyna, Maria, "Rossiya 24 pokazala kartu s 'territoriyami-podarkami' Ukraine" ("Russia 24 Showed a Map with 'Gift Territories' to Ukraine"), *RBC*, 23 February 2022, https://www.rbc.ru/politics/23/02/2022/6216280c9a794717da17a93d [accessed: 23.07.2024].

Makhortykh, Myloka, and Juan Manuel González Aguilar, "Memory, politics and emotions: internet memes and protests in Venezuela and Ukraine", *Continuum* 34/3, 2020, 342–362.

Makhortykh, Mykola, and Maryna Sydorova, "Social media and visual framing of the conflict in Eastern Ukraine", *Media, War & Conflict* 10/3, 2017, 359–381, https://doi.org/10.1177/1750635217702539.

Manor, Ilan, "Do memes matter for the Russia–Ukraine War?", *Medium*,13 July 2022, https://medium.com/international-affairs-blog/do-memes-matter-for-the-russia-ukraine-war-c86887b5b7f5 [accessed: 23.07.2024].

Ministry of Defence 🇬🇧 (@DefenceHQ), https://twitter.com/DefenceHQ, X page, [accessed: 23.07.2024].

Ministry of Defence 🇬🇧 (@DefenceHQ), "The illegal and unprovoked invasion…", X post, 15 May 2022, https://twitter.com/DefenceHQ/status/1525767592316747776 [accessed: 23.07.2024].

The Moscow Times, "Crimean Map Scandals: Choice Between Offending Russia or Ukraine", 29 July 2016, https://www.themoscowtimes.com/2016/07/29/map-scandals-topography-after-annexations-a54796 [accessed: 23.07.2024].

Pop, Rebeca, "Similar Stories, Different Maps – A Visual Narrative of the War in Ukraine", *Everviz*, 10 May 2022, https://www.everviz.com/blog/similar-stories-different-maps-a-visual-narrative-of-the-war-in-ukraine/ [accessed: 23.07.2024].

Prezidentpress.ru, https://prezidentpress.ru/news/2816-ukraina-podarki-russkih-carey.html [accessed: 14.03.2024].

Pupkova, Natalya, "Territorialnyy pazl Dlya Ukrainy on slozhilsya blagodarya 'okkupantam' – rossiyskim tsaryam i bolshevikam" ("The Territorial Puzzle: For Ukraine, It Was Formed Thanks to the 'Occupiers' – the Russian Tsars and Bolsheviks"), *Krymskaya Pravda* (*Crimean Truth*), 10 July 2014, https://c-pravda.ru/news/2014-07-10/territorialnyjj-pazl [accessed: 23.07.2024].

Radio Svoboda (Radio Freedom), "MZS Ukrainy bude monitoryty, yak poznachaiut Krym na kartakh svitu" ("Ukraine's Foreign Ministry Will Monitor How Crimea Is Marked on World Maps"), 02 December 2015, https://www.radiosvoboda.org/a/27402854.html [accessed: 23.07.2024].

Romano, Aja, "Reckoning with the war meme in wartime: Is it ever okay to meme at a war?", *Vox*, 25 February 2022, https://www.vox.com/culture/2022/2/25/22950655/ukrainian-invasion-memes-political-cartoons-controversy [accessed: 23.07.2024].

Samsonov, Alexander, "Pohoronit antiruskiy proyekt 'Ukraina'" ("Bury the Anti-Russian Project 'Ukraine'"), *Voennoe Obozrenie* (*Military Review*), 2022, https://topwar.ru/192827-pohoronit-antirusskij-proekt-ukraina.html [accessed: 23.07.2024].

Sevastopol.su, "V GD predlozhili vernut' Rossii pol-Ukrainy posle slov ob 'okkupatsii'" ("In the State Duma, They Proposed to Return Half of Ukraine to Russia after Talk about 'Occupation'"), 08 January 2018, https://sevastopol.su/news/v-gd-predlozhili-vernut-rossii-pol-ukrainy-posle-slov-ob-okkupacii [accessed: 23.07.2024].

Somov, Kirill, "Ukraina na tret sostoit iz rossiyskikh 'podarkov'" ("Ukraine is One-Third Comprised of Russian 'Gifts'"), *Federalcity.ru*, 19 March 2021, https://feder

alcity.ru/10283-ukraina-na-tret-sostoit-iz-rossijskih-podarkov-jekspert.html [accessed: 23.07.2024].

Stalinskii Polk – Sovinformbyuro (Stalin's Regiment – the Soviet Information Bureau), VKontakte page, https://vk.com/sovinformburo [accessed: 23.07.2024].

Ulyanov, Alexander, "esli USSR vykhodit iz sostava..." ("if the Ukrainian SSR leaves..."), VKontakte post, 01 April 2022, https://vk.com/wall249749579_8993 [accessed: 23.07.2024].

Ushchyna, Valentyna, "From conflict of discourses to military conflict: multimodality of identity construction in Russo–Ukrainian war discourse", *East European Journal of Psycholinguistics* 9/2, 2022, 130–143, https://doi.org/10.29038/eejpl.2022.9.2.ush.

Wiggins, Bradley E., "Crimea River: Directionality in Memes from the Russia–Ukraine Conflict", *International Journal of Communication* 10, 2016, 451–485.

Zapadenets News, VKontakte page, https://vk.com/zapadeneznews [accessed: 23.07.2024].

Zhytomyrska oblasna derzhavna administratsiia (Zhytomyr Oblast State Administration), "V Ukraini startuvala komunikatsiina kampaniia 'Krym – tse Ukraina'" ("Communication Campaign 'Crimea is Ukraine' Launched in Ukraine"), 01 March 2016, https://oda.zht.gov.ua/news/v-ukrayini-startuvala-komunikatsijna-k/ [accessed: 23.07.2024].

The Postsecular Sacred

Religious Imagery in the Secular Context of War in Ukraine

Yuliya Yurchuk

Since the beginning of the full-scale invasion of Ukraine on 24 February 2022, images of Ukrainian resistance have been going viral throughout the world's media. Not many commentators outside Ukraine believed that Ukraine would resist and endure the assault of the Russian Army during the first days of the invasion. For this reason, pictures of the Ukrainian president not leaving the country and images of Ukrainian people showing their will to defend their state with weapons or by any other means made headlines worldwide. At the same time, images of resistance produced by Ukrainians on the ground flooded social media.[1] These images were spontaneous reactions to the war. One could distinguish several themes in this imagery. These themes pointed to historical events or topics that could evoke specific emotions among those who share the same culture and history.[2] Selling collections of such posters even became a way that the creative community gathered funds for Ukraine.[3]

Religion is one of the resources used to create this imagery of resistance. Thousands of images circulating on social media employ religious symbolism. But what does this imagery reveal about people's perceptions of the war? And which messages are encoded in these images? This paper approaches these questions by analysing the religious imagery in the secular context of the Russo–Ukrainian War. I argue that secular actors use well-recognisable images to convey messages of hope and resistance to broader audiences and that these images cross cultures, nations, and

1 Roman Horbyk and Daria Orlova, "Transmedia storytelling and memetic warfare: Ukraine's wartime public diplomacy", *Public Diplomacy and Place Branding* 19, 2023 (original article published online 19 November 2022), 228–231.

2 Kateryna Boyko, "Valkyries & Madonnas: Constructing femininity during the Russo–Ukrainian War", in: Ann-Mari Sätre, Yulia Gradskova, and Vladislava Vladimirova (eds.), *Post-Soviet Women: New Challenges and Ways to Empowerment*, New York: Palgrave MacMillan, 2023, 203–224.

3 See, for example: Baza creatyvnykh posteriv (Database of Creative Posters), "Stand with Ukraine Visuals", https://prjctr.notion.site/a441535fb4fb4a9cab4cda445ee3a869 [accessed: 31.07.2024].

languages. At the same time, these images go beyond the temporal dimension of the war and blur the boundaries of a temporal axis, presenting the war as an eternal struggle between good and evil. On the one hand, this imagery mixes secular and religious symbols in assemblages that reveal traces of a specifically Ukrainian past and present. On the other hand, these traces become universally recognisable thanks to the religious symbolism. The paper approaches these images as examples of the 'postsecular sacred', which is produced by a specific condition of postmodernity that erases boundaries between the secular and the religious, and between the sacred and the profane. Methodologically, the paper is based on a semiotic analysis of images circulating on social media. These images can be better understood through the theory of premediation and remediation, which argues that new cultural meanings are produced through the reshaping and renegotiating of meanings that already exist in a given culture.[4] By analysing these images, we can better understand how people make sense of the war and to which resources they turn in the most critical moments of history.

Remediated Images of Resistance: Methodological Considerations

For this study, I analyse images that circulated on social media (i.e., Facebook, X (formerly known as Twitter), Telegram, and Instagram) from 24 February 2022 to 23 February 2023. I carried out this analysis in three steps: 1. collecting images with religious themes; 2. dividing the images into groups according to repeating patterns; 3. and conducting a semiotic analysis of the groups of images to decode the messages therein.[5] In decoding the messages, I seek preestablished meanings in the images in accordance with the theory of premediation and remediation. As I argue above, this imagery is created with tools that already exist in the culture of the creators.

Literature and media scholars Astrid Erll and Ann Rigney explain pre- and remediation through the example of cultural memory formation: "[s]haping cultural memory is a work of refashioning, reconfiguring, formatting, absorbing, incorporating, selecting, and editing from the reservoir of available meanings in a given culture".[6] Thus, studying these images involves looking for previously established meanings that can shape new images. In a way, this is a search for the 'pre-life' of representations to understand how the new representations are established. In Erll and

---

4 Astrid Erll and Ann Rigney (eds.), *Mediation, Remediation, and the Dynamics of Cultural Memory*, Berlin, Boston: De Gruyter, 2009.

5 Stuart Hall, *Encoding and Decoding in the Television Discourse*, Birmingham: Centre for Contemporary Cultural Studies, 1973.

6 Astrid Erll and Ann Rigney (eds.), *Mediation, Remediation, and the Dynamics of Cultural Memory*, 8.

Rigney's conceptualisation, premediation can be seen in the diachronic axis of representation and it refers to "the cognitive schemata and patterns of representation that are available in a given media culture [...] and which already preform the events that we later remember through remediation".[7] We can view remediation through the synchronic axis of representation, as the patterns of representations, according to Erll and Rigney, "realized, over and over, by means of those media technologies that a community has at its disposal and to which it ascribes the potential of creating ever greater immediacy and memorial truth".[8] However, it is not only representations of earlier events that shape understandings of a later event. Rather, art, mythology, and religion can exert great potential as premediators that shape our understanding of reality. In this specific context, religion and culture are premediators that shape people's understanding of war and resistance.

Postsecular Sacred Images

This study contributes to discussions on postsecularity and the transformation of religion in a postsecular context. I define postsecularity as the 'intertwinement' of the secular and the religious in new forms.[9] Following scholars who encourage a critical exploration of the limits of secularity and who criticise secularity's normative status,[10] this study focuses on hybrid forms of representation that simultaneously draw on religious and secular spheres. Meanwhile, religion is closely connected to nationalism, especially in Eastern Europe, where religion was suppressed for decades during the Soviet Union.[11] However, the analysed images cannot be simply explained by the political agenda and nationalist feelings of their creators, as the images were very often created spontaneously, without instruction from any institution or authority, and refer not only to national but also to broader Christian traditions and symbols.

Postsecularity, as a specific cultural and historical condition, allows for the creation of new forms of coexistence between the secular and the religious. Andrii Fert and I refer to this elsewhere as the postsecular sacred in relation to the religious

7 Ibid.

8 Ibid., 8–9.

9 Arie L. Molendijk, "In pursuit of the postsecular", *International Journal of Philosophy and Theology* 76/2, 2015, 100–115, here 110.

10 Mario Rosati and Kristina Stoeckl (eds.), *Multiple Modernities and Postsecular Societies*, Farnham: Ashgate, 2012.

11 Liliya Berezhnaya and Schmitt Christian (eds.), Iconic Turns: Nation and Religion in Easter n European Cinema since 1989, Leiden: Brill, 2013; and Uilleam Blacker, "Martyrdom, Spectacle, and Public Space: Ukraine's National Martyrology from Shevchenko to the Maidan", *Journal of Soviet and Post-Soviet Politics and Society* 1/2, 2015, 257–292.

commemoration of the Euromaidan revolution.[12] The term postsecular sacred is also based on the understanding of postsecularity in relation to postmodernity. Gianni Vattimo argues that in postmodernity, we enter an era in which Christianity does not need to lead a polemic with rationalism and Enlightenment.[13] Christian symbols can be used not as religious but as part of a broader culture and tradition. In such a way, postmodernity produces new hybrid forms of representation that result in combinations of different elements of culture, with religion being a part of it.

The Symbol of the Protection ('Pokrova') of Our Most Holy Lady Theotokos

The Virgin Mary is the most widely used religious figure in images of resistance. For instance, Nikita Titov's picture depicts the Holy Lady Theotokos holding a Ukrainian flag over soldiers in trenches and protecting them under a starry sky.[14] This and similar visuals have parallels to another set of images that went viral during the first months of the invasion and that formulated the demands of Ukrainians to close or shelter the sky.[15] In this way, religious symbols of protection are products of remediation from nonreligious images. Importantly, the images asking for sky shelter explicitly addressed countries and people outside of Ukraine, as Ukraine did not have the military capacity to protect itself and relied on the support of other states.

At the same time, the symbols of 'Pokrova' are premediated by well-known symbols of Orthodox iconography. Pokrova (or the Feast of Protection or the Intersession of Theotokos) venerates the Mother of God and is one of the biggest holidays in Orthodox Christianity. According to legend, the apparition of Mary the Theotokos occurred at the Blachernae Church during one of the sieges of Constantinople, where she spread her veil over the people as a protection against their enemies. As a result, the enemies withdrew, and the city was rescued. On icons, the Intersession of Theotokos is depicted as the Mother of God holding a cover, or veil, over people who seek protection. Pokrova derives from the word *pokrov*, which literally means 'cover'.

---

12 Yuliya Yurchuk and Andrii Fert, "Sacralization of Memory of Euromaidan Protests from a Post-secular Perspective", in: Hanna Meisel and Liliya Berezhnaya (eds.), *Sacralization of History: Actors – Networks – Topics in Eastern Europe*, Budapest: CEU Press, forthcoming.

13 Gianni Vattimo, *After Christianity*, New York City: Columbia University Press, 2002.

14 *Pokrova*, image from Nikita Titov, "Davno zrobyv tsei maliunok na Pokrova..." ("I made this drawing for the Intercession a long time ago..."), Facebook post, 06 March 2022, https://www.facebook.com/photo.php?fbid=4950682488332199 [accessed: 31.07.2024].

15 See, for example, *Shelter our Sky*, image from Andriy Yermolenko, "Shelter our sky – we will handle the rest!", ArtDopomoga | Help Ukraine, https://artdopomoga.com/shop/prints-on-fabric-and-textiles/shelter-our-sky-we-will-handle-the-rest-art-by-andriy-yermolenko/ [accessed: 31.07.2024]. "Close the Sky" was not only represented in visual culture, but also in music. See, for example: TARABAROVAcom, "Close the Sky", YouTube, 17 March 2022, https://music.youtube.com/watch?v=ouHIAUkikQc [accessed: 31.07.2024].

Often, the cover has the colours of the Ukrainian flag, articulating clear national symbolism.[16] This is not a coincidence, as Pokrova is a well-established symbol in Ukrainian national culture. The veneration of Pokrova as a patroness of the Cossacks took root in the 17th century, when her status as the protectress of Cossacks was established. In the 20th century, nationally minded Ukrainians venerated Pokrova as the protectress of the soldiers of the Ukrainian Insurgent Army (UPA), the military arm of the Organisation of Ukrainian Nationalists (OUN), active between 1942 and 1956. Since 1947, the UPA celebrated the day of its creation on the same day as the Pokrova. And, since 2014, this day has been officially celebrated as the Day of the Defenders of Ukraine in the national calendar. Accordingly, Pokrova is part of both the religious and national calendars: Since 1 January 2023, the 14 October marks the Orthodox Feast of Protection, the Day of the Cossacks, the Day of the Creation of the UPA, and the Day of the Defenders of Ukraine.[17]

If we consider the premediated images of Pokrova, then we can go back as far as the 17th century. One of the best known Pokrova icons is the Deshky village icon from the late 17th century, which is connected to the revival of the cult of the Cossack Hetman Bohdan Kmelnytsky (1596–1657).[18] Pokrova iconography is also widely used in the commemoration of the protestors – commonly known as the Heavenly Hundred – killed during the Revolution of Dignity (November 2013–February 2014) and of the soldiers fallen in the war in the east of the country since spring 2014, as seen for instance on the icon in the Askold Grave Chapel in Kyiv (Figure 9).[19]

The images that implement the symbols of Pokrova inscribe the war and Ukrainian resistance into a longer history that stretches from the 17th century until today. These images contribute to a sense of historical continuity that shapes and strengthens the image of Ukraine as a country with a long history as well as a country under the protection of the Mother of God. It is worth mentioning that a nationwide electronic warfare system, which Ukraine launched as the new strategy

16 See, for example: Nikita Titov, "Davno zrobyv tsei maliunok na Pokrova..." ("I made this drawing for the Intercession a long time ago..."), Facebook post, 06 March 2022, https://www.facebook.com/photo.php?fbid=4950682488332199 [accessed: 31.07.2024].

17 Yuliya Yurchuk, *Reordering of Meaningful Worlds: Memory of the Organization of Ukrainian Nationalists and the Ukrainian Insurgent Army in Post-Soviet Ukraine*, Stockholm: Acta, 2014; and Yuliya Yurchuk, "Global Symbols Local Meanings: The 'Day of Victory' after Euromaidan", in: Timm Beichelt and Susann Worschech (eds.), *Transnational Ukraine? Networks and Ties that Influence(d) Contemporary Ukraine*, Stuttgart: ibidem, 2017, 66–89.

18 On the cult of Khmelnytsky and Pokrova see: Serhii Plokhy, *Tsars and Cossacks: A Study in Iconography*, Cambridge, MA: HURI, 2002.

19 Yurchuk and Fert, "Sacralization".

in air defence, is called Pokrova, as announced by the Commander-in-Chief of the Armed Forces of Ukraine, Valerii Zaluzhnyi.[20]

Figure 9: Pokrova icon in the Askold Grave Chapel

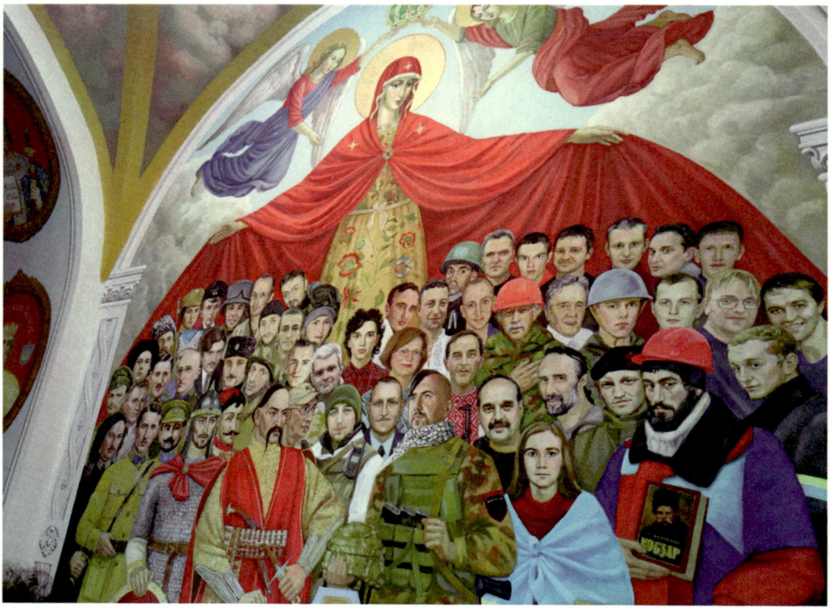

Pokrova icon, Askold Grave Chapel, Kyiv, 2021, photo courtesy of Andrii Fert.

Saint Javelin: Militarised Icons

Perhaps the best globally known symbol of Ukrainian resistance is the image of Saint Javelin, which depicts a saint carrying a Javelin, or an Advanced Antitank Weapon System-Medium.[21] Saint Javelin was created by the Canadian marketing executive and filmmaker Christian Borys as the label for a charity campaign to help Ukraine at the beginning of the full-scale invasion.[22] It can be read as a remediation of Chris

20 Valerii Zaluzhnyi, "Modern Positional Warfare and How to Win it", *The Economist*, 01 November 2023, https://infographics.economist.com/2023/ExternalContent/ZALUZHNYI_FULL_VERSION.pdf, [accessed: 31.07.2024].

21 See, for example, *Saint Javelin*, image from Saint Javelin, "Saint Javelin Sticker", official website, https://www.saintjavelin.com/products/saint-javelin-sticker-1 [accessed: 31.07.2024]. See also the analysis of the feminine iconography of Saint Javelin in Boyko, "Valkyries".

22 Saint Javelin, official website, https://www.saintjavelin.com/ [accessed: 31.07.2024].

Shaw's 2012 painting *Madonna Kalashnikov*, in which the Holy Mary holds an AK-47.[23] For Shaw, this weapon was both a symbol of "the official weapon of conservative Islamic terrorists, and a symbol of freedom and democracy during the Arab Spring".[24] It is worth mentioning that in 2007, the anonymous England-based street artist Banksy created the famous graffiti *Mona Lisa Bazooka*, which may also be a premeditation of Shaw's image.[25] In 2022, in the Ukrainian context, the Holy Mary holds a symbol of the Ukrainian struggle, revealing the hopes invested in the weapon. For Ukraine, the struggle for this weapon and the country's right to defend itself became as important as the combat itself.

The Saint Javelin image has already become a source of remediation itself, in this way serving as a premediated image. Different artists have rearticulated the image in their own art, imbuing new meanings into it. For instance, one remediation depicts a female saint in a Ukrainian military uniform with a Malyuk rifle.[26] The artist explains that they picked specifically the Malyuk rifle for "reimagining of the Saint Javelin art that had became [sic] one of the symbol [sic] of Ukrainian resistance" because the Malyuk rifle is "the Ukrainian home growth [sic] rifle, used by their special forces".[27]

Through this remediation, the original image became more localised and nationalised. It might not work for an international audience in the same way as the original Saint Javelin, but it reveals the high potential of such images to produce new manifestations of resistance. The original Saint Javelin, on the other hand, evokes a more recognisable (and perhaps more transnational) image, which worked on the global market and helped collect 1 million Canadian dollars during the first month of the campaign.[28] Interestingly, the Malyuk rifle, also known as the Vulcan or Vulcan-M, is itself reconfigured from the Kalashnikov rifle into a bullpup layout. In this case, multiple remediations exist not only in the different representations but also in the refiguration of the material world.

---

23 See, for example, *Madonna Kalashnikov*, 30 inch x 40 inch, acrylic on canvas, 2012, image from Chris Shaw: Rock Posters & Art, "Chris Shaw at the San Francisco Museum of Modern Art", 18 April 2013, https://chrisshawstudio.com/2013/04/chris-shaw-at-the-san-francisco-museum-of-modern-art/ [accessed: 31.07.2024].

24 Shaw as cited in Boyko, "Valkyries", 213.

25 The author is grateful to Rostyslav Semkiv for drawing her attention to Banksy's image, which is a great example of postmodern collage and the postsecular sacred.

26 See, for example, *Saint Javelin*, image from Luches, *Saint Javelin*, DeviantArt, 11 April 2022, https://www.deviantart.com/luches/art/Saint-Javelin-912697865 [accessed: 31.07.2024].

27 Luches, "Saint Javelin", DeviantArt, 11 April 2022, https://www.deviantart.com/luches/art/Saint-Javelin-912697865 [accessed: 23.07.2024].

28 Bernd Debusmann Jr., "How 'Saint Javelin' raised over $1m for Ukraine", *BBC*, 10 March 2022, https://www.bbc.com/news/world-us-canada-60700906 [accessed: 23.07.2024].

Madonna and Pieta Iconography

Most of the images that use religious themes concentrate on the image of Madonna. This is not surprising, considering the photos of Ukrainian women and children on the covers of international newspapers, starting from the first moments of the full-scale invasion. Madonna imagery serves as the direct source of this remediation. One of such images depicts a young woman with a child in a Kyiv metro station. It is only one of many examples of such remediations.[29]

The picture was published by the Tubik Agency, a Ukrainian graphic design company. In the description, the agency wrote:

> "Mother is the name for God in the lips and hearts of little children," William Makepeace Thackeray once wrote, and now facing war in Ukraine, with thousands of civilians living in horror and not knowing if they have tomorrow, we also see thousands of expressions of mother's love.
> This artwork is one of them, and it is inspired by the real photo of the real mother hiding with her baby in the Kyiv subway while the city was under shelling. Sadly, that's the look of Kyivan Madonna in 2022.[30]

The post ended with the words: "Please, stop the war. Stand with Ukraine. Children shouldn't suffer".[31] By citing the British writer and explicitly asking for support in the last sentence, the image and the message are created with the intention to reach an international audience. It seems that most of the images analysed in this study are created with the belief that a Ukrainian audience is convinced of the importance of support for their resistance, while it is an international audience that should be persuaded that Ukraine and its people should be supported. The postsecular sacred is used here to reach audiences both within and outside of Ukraine.

Another distinguished feature of such images is that they are inspired by photos (and stories) of real women and their children that were shown in the news.[32]

---

29 *Kyivan Madonna*, image from tubik shop, "Kyivan Madonna Illustration HIGH RES", Creative Market, 12 March 2022, https://creativemarket.com/tubik/7056439-Kyivan-Madonna-Illustration-HIGH-RES [accessed: 24.07.2024].

30 tubik shop, "Kyivan Madonna Illustration HIGH RES", Creative Market, 12 March 2022, https://creativemarket.com/tubik/7056439-Kyivan-Madonna-Illustration-HIGH-RES [accessed: 24.07.2024].

31 Ibid.

32 For more examples of similar images, see: Boyko, "Valkyries"; and Anna Shykanova, "Ukrainska Madonna: u Kyevi maty vrianuvala dytynu, zakryvshy ii svoim tilom vid obstriliv" ("Ukrainian Madonna: In Kyiv, a Mother Saved Her Child from Shelling by Covering It with Her Body"), *RBK-Ukraina*, 19 March 2022, https://www.rbc.ua/ukr/styler/ukrainskaya-madonna-kieve-mat-spasla-rebenka-1647684163.html [accessed: 31.07.2024].

These photos serve as premediated images later used for creating iconic, less personalised, and thus more recognisable images that transcend national boundaries. This implementation of photography has become a significant feature in the creation of the postsecular sacred in commemorative culture in Ukraine since 2014, as we argue elsewhere.[33]

Notably, on 25 March 2022, Pope Francis evoked the Holy Mary when he consecrated Russia and Ukraine to the Immaculate Heart of Mary. He prayed the Act of Communion with all Catholic Bishops across the globe. After finishing the prayer of the Act of Consecration, the Pope commented:

> This is no magic formula but a spiritual act. It is an act of complete trust on the part of children who, amid the tribulation of this cruel and senseless war that threatens our world, turn to their Mother, reposing all their fears and pain in her heart and abandoning themselves to her.[34]

Although Ukrainians (both part of and outside the church) largely criticise the acts of Pope Francis,[35] it is worth mentioning that in the transnational context, the figure of the Virgin Mary is central not only in Ukrainian popular culture but also for the Catholic Church. The Pope's evocations of the Mother of God in the context of the war show that the war, too, has a central place in the Catholic Church. In this way, the Madonna, in relation to the war, is an essential element not only in the images created by Ukrainians on the ground but also as a symbol referred to by the Pope, a transnational actor representing the Catholic Church.

Icons and Ruins

A final grouping of images that depict the horrors of the war in Ukraine combine photos of war scenes and ruination with the well-known icons. This group of images differs from those discussed above. In contrast to art that imitates icons, here we see less of an imitation and more of an incorporation of the contemporary war into traditional iconography. For example, Ireneaus Yurchuk, an American artist of

33 Yurchuk and Fert, "Sacralization".

34 Devin Watkins, "Pope consecrates Russia & Ukraine: 'Spiritual act of trust amid cruel war'", *Vatican News*, 25 March 2022, https://www.vaticannews.va/en/pope/news/2022-03/pope-francis-consecration-russia-ukraine-mary-war-lent.html [accessed: 31.07.2024].

35 Tania Matiash, "Papa Rymskyi neuvazhno chytav Dostoievskoho, inakshe ne dyvuvavsia by zhorstoki rosiian, – Markarova" ("The Pope of Rome Did Not Carefully Read Dostoyevsky, Otherwise He Would Not Be Surprised by the Cruelty of the Russians – Markarova"), *LB.ua*, 07 November 2022, https://lb.ua/world/2022/11/07/535034_papa_rimskiy_neuvazhno_chitav.html [accessed: 31.07.2024].

Ukrainian origin, creates pictures that merge the genres of documentary photography and icon painting.[36] In his images – for instance, *Nativity* or *Saint Nicholas – help us in this time of need* – the artist placed the easily recognisable religious images of Christ's birth and of Saint Nicholas among the chaos of war and ruins.[37] He created both images specifically around Christmas of 2022.

Looking at the images, I could not help but shift between the joyful time of Christmas in places where there is no war and this same time in Ukraine, which is under the constant threat of destruction. Furthermore, the image of the birth of Christ in the middle of images of the war draws parallels to the very essence of Christianity: Christ's life was threatened from his very birth, but at the same time, his birth made the salvation of all of humankind possible. The artist might also be conveying a hopeful message for Ukraine. He created the image of Saint Nicholas during the time when the saint is venerated. Fittingly, these images, created during commemorative days of the religious calendar, add to the calendar actual images from the present. In the latter image, the symbolism of Saint Nicholas is central, as he is thought to be a protector of all children and has the power of enacting miracles. In the context of a war that has claimed the lives of at least 501 children in Ukraine, this potent symbolism cannot go unnoticed.[38]

Merging artistic genres, these images address the emotions of not only believers but also of humanity generally, as the reality of the photographs turns the audience into (co)witnesses. The religious symbols are also imbued with hope for justice and salvation, key themes in Christianity. In this way, the hybrid postsecular sacred imagery works on both religious and secular levels. The viewer does not need to decide whether these images are religious icons or not, as they are both at the same time

36 Ukrainian Institute of America, "Peripheral Visions: Recent Art by Irenaeus and Dorian Yurchuk, February 21, 2020–March 29, 2020", https://ukrainianinstitute.org/event/peripheral-visions-recent-art-by-irenaeus-and-dorian-yurchuk/ [accessed: 31.07.2024]. The artist has worked in this style for many years, erasing the boundaries between photography and painting. See: Delaware Valley Arts Alliance, "IRENAEUS YURCHUK | Visual Reassessments, Jul 13, 2019–Aug 11, 2019", https://delawarevalleyartsalliance.org/exhibition/irenaeus-yurchuk-visual-reassessments/ [accessed: 31.07.2024].

37 *Nativity*, image from Ireneaus Yurchuk, "Irynei Yurchuk: 'Rizdvo' (Nativity) 2022", Facebook post, 14 December 2022, https://www.facebook.com/photo.php?fbid=2701372876663386&set=pb.100003721015322.-2207520000&type=3 [accessed: 31.07.2024] and *Saint Nicholas – help us in this time of need*, image from Ireneaus Yurchuk, "Irynei Yurchuk: 'Sviatyi Mykolai – na vsiakyi chas pomahai...'..." ("Ireneaus Yurchuk: 'St. Nicholas – help at all times...'..."), Facebook post, 06 December 2022, https://www.facebook.com/photo.php?fbid=2693305017470172 [accessed: 31.07.2024].

38 This estimated number refers to the period between 24 February 2022 and 31 March 2023. United Nations, "Child deaths hit 'tragic milestone' in Ukraine", 03 April 2023, https://news.un.org/en/story/2023/04/1135322 [accessed: 31.07.2024].

and they are open to interpretation. The main, unambiguous message of the images is the horror of war and its consequences.

The artistic project "Icons on Ammunition Boxes" by Sonia Atlantova and Oleksandr Klymenko also fits within this context. The artists initiated it in 2014, when they started painting icons on boxes that came directly from the frontline in the Donbas. As the artists explain, these icons on ammunition boxes are not only witnesses of war but also symbols of the victory of life over death. This project contributes to such a victory not only symbolically but also practically, as, through the project, the artists collect money for a mobile hospital.[39]

Conclusions

Religious symbols are actively used in the imagery of resistance in Ukraine. The use of such symbolism, however, does not show that Ukrainians are especially religious. Rather, these images serve as vehicles of representation that evoke positive emotional responses both locally (in Ukraine) and internationally, as they can be recognised by other people who share or are familiar with Christian iconography and traditions. Importantly, Christianity here functions more as a cultural tradition than a religion.[40] These well-known images are used to convey messages of hope and resistance to broader audiences and can cross cultures, nations, and languages. At the same time, these images cross beyond the temporality of the current war and blur boundaries between the past and present. The postsecular sacred produced by these images, with help of postmodern cultural tools, enables an erasure of boundaries between the secular and the religious, and between the sacred and the profane. Remediated in different times and contexts, these images are intrinsically hybrid, and thus open to interpretation by many groups and in many situations.

Bibliography

Baza creatyvnykh posteriv (Database of Creative Posters), "Stand with Ukraine Visuals", https://prjctr.notion.site/a441535fb4fb4a9cab4cda445ee3a869 [accessed: 23.07.2024].

39 *New Lib*, "Ikony na iashchykakh z-pid naboiv: Knihi, Oleksandr Klymenko, Sonia Antalantova" ("Icons on Ammo Boxes: Books, Oleksandr Klymenko, Sonia Antalantova"), https://www.newlib.org.ua/ikony-na-iashchykakh-z-pid-naboiv/ [accessed: 31.07.2024].

40 On religion as a cultural tradition, see: Danielle Hervieu-Léger, *Religion as a Chain of Memory*, Cambridge: Polity, 2000.

Berezhnaya, Liliya, and Schmitt Christian (eds.), Iconic Turns: Nation and Religion in Eastern European Cinema since 1989, Leiden: Brill, 2013.

Blacker, Uilleam, "Martyrdom, Spectacle, and Public Space: Ukraine's National Martyrology from Shevchenko to the Maidan", *Journal of Soviet and Post-Soviet Politics and Society* 1/2, 2015, 257–292.

Boyko, Kateryna, "Valkyries & Madonnas: Constructing femininity during the Russo–Ukrainian War", in: Ann-Mari Sätre, Yulia Gradskova, and Vladislava Vladimirova (eds.), *Post-Soviet Women: New Challenges and Ways to Empowerment*, New York: Palgrave MacMillan, 2023, 203–224.

Chris Shaw: Rock Posters & Art, official website, https://chrisshawstudio.com/2013/04/chris-shaw-at-the-san-francisco-museum-of-modern-art/ [accessed: 23.07.2024].

Debusmann Jr., Bernd, "How 'Saint Javelin' raised over $1m for Ukraine", *BBC*, 10 March 2022, https://www.bbc.com/news/world-us-canada-60700906 [accessed: 23.07.2024].

Delaware Valley Arts Alliance, "IRENAEUS YURCHUK | Visual Reassessments, Jul 13, 2019–Aug 11, 2019", https://delawarevalleyartsalliance.org/exhibition/irenaeus-yurchuk-visual-reassessments/ [accessed: 23.07.2024].

Erll, Astrid, and Ann Rigney (eds.), *Mediation, Remediation, and the Dynamics of Cultural Memory*, Berlin, Boston: De Gruyter, 2009.

Hall, Stuart, *Encoding and Decoding in the Television Discourse*, Birmingham: Centre for Contemporary Cultural Studies, 1973.

Hervieu-Léger, Danielle, *Religion as a Chain of Memory*, Cambridge: Polity, 2000.

Horbyk, Roman, and Daria Orlova, "Transmedia storytelling and memetic warfare: Ukraine's wartime public diplomacy", *Public Diplomacy and Place Branding* 19, 2023 (original article published online 19 November 2022), 228–231.

Luches, "Saint Javelin", DeviantArt, 11 April 2022, https://www.deviantart.com/luches/art/Saint-Javelin-912697865 [accessed: 23.07.2024].

Matiash, Tania, "Papa Rymskyi neuvazhno chytav Dostoievskoho, inakshe ne dyvuvavsia by zhorstoki rosiian, – Markarova" ("The Pope of Rome Did Not Carefully Read Dostoyevsky, Otherwise He Would Not Be Surprised by the Cruelty of the Russians – Markarova"), *LB.ua*, 07 November 2022, https://lb.ua/world/2022/11/07/535034_papa_rimskiy_neuvazhno_chitav.html [accessed: 23.07.2024].

Molendijk, Arie L., "In pursuit of the postsecular", *International Journal of Philosophy and Theology* 76/2, 2015, 100–115.

New Lib, "Ikony na iashchykakh z-pid naboiv: Knihi, Oleksandr Klymenko, Sonia Antalantova" ("Icons on Ammo Boxes: Books, Oleksandr Klymenko, Sonia Antalantova"), https://www.newlib.org.ua/ikony-na-iashchykakh-z-pid-naboiv/ [accessed: 23.07.2024].

Rosati, Mario, and Kristina Stoeckl (eds.), *Multiple Modernities and Postsecular Societies*, Farnham: Ashgate, 2012.

Plokhy, Serhii, *Tsars and Cossacks: A Study in Iconography*, Cambridge, MA: HURI, 2002.

Saint Javelin, official website, https://www.saintjavelin.com/ [accessed: 23.07.2024].

Shykanova, Anna, "Ukrainska Madonna: u Kyevi maty vrianuvala dytynu, zakryvshy ii svoim tilom vid obstriliv" ("Ukrainian Madonna: In Kyiv, a Mother Saved Her Child from Shelling by Covering It with Her Body"), *RBK-Ukraina*, 19 March 2022, https://www.rbc.ua/ukr/styler/ukrainskaya-madonna-kieve-mat-spasla-rebenka-1647684163.html [accessed: 23.07.2024].

TARABAROVAcom, "Close the Sky", YouTube, 17 March 2022, https://music.youtube.com/watch?v=0uHlAUkikQc [accessed: 23.07.2024].

tubik shop, "Kyivan Madonna Illustration HIGH RES", Creative Market, 12 March 2022, https://creativemarket.com/tubik/7056439-Kyivan-Madonna-Illustration-HIGH-RES [accessed: 23.07.2024].

Ukrainian Institute of America, "Peripheral Visions: Recent Art by Irenaeus and Dorian Yurchuk, February 21, 2020–March 29, 2020", https://ukrainianinstitute.org/event/peripheral-visions-recent-art-by-irenaeus-and-dorian-yurchuk/ [accessed: 23.07.2024].

United Nations, "Child deaths hit 'tragic milestone' in Ukraine", 03 April 2023, https://news.un.org/en/story/2023/04/1135322 [accessed: 23.07.2024].

Vattimo, Gianni, *After Christianity*, New York City: Columbia University Press, 2002.

Watkins, Devin, "Pope consecrates Russia & Ukraine: 'Spiritual act of trust amid cruel war'", *Vatican News*, 25 March 2022, https://www.vaticannews.va/en/pope/news/2022-03/pope-francis-consecration-russia-ukraine-mary-war-lent.html [accessed: 23.07.2024].

Yurchuk, Yuliya, "Global Symbols Local Meanings: The 'Day of Victory' after Euromaidan", in: Timm Beichelt and Susann Worschech (eds.), *Transnational Ukraine? Networks and Ties that Influence(d) Contemporary Ukraine*, Stuttgart: ibidem, 2017, 66–89.

Yurchuk, Yuliya, *Reordering of Meaningful Worlds: Memory of the Organization of Ukrainian Nationalists and the Ukrainian Insurgent Army in Post-Soviet Ukraine*, Stockholm: Acta, 2014.

Yurchuk, Yuliya, and Andrii Fert, "Sacralization of Memory of Euromaidan Protests from a Post-secular Perspective", in: Hanna Meisel and Liliya Berezhnaya (eds.), *Sacralization of History: Actors – Networks – Topics in Eastern Europe*, Budapest: CEU Press, forthcoming.

Zaluzhnyi, Valerii, "Modern Positional Warfare and How to Win it", *The Economist*, 01 November 2023, https://infographics.economist.com/2023/ExternalContent/ZALUZHNYI_FULL_VERSION.pdf, [accessed: 23.07.2024].

Zombies, Orcs, and Fascists

Naming the Other in the Context of Russia's War against Ukraine

Oleksandr Zabirko

The dehumanisation of the enemy is a common feature of any armed conflict and the ongoing Russo–Ukrainian War is no exception. This paper explores the rhetorical strategies of naming the enemy employed by both sides of the conflict, focusing on ideologically charged descriptions (e.g., 'fascists') and on utterly fantastic images from literature and mass culture (e.g., 'orcs', 'zombies', or 'witches'), which have circulated on media and in literary texts since the beginning of the Russian full-scale invasion of Ukraine in February 2022.

This new phase of the Russo–Ukrainian War led not only to a new and unprecedented level of violence, but also marked a shift in the war rhetoric. Between 2014 and 2022, war semantics – that is, the understanding of who is fighting whom, how, and why – remained largely frozen. The situation changed dramatically in February 2022, after the explicit attack by the Russian Army on Ukraine following an official statement by the Russian head of state. This rendered the former rhetoric and vocabulary of both sides outdated. The Russian side could no longer feign that the war was a domestic Ukrainian issue, or a 'civil war', which was Russia's official stance since 2014. Ukraine, in turn, also had to acknowledge that the armed conflicts were no longer limited to a specific region but instead represented a full-fledged assault of a foreign power on the Ukrainian state and its people.[1] This new situation required the development of a new language and a new understanding, including a new identification of the enemy, a pivotal element of any war rhetoric.

Obviously, this type of naming often serves as a mechanism for affective relief through verbal insults and denigration of the foe. However, in cases of more complex metaphors and allegories, such rhetoric also acts as a cognitive tool for conceptualising the complexities of war. This is precisely the point at which literature and culture become significant in modern conflicts, since here, the figures and narratives from

1 Serhy Yekelchyk, "Naming the war: Russian aggression in Ukrainian official discourse and mass culture", *Canadian Slavonic Papers* 64/2–3, 2022, 232–246, here 233.

popular culture play an increasingly critical role alongside national stereotypes and ideological clichés. In this context, literature and popular culture deserve close examination, as they provide the testing grounds for new political metaphors and a new vocabulary.

Zombification: From Literary Trope to Media Cliché

At the end of February 2022, a few days before Russian forces invaded Ukraine, videos and photos of Russian tanks and military vehicles painted with the letter 'Z' circulated on social media. Initially intended to identify specific task forces or squadrons, the letter Z (which does not even exist in the Cyrillic alphabet) soon became a symbol for active support of the Russian 'special military operation' in Ukraine.

For those opposing the war, the sign was interpreted on social media differently than intended, with users immediately contextualising it in Marc Foster's action-horror film *World War Z* (2013). The film is about a sudden zombie apocalypse that threatens all of humanity. Such decontextualisation of the Z as a rallying symbol allowed for conceptualising the invading Russian Army as a horde of aggressive zombies.

However, official Ukrainian media and government channels initially ignored these allusions. As Serhy Yekelchyk persuasively shows, in the first days of the invasion, the propaganda strategies of the Ukrainian state drew on the Soviet commemorative tradition. For example, President Volodomyr Zelenskyy used the term 'the Patriotic War' in his first video speeches in February 2022 and his administration took the initiative to reintroduce the honorary title of 'Hero City' and award it to cities whose defenders offered a particularly stubborn resistance against the Russian onslaught.[2] Yet, this challenging of Russia on the field of commemoration of the Second World War soon gave way to using characters and symbols from globalised Western popular culture.

Already in March, the president's advisor Oleksiy Arestovych, who gradually monopolised the media coverage of the war during that time, referred to the zombie comparison by calling the Russian troops "an army of doomed zombies"[3] and their march towards Kyiv "a zombie incursion".[4] On the Russian side, the first references

2 Ibid., 237–238.

3 Oleksii Arestovych, "Rosiiska armiia – tse armiia pryrechenykh zombie" ("The Russian Army is an Army of Doomed Zombies"), *Glavkom*, 10 March 2022, https://glavcom.ua/columns/arestovich/rosiyska-armiya-ce-armiya-prirechenih-zombi-828505.html [accessed: 31.07.2024] [author's trans.].

4 bigimir.net, "Arestovich: 'Zombi-nashestvie' RF konchitsia cherez 2–3 nedeli" ("Arestovich: The 'Zombie-Incursion' of the Russian Federation Will Be Over in 2 or 3 Weeks"), 22 March

to the Ukrainian 'zombie-warriors' were usually made in relation to the narrative of secret US biological laboratories on the territory of Ukraine and the supposed excessive drug use by Ukrainian military personnel.[5] While intended as a way to dehumanise the enemy, this naming created rhetorical implications that went beyond a mere insult.

Starting with George Romero's seminal film *Night of the Living Dead* (1968), the trope of a zombie apocalypse has always been a strong political metaphor in Western mass culture. At first glance, zombies do not necessarily have anything to do with war, in the sense of a conventional military conflict. However, if we define 'war' as a situation in which normality is programmatically suspended, then a zombie apocalypse offers precisely this kind of crisis – a collapse of modern society caused by the pandemic rise of a hostile species united in an attack on humanity. While in fiction the cause of a zombie epidemic varies significantly, ranging from voodoo sorcery to the spread of a virus, a zombie infestation is typically conceptualised as a kind of plague and not as a result of conscious decision-making, which traditional zombies are not capable of. Naturally, the idea of negotiating with such an enemy is absurd.

Similarly, for post-Soviet societies, the trope of a zombie apocalypse provides a narrative framework for stories about an unexpected and unstoppable transformation of society, in which one's neighbour suddenly turns into a hostile and aggressive 'Other'. Following the genre conventions of Western fiction, the post-Soviet zombie apocalypse, however, has its own literary pedigree and several distinct features.

First and foremost, a post-Soviet zombie is less an imaginary creature than it is a state of mind. The genealogy of this view can be traced back to Viktor Pelevin's seminal essay "The Zombification of the Soviet Person", first published in 1990.[6] After a lengthy overview of the voodoo tradition, Pelevin makes a rather straightforward argument that everyday life in the Soviet Union (with its ideologically charged, propagandistic rituals) was, in itself, an ongoing project of zombification. Pelevin, however, quickly adapts zombification to a post-Soviet reality (or, at least, for what

2022, https://news.bigmir.net/ukraine/6262594-arestovich-zombi-nashestvie-rf-konchitsya-cherez-2-3-nedeli [accessed: 31.07.2024] [author's trans.].

5 See for example: Liudmila Chertkova, "Ukraina prevratila VSU v 'zombi-armiiu': prut na uboi" ("Ukraine Turned its Armed Forces into a 'Zombie Army': They're Roaring to Slaughter"), *Pravda.Ru*, 25 October 2022, https://www.pravda.ru/society/1763348-narkogosudarstvo_ukraina/ [accessed: 31.07.2024]; and *Luganskii Informatsionnyi Tsentr (Lugansk Information Centre)*, "Boitsy VSU v Rubezhnom voiuiut 'v sostoianii zombi' pod vozdeistviem narkotikov – Miroshnik" ("The Soldiers of the Ukrainian Armed Forces in Rubezhnoye Fight 'in a Zombie State' under the Influence of Drugs – Miroshnik"), 07 April 2022, https://lug-info.com/news/bojcy-vsu-v-rubezhnom-voyuyut-v-sostoyanii-zombi-pod-vozdejstviem-narkotikov-miroshnik [accessed: 31.07.2024].

6 Viktor Pelevin, "Zombifikatsiia sovetskogo cheloveka" ("The Zombification of the Soviet Person"), *Novyi Zhurnal (New Journal)* 179, 1990, 324–338.

passes as reality in Pelevin's deliberately elusive fiction). Thus, following Eliot Borenstein's insightful analysis, it's possible to argue that,

> as in the West, [post-Soviet] zombies are the product of contagion, but along a completely different disease vector. The post-Soviet discourse is less concerned with zombie as thing than it is with zombie as process: not zombies, but zombification.[7]

This observation is not only applicable to highbrow literary texts but is also a stable stereotype in post-Soviet mass culture.[8]

Pelevin's idea of 'zombification' assumes a certain view of human nature, shaped by widely accepted beliefs about the influence of technology, media, and propaganda on an individual's identity. This perspective implies that individuals are highly receptive to external stimuli and lack agency in their consumption of information. In colloquial Russian, this idea is often associated with the use of television, dubbed the 'zombie box' (Russian: *zomboyashchik*), as the primary tool for zombification.

Thus, invoking zombification is an inherently political gesture. It turns 'zombie' into a collective noun describing stupid, lumpen masses, whose gullibility allows the regime to control the country. This can be connected to the frequent accusation that the majority of the population that allegedly supports Putin's regime are victims of zombification. For instance, the Russian opposition leader Boris Nemtsov asserted only two months before his assassination that "zombifying people is the main attribute of Putin's regime".[9] Putinists, in turn, hurl the same accusation at the supporters of the protest movements in Russia, Ukraine, and Belarus, essentially conflating crowds at a street protest with the proverbial zombie hordes. Since 2014 – that is, since the beginning of the so-called 'Ukrainian crisis' – the metaphor of zombification has been equally applied both to the supporters of the Euromaidan and the participants of the anti-Maidan rallies in Ukraine and Rus-

---

7 Eliot Borenstein, *Plots against Russia: Conspiracy and Fantasy after Socialism*, Ithaca, NY: Cornell University Press, 2019, 184.

8 This is, for example, the case in the highly popular S.T.A.L.K.E.R. game series, which the Ukrainian studio GSC Game World developed. The game is a mixture of an ego-shooter and a survival horror and takes place in the Chernobyl exclusion zone, where the player encounters different physical anomalies, but also mutants and 'zombified soldiers', whose consciousness was corrupted and ultimately destroyed by the radiation.

9 Borenstein, *Plots against Russia*, 196.

sia.[10] Thus, the zombie metaphor effectively takes us back to the very beginning of the Russo–Ukrainian armed conflict, which started in the spring of 2014.

An informationally 'zombified' person ceases to be a valid interlocutor and cannot engage in a meaningful discussion. Yet, unlike the 'traditional' zombies of Hollywood blockbusters, they cannot be simply annihilated – thus, one needs to look for strategies for coming to terms with such 'zombified' compatriots. Ukrainian and Russian literatures reacted to this challenge almost simultaneously with two important novels: Sergei Lukianenko's *Kvazi* (2016; the original Russian spelling is КВАZИ) and Volodymyr Rafeyenko's *The Length of the Days: An Urban Ballad* (*Dolgota dnei: Gorodskaya ballada*, 2017).[11]

Lukianenko, one of the most commercially successful Russian writers of the last decades and an ardent proponent of Putin's regime, sets his novel in 2027. The story unfolds in a world where a mysterious catastrophe occurred ten years prior, causing humans to coexist with the resurrected dead who evolved beyond their initial zombie state into intelligent and unemotional beings known as 'kvazis'. The narrative follows a Moscow police officer whose wife and son were killed by the undead. He attempts to uncover a conspiracy that aims to destroy the fragile peace between humans and kvazis. To succeed, the hero must overcome his grief and desire for vengeance and collaborate with some of the kvazis, learning to see his former foes as allies. However, the novel depicts this mutual understanding as limited and constantly overshadowed by suspicion.

The subtext of *Kvazi* can be interpreted as a political commentary on the ideological division between pro-European, liberal segments of post-Soviet society and their conservative, Soviet-nostalgic counterparts. The human society depicted in the novel seeks to preserve its identity by rejecting modern technologies such as radios and computers and reverting to an archaic lifestyle to protect itself from possible 'zombification'. In contrast, the novel portrays the kvazis as highly rational, tolerant, technologically advanced, and bicycle-riding vegetarians. Therefore, Lukianenko's novel presents a terrifying vision of a future where a liberal society of 'quasi-humans' may reign supreme.

The Ukrainian response to these newly drawn frontlines came in 2017 from the award-winning Ukrainian writer Rafeyenko. A native of Donetsk, Rafeyenko

10 For corresponding examples, see Triin Vihalemm and Jānis Juzefovičs, "'They say we are all zombies': Rethinking the role of audiences in a mediatized international conflict", *Global Media and Communication* 19/1, 2023, 3–28; Bradley E. Wiggins, "Crimea River: Directionality in Memes from the Russia–Ukraine Conflict", *International Journal of Communication* 10, 2016, 451–485; and William Jay Risch, "Prelude to War?", in: David. R. Marples (ed.), *The War in Ukraine's Donbas: Origins, Contexts, and the Future*, Budapest: Central European University Press, 7–28.

11 Sergei Lukianenko, *Kvazi*, Moscow: AST, 2016; and Vladimir Rafeyenko, *Dolgota dnei: Gorodskaya ballada* (*The Length of the Days: An Urban Ballad*), Kharkiv: Fabula, 2017.

wrote most of his prose fiction in Russian and, until the outbreak of the war in 2014, enjoyed more popularity in the Russian Federation than in Ukraine. In July 2014, however, he had to leave his hometown of Donetsk and moved to a town near Kyiv because of the incompatibility of his political views with those of the self-proclaimed Donetsk People's Republic. As an eyewitness of the first months of the war, Rafeyenko captured his experience in *The Length of the Days*, which depicts the occupied city of Z (recognisable as Donetsk) during the spring of 2014.

In the novel, the restoration of the Soviet Union in Z creates a tectonic shift in the structure of reality, letting irrational black matter devour the entire region. The city becomes an antiworld inhabited by bizarre images: the ghost of Rosa Luxemburg wandering the streets and giant flying beetles that carve up people, among other things.[12] The protagonists of the novel, two elderly men and a young girl, can only return and restore peace in the city if they find a statue of the elephant-headed Ganesha dressed in a Ukrainian embroidered shirt. Then they need to rub the statue's belly while performing three different mantras that will break the link between the city of Z and the Soviet legacy. In the final part of the novel, titled "The Displaced Persons", only the young girl manages to accomplish this, thus escaping the bizarre city. The two male protagonists, the representatives of the older generation, find themselves completely oblivious to their past and fail to escape.

Despite the novel's ironic tone, humour, and surreal plot twists, its message can be easily interpreted as nationalist. That is, it is a plea to abandon Soviet Russian culture in favour of a national Ukrainian one. However, the novel's narration from the point of view of supposedly zombified people resists straightforward interpretation. The so-called 'Z people' are recognisable as a Russian-speaking population of Eastern Ukraine, nostalgic for the Soviet Union. The novel presents them as both the reason for the war (they are literally the Kremlin's *casus belli*) and as its first victims, who deserve sympathy and solidarity.

Although in the current war discourse (shaped more by mass media than by works of literature) the collective images of zombified people are far less sophisticated and ambivalent, their literary genealogy should still be kept in mind, since the trope of zombification is implicitly present in the stories of the assaults of the 'zombified enemy soldiers', which circulate on both sides of the conflict.[13] Even if

---

12 Yuliya Ilchuk, "Memory as Forgetting in the Prose Fiction of Serhiy Zhadan and Volodymyr Rafieienko", *The Slavic and East European Journal* 65/2, 2021, 334–353, here 344.

13 Radio Svoboda (Radio Freedom) interview with Oleksandr Iabchanka, "'Ia takoho ne bachyv! Khiba shcho v filmach pro zombi-apokalipsys' – Oleksandr Iabchanka pro Bakhmut" ("'I Have Never Seen Anything Like This! Except in Films about the Zombie Apocalypse' – Oleksander Iabchanka about Bakhmut"), 11 April 2023, https://www.radiosvoboda.org/a/oleksandr-yabchanka-bahmut/32358371.html [accessed: 31.07.2024]; and Elena Proshina, "SMI rasskazali o 'zombie-atakakh' boicov VSU" ("The Media Reported about the 'Zombie-Attacks' by the Soldiers of the Armed Forces of Ukraine"), *Rambler*, 31 October

the zombie imagery is inspired first and foremost by Hollywood movies or popular TV series about zombie apocalypses (which effectively place the devastated towns of Eastern Ukraine in the globally recognisable narrative about the breakdown of human civilisation), a zombified person as such is not necessarily a braindead, flesh-eating monster from a blockbuster but rather any person whose state of mind is corrupt. According to this logic, a heavily armed enemy soldier on steroids or a civilian who unconsciously consumes and reproduces 'enemy propaganda' on the internet can both be described as 'zombies'. Thus, rhetorically, the zombification trope bridges the gap between the battles on the real frontline and the outbursts of 'informational warfare' on the home front. If zombies are everywhere, so is the war.

Fascists and Witches

The intrinsic totality of 'zombification' means that this trope is open to a vast variety of images of the enemy, which spread in the context of the ongoing Russo–Ukrainian War. On the Russian side of the propaganda frontline, this zombified enemy is epitomised by the figure of a 'Ukrainian fascist', which comprises the core of Russian war rhetoric.

Since at least 2014, scholarly publications have discussed the propaganda tropes of Ukrainian Nazis or fascists. Most of these studies focus on ideology and history to debunk the myth of Ukraine as a country ruled by a Nazi junta.[14] While a legitimate scholarly endeavour, these analyses often obfuscate the fact that, in Russian war rhetoric, a Ukrainian fascist is not an ideological but an utterly fantastic figure – a person with a corrupted or manipulated consciousness and a representative of absolute evil. This type of person rejects or even undoes the common Soviet heritage of victory in the so-called Great Patriotic War (1941–1945) and thus rejects the central founding myth of the late USSR and contemporary Russia. In this regard, a

---

2022, https://news.rambler.ru/army/49607507-smi-rasskazali-o-zombi-atakah-boytsov-vsu / [accessed: 31.07.2024].

14 See, for instance, Timothy Snyder, "Fascism, Russia, and Ukraine", *The New York Review of Books*, 20 March 2014, https://www.nybooks.com/articles/2014/03/20/fascism-russia-and-ukraine/ [accessed 31.07.2024]; Oksana Dudko, "A Conceptual Limbo of Genocide: Russian Rhetoric, Mass Atrocities in Ukraine, and the Current Definition's Limits", *Canadian Slavonic Papers* 64/2–3, 2022, 133–145; Myroslav Shkandrij, "Living with Ambiguities: Meanings of Nationalism in the Russian–Ukrainian War", in: Olga Bertelsen (ed.): *Revolution and War in Contemporary Ukraine: The Challenge of Change*, Stuttgart: Ibidem, 2016, 121–138; and Tatiana Zhurzhenko, "Russia's Never-ending War Against 'Fascism': Memory Politics in the Russian–Ukrainian Conflict", *Eurozine*, 08 May 2015, https://www.eurozine.com/russias-never-ending-war-against-fascism/ [accessed 31.07.2024].

Ukrainian fascist is less a bearer of a certain ideology but, rather, a heretic, an apostate, and a Judas.[15]

Like the zombie apocalypse, the war of apostasy is always an existential conflict, a war of annihilation. In the case of Russian aggression against Ukraine, it is also a war for the purity of the imagined Russian community, a deadly quest for consolidation in the face of the 'Global West'. The discursive continuity between the sacralisation of the victory in the Great Patriotic War and the immortality of the fallen heroes makes the boundary between the ideological and pseudo-religious dimensions of the Russian war narrative blurred and permeable. Accordingly, Russian war rhetoric easily swings from the 'denazification' of Ukraine (as an officially declared *casus belli*) to the 'de-Satanisation' of the country – that is, to a holy war against Satanism and occultism, which, according to Russian officials, are flourishing in Ukraine.[16]

On this point, Russian and Ukrainian war rhetoric seem to reinforce each other in a paradoxical way, specifically when considering Ukrainian war narratives that present Ukraine as a land protected by powerful sorcerers and, above all, by witches. The image of Ukraine as a land inhabited by various demonic beings has its origins in Russian and Polish literature of the Romantic period.[17] In this literature, Ukraine was exoticised and represented as an object to be both tamed and admired. The reactivation of this image in the context of the current military conflict can be

15 The trope of this Ukrainian apostasy or treason is firmly anchored in the Russian master narrative. Its genealogy can be traced back to the Ukrainian Hetman Ivan Mazepa, who, during the Great Nordic War (1700–1721), defected from the Russian Army and sided with King Charles XII of Sweden. The Russian Orthodox Church laid an anathema on Mazepa's name in 1708. In the Russian imperial discourse, the term 'mazepinstvo' became an established rhetorical device for presenting Ukraine as being substantially a part of non-Orthodox or Catholic (Polish or 'Jesuit') culture that has been treacherously driven into the body of Russia to undermine its stability. In the genealogical tree of 'Ukrainian betrayal', the place of Mazepa was later taken by Symon Petliura, the military leader of the Ukrainian People's Republic during Ukraine's short-lived sovereignty from 1918 to 1921, and finally by Stepan Bandera (1909–1959), the head of the Organisation of Ukrainian Nationalists. Today, in the Russian patriotic discourse, these three historical figures (as well as their followers) comprise a collective image of the 'Ukrainian Judas'. For more information, see: Alfred Sproede, "'Mazepinstvo' and Other Ukrainian Vexations Featured in Russian Conspiracy Theories (from Poltava 1709 to the Maidan Revolt and After)", *Philologie im Netz* (*Philology Online*) 93, 2022, 83–112.

16 See, for example, the article by Aleksei Pavlov, the Assistant Secretary of the Russian Security Council: Aleksei Pavlov, "Chto variat v vedminom kotle. Na Ukraine nabrali silu neoiazycheskie kulty" ("What is Brewing in the Witch's Cauldron: Neo-Pagan Cults Have Gained Strength in Ukraine"), *Argumenty i fakty* (*Arguments and Facts*), 25 October 2022, https://aif.ru/society/religion/chto_varyat_v_vedminom_kotle_na_ukraine_nabrali_silu_neoyazycheskie_kulty [accessed: 31.07.2024].

17 E.g., the poem *Rusałki* (*Mermaids*, 1829) by Józef Bohdan Zaleski or Gogol's collection *Vechera na hutore bliz Dikanki* (*Evenings on a Farm Near Dikank*, 1829–1832).

traced to a video from March 2022, in which an unarmed Ukrainian woman from the town of Konotop addresses an armed Russian soldier, threatening him with the spell of impotence.[18] Konotop as the unofficial 'capital' of Ukrainian witches has its origins in Hryhorii Kvitka-Osnovianenko's satirical novella *The Witch of Konotop* (*Konotopska Vidma*, 1837), which belongs to the Ukrainian literary canon. Yet, the figure of a Ukrainian witch is also firmly anchored within the Russian literary tradition, where it prominently features in the texts of famous writers like Nikolai Gogol, Orest Somov, and Mikhail Bulgakov.[19] The Ukrainian witch of these texts is a liminal figure who is both attractive and dangerous and is, therefore, a sexualised and exotic Other, but also a symbol of empowerment and independence.

This liminality explains the popularity of the witch as an allegory for contemporary Ukraine as a country at war. In the war context, a witch represents a frightening but undoubtedly positive figure – one that stimulates resilience and a persistent belief in the triumph of justice. For instance, a popular comic book, *Father: The Forge of Armour* (*Tato. Kuznia zbroii*, 2021), by Oleksandr Komiakhov features the Iron Witch. This character appears in the dreams of the book's protagonist, 14-year-old Marina, during the events of the Euromaidan and the first armed clashes in the Donbas.[20] In Marina's nightmares, the Iron Witch prophesises a terrible future for Ukraine. However, Marina gradually understands that the Iron Witch is not only the herald of the upcoming war but also an avenger, a defender, and a female warrior who brings death to enemies and protects Ukrainians.

After Russia launched its full-scale invasion of Ukraine, the poet Liudmyla Horova wrote the poem "To the Enemy" ("Vrazhe"), a grim and macabre poetic monologue of a witch who foresees doom and misfortune for Ukraine's foes. Later, the Ukrainian band Angy Kreyda released a track and a video clip of the same name based on Horova's lyrics. Performed as a magic spell, the text suggests that the invaders will suffer the fate the witch has prepared for them: "As many steps as you take in Ukraine, so will that many of your kin lie in a coffin". Additionally, the video features young women performing rituals with needles, candles, sculls, and other witchcraft paraphernalia (see figure 10). The song was a massive hit in Ukraine.[21]

---

18 The video is available, for instance, on the X (formerly Twitter) account of Oleksandra Matviichuk: Oleksandra Matviichuk (@avalaina), "Woman from Konotop speaks to a Russian soldier…", X post, 02 March 2022, https://twitter.com/avalaina/status/1499117292545888260 [accessed: 31.07.2024] [author's trans].

19 E.g., the witch Solokha in Gogol's "Noch pered Rozhdestvom" ("Christmas Eve", 1832), Katrusia in Somov's *Kievskie vedmy* (*The Witches of Kyiv*, 1833), or Yavdokha in Bulgakov's *Belaya gvardiya* (*The White Guard*, 1925).

20 Oleksandr Komiakhov, *Tato. Kuznia Zbroii (The Father: The Forge of Armour)*, Kyiv: Liuta sprava, 2021.

21 The official YouTube video of the song got 13 million views by March 2023: Endzhi Kreyda / Angy Kreyda, "Endzhi Kreyda – Vrazhe (Ofitsiinyi Vydnohrai)", YouTube video,

Figure 10: Witches and witchcraft paraphernalia, screenshot from "Vrazhe" by Angy Kreyda

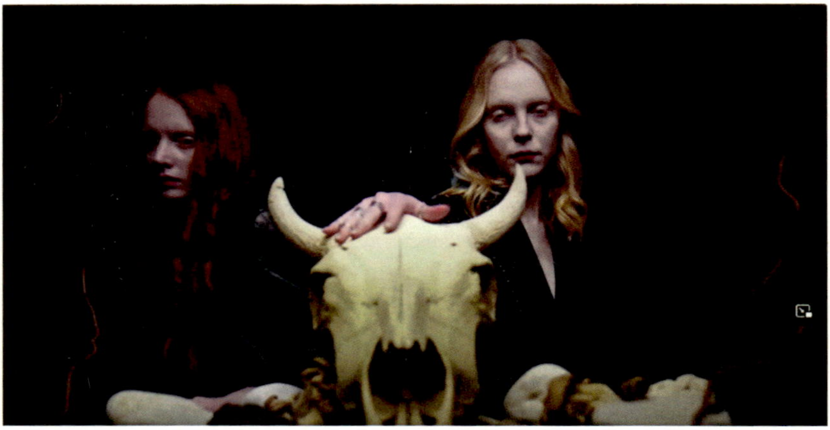

Endzhi Kreyda / Angy Kreyda, "Endzhi Kreyda – Vrazhe (Ofitsiinyi Vydnohrai)", YouTube video, 23 May 2022, 4:13, screenshot from 0:40, https://www.youtube.com/watch?v=cdEEffF7_rU [accessed: 23.07.2024].

Figure 11: A TV propagandist turns a human into a blood-thirsty orc

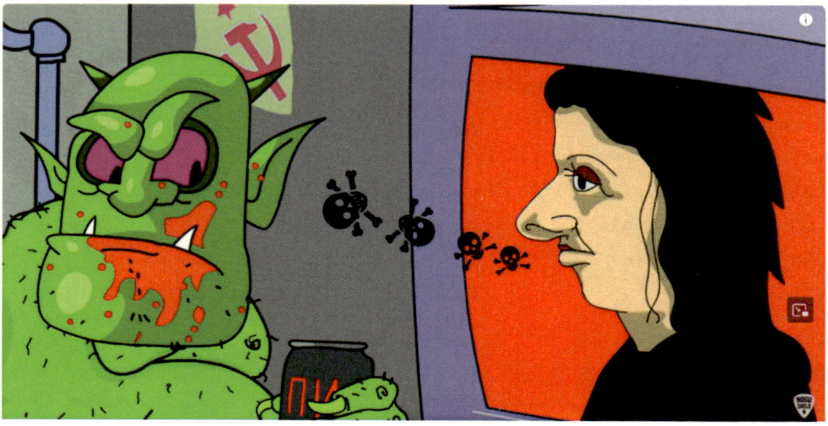

Nogu Sveló!, "Nogu Svelo! – Gimn Obrechennykh (Goida, Orki!)" ("Nogu Svelo! – Hymn of the Damned (Goida, Orcs!)"), YouTube video, 17 November 2022, 3:38, screenshot from 0:28, https://www.youtube.com/watch?v=q07dm6lPs2k [accessed: 23.07.2024].

23 May 2022, 4:13, https://www.youtube.com/watch?v=cdEEffF7_rU [accessed: 31.07.2024] [author's trans.].

Ukraine's Middle-earth

While the witch represents a 'home-grown' phenomenon, rooted in Ukrainian literary and cultural traditions, terminology borrowed from *The Lord of the Rings* film trilogy and from J. R. R. Tolkien's novels of the same name, on the contrary, refers to global mass culture. Specifically, *The Lord of the Rings* has provided Ukrainians with a universally understood vocabulary for naming the enemy.

Even prior to the Russian annexation of Crimea and the start of so-called hybrid warfare in the Donbas, Ukrainian and Russian social media occasionally referred to Russia, and particularly to its capital, Moscow, as 'Mordor'.[22] In literature, this rhetoric was first exploited by the Polish author Ziemowit Szczerek in his book *Mordor Will Come and Eat Us, or a Secret History of the Slavs* (*Przyjdzie Mordor i nas zje, czyli tajna historia Słowian*, 2013). Contrary to its title, the book does not provide a fantasy setting but offers a humorous account of the author's travels through Ukraine. Lying somewhere between a travelogue and gonzo journalism, *Mordor* primarily aims at a total deconstruction of a biased Polish cultural gaze at Ukraine and Ukrainians, but it also criticises the attitudes of Ukrainians towards themselves. This includes, among other things, the description of Russians and Russian-speaking Ukrainians as orcs from Mordor. Yet, in the book, the gaping abyss of Mordor is not a geopolitical entity but rather a metaphysical one, which is not synonymous with Russia. Although its localisation in Szczerek's book remains unclear, Mordor nevertheless offers a powerful metaphor for the vague but constant feeling of a threat coming from the 'East' – a threat of imperial revanche. While Szczerek tries to counter this anxiety with an ironic and humorous tone, he also provides a vivid example of the persistence of images from Tolkien's mythopoetic universe in the Ukrainian context and therefore offers a literary explanation for the popularity of *orky* (orcs) as a popular term for the invading Russian forces in 2022.

President Zelenskyy, his ministers, and government officials at all levels also used the term 'orcs' in reference to the Russian military onslaught against Ukraine. Numerous orc memes based on clips from *The Lord of the Rings* films also circulated on Ukrainian social media.[23] While the originator of this trend is hard to detect, most observers refer to a Facebook post that appeared on the official page of the Ukrainian Ground Forces on 25 February 2022 as a seminal moment for such

---

22 See, for example, Leonid Bershidskii, "Moskva pokhozha na Mordor" ("Moscow Resembles Mordor"), *Tsenzor.Net*, 02 May 2013, https://censor.net/ru/resonance/240801/moskva_pohoja_na_mordor_ukraina_na_stranu_hobbitov [accessed 31.07.2024]; and Ekaterina, "V sotssetiakh: Moskva okonchatelno ukrepilas v statuse Mordora" ("In the Social Networks: Moscow Has Finally Consolidated Its Status as Mordor"), *RB.RU*, 09 December 2014, https://rb.ru/article/v-sotssetyah-moskva-okonchatelno-ukrepilas-v-statuse-mordora/7418547.html [accessed 31.07.2024].

23 Yekelchyk, "Naming the war", 237.

memes.[24] Throughout 2022, state and mass media adopted the language of popular culture, leading to the meme's even greater popularity among the Ukrainian public. But what does this boom of the orc metaphor mean in the war context, and how do orcs function as rhetorical figures?

Orcs populate Tolkien's fantasy world of Middle-earth, where they serve as willing servants of Evil. In the books, they are humanoid, ugly, grey- or black-skinned, and bow-legged. Despite the emphasised fiction and fairy-tale 'unreality' of Tolkien's novels, the books convey a political categorisation based on different groups' physical characteristics and 'civilisational' contrasts. In the world of *The Lord of the Rings*, communities differ not only through skin colour and bodily size and appearance but also in terms of moral integrity and political righteousness: they are either benevolent and wise, as is the case with the Elves, or they are brutish, ruthless, and aggressive, like the Orcs. The absolute and insurmountable hatred between Elves and Orcs in *The Lord of the Rings* is thus not presented as the result of political decisions but is essential and existential in nature: warfare is the 'natural' fate of these two races, while peace between them is to be understood as only a temporary truce, a respite before the next conflict.

As Niels Werber observes, the totality of warfare in Middle-earth also denies the possibility of any neutral positions or moral and legal boundaries in the extermination of the enemy. The destruction of the Orcs, in the view of the Elves, must be on the same scale as they are produced by the Dark Lord Sauron. Meanwhile, Tolkien does not portray his protagonists in a worse light when they continue to massacre Orcs, even if the latter flee, are wounded, or surrender on the battlefield.[25] The classic *ius belli* of sovereign states, which defines the opponent as an honourable enemy, is programmatically suspended in this world and replaced by a biopolitical image of the absolute Other, who deserves neither mercy nor respect.

It is precisely this Manichean totality of the conflict between absolute Good and absolute Evil that makes Tolkien's universe a popular model for conceptualising armed conflicts, although the author himself rejected any allusions to real-world politics. In his theoretical essay "On Fairy Stories", Tolkien highlights the programmatic importance of distancing effects when he defines fantasy as occurring entirely in a separate "secondary world".[26] This does not mean, however, that the two worlds do not connect to each other, even if against the author's will. This connection is especially true for post-Soviet Russian fantasy fanfiction, which often deliberately tries to bridge the gap between the real and the fantastic, to deliver a

24 Ibid.

25 Niels Werber, "Geo- and Biopolitics of Middle-Earth: A German Reading of Tolkien's *The Lord of the Rings*", *New Literary History* 36/2, 2005, 227–246, here 231.

26 Carpenter, Humphrey (ed.), *The Letters of J. R. R. Tolkien*, London: George Allen & Unwin, 1981, 216.

geopolitical message. One of the most striking outcomes of this literary production was the reversal of Tolkien's dualistic worldview in *The Black Book of Arda* (*Chernaya kniga Ardy*, 1995), a novel by Nataliia Vasilieva and Nataliia Nekrasova, based on Tolkien's *The Silmarillion*, as well as in *The Last Ringbearer* (*Poslednii koltsenosets*, 1999) by Kirill Eskov, based on *The Lord of the Rings*. In both novels, the authors unequivocally take the side of the dark forces, thus portraying either the evil spirit Melkor as a kind of Promethean hero (as done in *The Black Book of Arda*) or the aggressive empire of Mordor as an advanced, multinational high-tech civilisation (as in *The Last Ringbearer*). Although these obvious geopolitical reminiscences of the demise of the Communist utopia and the collapse of the Soviet Union circulated in the limited sphere of fantasy subculture, the war against Ukraine and Russia's escalating contestation with the West certainly facilitate further revisions of the categories of 'good' and 'evil' (i.e., the norms of acceptable sociopolitical behaviour) in the Russian cultural landscape.[27] The resemanticisation of the central figures and concepts from Tolkien's literary universe may serve as an important indicator of these tectonic shifts.

Unsurprisingly, in the preface to the new edition of *The Black Book of Arda* (2022), Anna Dolgareva, an active supporter of the Russian invasion of Ukraine, deliberately places the book's plot in the context of the war in the Donbas by comparing the local pro-Russian separatists with smart and modest Orcs, who supposedly had always been suppressed and slandered by arrogant Elves.[28] This positive reversal of the orc figure resonates with official Russian propaganda on many levels, including the Kremlin's official claim that they launched the invasion to prevent the imminent "genocide of the population of the Donbas".[29]

In contrast, Ukrainian war rhetoric adheres to Tolkien's dichotomy of good and evil when it refers to the Orcs as aggressive and ultimately stupid creatures – an epitome of brute force. However, the term itself is applied almost exclusively to the officers and soldiers of the invading army and not to Russians as a nation. For instance, in the popular electro song "The Orc's Body Goes into the Ground, the Armed Forces of Ukraine Will Take Care of That" ("Orka tilo liazhe v grunt, dopomozhe ZSU") by

---

27 Iurii Saprykin, "Reviziya zla: Kak russkaya literature postsovetskogo perioda razbiralas, gde svet, a gde tma, i ne razobralas" ("Revision of Evil: How Russian Literature of the Post-Soviet Period Sorted Out Where the Light Is, Where the Darkness Is, and Failed to Do So"), *Kommersant* (*Merchant*), 16 December 2022, https://www.kommersant.ru/doc/5721611 [accessed: 31.07.2024].

28 Nataliia Vassilieva and Nataliia Nekrasova, *Chernaya kniga Ardy* (*The Black Book of Arda*), Saint Petersburg: Acta Diurna, 2022, 6–7.

29 Vladimir Putin, "Obrashchenie prezidenta Rossiiskoi Federacii 'O provedenii spetsialnoi voyennoi operatsii'" ("The Address of the President of the Russian Federation 'On Conducting a Special Military Operation'"), *Prezident Rossii* (*The President of Russia*), 24 February 2022, http://kremlin.ru/events/president/news/67843 [accessed 31.07.2024].

the artists Chico and Qatoshi, the orc is clearly identifiable as a Russian soldier. The song "The Armed Forces of Ukraine Are Close" ("ZSU blyzko") by The Butcherzz Band follows the transformation of simple Russian Vanias and Vovas into an army of orcs and ultimately celebrates their inevitable death in the fields of Ukraine. The macabre allusions notwithstanding, it is important to note that the latter song text assumes that one is not born an orc but can only 'become' one. This limitation also allows Russian artists, who oppose Putin's regime, to invoke the figure of the hostile orc as a primary enemy image. For example, in the song "Anthem of the Doomed" ("Gimn obrechennykh") by the Russian punk band Nogu Svelo! (Cramp in the Leg!), hordes of orcs invade – or rather infest – Moscow and subjugate it to their cruel and bizarre rule before marching further west (i.e., in the direction of Ukraine and Europe). However, the animated video clip for the song suggests that the orcs themselves are, first and foremost, the products of TV propaganda. In one episode, a TV propagandist, reminiscent of the notorious Russian media executive Margarita Simonyan, "transforms" ordinary TV viewers into orcs (see figure 11).

The image of a Russian soldier as an orc is a means of dehumanisation, yet it functions differently than its propagandistic counterpart, that of a Ukrainian Nazi (or fascist). While orc, as a pejorative label, refers predominantly to the members of the Russian military, Nazi does not have a clear referent and functions rather as a floating signifier (in the structuralist sense). That is, it can be applied to virtually any Ukrainian, regardless of their political and ideological views.

Conclusions

Images and figures from literature and popular culture shift the context and the discursive framing of the ongoing war and overlay it with additional, often unintended, meanings and connotations. This shift can, at least potentially, provide new models for the interpretation of events in Ukraine since the start of the Russian full-scale invasion. If we define 'model' as a simplified representation of reality, then a zombie apocalypse or an onslaught of orcs seem to indeed provide a relatively simple, abridged, and decontextualised understanding of war. While it is legitimate to view the spread and popularity of such perceptions as signs of infantilising or even trivialising the military conflict,[30] they can also be interpreted as means of stress management and morale boosters. More importantly, for the Ukrainian side, the active use of globally recognisable imagery remains an important factor for strengthening worldwide solidarity with Ukraine as a victim of unprovoked military aggression.

30 Mikhail Yampolskii, "Rezhim imperskoi paranoi: voina v epokhu pustosloviia" ("The Regime of Imperial Paranoia: War in the Age of Empty Words"), *Re: Russia*, 26 December 2022, https://re-russia.net/expertise/043/ [accessed: 31.07.2024].

While the content of this cultural production may not conform to principles of political correctness and can raise some justified ethical concerns, it also helps to strengthen the bond between the armed forces and society by fostering the shared sense of determination necessary for effective national defence. Thus, the German military analysts Nico Lange and Carlo Masala highlight Ukrainian popular cultural production as one of the key factors of Ukraine's resilience:

> Through music, culture, and humor, Ukrainian society is strengthening its cohesion, consoling itself over difficult situations, and bolstering its military motivation. This factor cannot be overestimated for total defense.
>
> It was precisely these cultural factors and opportunities for civil society to participate in defense through the provision of equipment, information, and/or data analysis that has seen Ukraine manage to form a global community of support and leverage it as a resource. This global backing has contributed significantly to Ukrainian military successes to this day.[31]

This kind of cultural response to Russian aggression, however, requires constant exchange and cultural negotiation between the state and society and thus reveals the highly decentralised structure of Ukrainian war rhetoric. In this structure, authorities often borrow images and vocabulary from popular songs, texts, and internet memes. This contrasts sharply with the highly centralised and state-controlled propaganda in Russia, which draws heavily on the memory of the Second World War and corresponding literary and cultural production. In Russian propaganda, references to Ukrainian Nazis (or even Satanists) construct the image of an absolute Other, thus enabling the presentation of a cosmogonic war between Good and Evil. Indeed, zombies and orcs are also examples of pejorative Othering, but unlike these fantastical figures, the notion of fascism is charged both historically and politically. It constitutes a discursive framework, in which, on the one hand, the war against Ukraine echoes the historical example of the Red Army's fight in the Great Patriotic War; on the other hand, this fight can only ever be a copy, or an imitation, of that truly 'cosmogonic' world war. Moreover, the propagandistic cliché of the 'fight against fascism' makes current Russian war rhetoric entirely retrospective: the Russian 'military operation' against Ukraine appears primarily as a war for a better past.

This past-oriented rhetoric often remains deadly serious in its tone, while its Ukrainian counterpart is open to irony, humour, and sarcasm, thus providing a truly postmodern framing of the conflict. Despite the overall grim context, references to

31 Nico Lange, "How to beat Russia: What armed forces in NATO should learn from Ukraine's homeland defense", *GLOBSEC*, February 2023, https://www.globsec.org/sites/default/files/2023-02/How%20to%20beat%20Russia%20by%20Nico%20Lange%20v7%20web.pdf, 10 [accessed: 31.07.2024].

the fantastical figures of zombies, orcs, or witches are often playful. If only for a moment, they alienate and downgrade the gloomy seriousness of war, thus highlighting its temporary nature and loosening the war's deadly grip on Ukrainian society.

Bibliography

Arestovych, Oleksii, "Rosiiska armiia – tse armiia pryrechenykh zombie" ("The Russian Army is an Army of Doomed Zombies"), *Glavkom*, 10 March 2022, https://glavcom.ua/columns/arestovich/rosiyska-armiya-ce-armiya-prirechenih-zombi-828505.html [accessed: 23.07.2024].

Bershidskii, Leonid, "Moskva pokhozha na Mordor" ("Moscow Resembles Mordor"), *Tsenzor.Net*, 2013, https://censor.net/ru/resonance/240801/moskva_pohoja_na_mordor_ukraina_na_stranu_hobbitov [accessed 23.07.2024].

bigimir.net, "Arestovich: 'Zombi-nashestvie' RF konchitsia cherez 2–3 nedeli" ("Arestovich: The 'Zombie-Incursion' of the Russian Federation Will Be Over in 2 or 3 Weeks"), 22 March 2022, https://news.bigmir.net/ukraine/6262594-arestovich-zombi-nashestvie-rf-konchitsya-cherez-2-3-nedeli [accessed: 23.07.2024].

Borenstein, Eliot, *Plots against Russia: Conspiracy and Fantasy after Socialism*, Ithaca, NY: Cornell University Press, 2019.

Carpenter, Humphrey (ed.), *The Letters of J. R. R. Tolkien*, London: George Allen & Unwin, 1981.

Chertkova, Liudmila, "Ukraina prevratila VSU v 'zombi-armiiu': prut na uboi" ("Ukraine Turned its Armed Forces into a 'Zombie Army': They're Roaring to Slaughter"), *Pravda.Ru*, 25 October 2022, https://www.pravda.ru/society/1763348-narkogosudarstvo_ukraina/ [accessed: 23.07.2024].

Dudko, Oksana, "A Conceptual Limbo of Genocide: Russian Rhetoric, Mass Atrocities in Ukraine, and the Current Definition's Limits", *Canadian Slavonic Papers* 64/2–3, 2022, 133–145.

Ekaterina, "V sotssetiakh: Moskva okonchatelno ukrepilas v statuse Mordora" ("In the Social Networks: Moscow Has Finally Consolidated Its Status as Mordor"), *RB.RU*, 09 December 2014, https://rb.ru/article/v-sotssetyah-moskva-okonchatelno-ukrepilas-v-statuse-mordora/7418547.html [accessed 23.07.2024].

Endzhi Kreyda / Angy Kreyda, "Endzhi Kreyda – Vrazhe (Ofitsiinyi Vydnohrai)", YouTube video, 23 May 2022, 4:13, https://www.youtube.com/watch?v=cdEEffF7_rU [accessed: 23.07.2024].

Ilchuk, Yuliya, "Memory as Forgetting in the Prose Fiction of Serhiy Zhadan and Volodymyr Rafieienko", *The Slavic and East European Journal* 65/2, 2021, 334–353.

Komiakhov, Oleksandr, *Tato. Kuznia Zbroii* (*The Father: The Forge of Armour*), Kyiv: Liuta sprava, 2021.

Lange, Nico, "How to beat Russia: What armed forces in NATO should learn from Ukraine's homeland defense", *GLOBSEC*, February 2023, https://www.globsec.org/sites/default/files/2023-02/How%20to%20beat%20Russia%20by%20Nico%20Lange%20v7%20web.pdf [accessed: 23.07.2024].

Luganskii Informatsionnyi Tsentr (Lugansk Information Centre), "Boitsy VSU v Rubezhnom voiuiut 'v sostoianii zombi' pod vozdeistviem narkotikov – Miroshnik" ("The Soldiers of the Ukrainian Armed Forces in Rubezhnoye Fight 'in a Zombie State' under the Influence of Drugs – Miroshnik"), 07 April 2022, https://lug-info.com/news/bojcy-vsu-v-rubezhnom-voyuyut-v-sostoyanii-zombi-pod-vozdejstviem-narkotikov-miroshnik [accessed: 23.07.2024].

Lukianenko, Sergei, *Kvazi*, Moscow: AST, 2016.

Matviichuk, Oleksandra, (@avalaina), "Woman from Konotop speaks to a Russian soldier...", X post, 02 March 2022, https://twitter.com/avalaina/status/1499117292545888260 [accessed: 23.07.2024].

Pavlov, Aleksei, "Chto variat v vedminom kotle. Na Ukraine nabrali silu neoiazycheskie kulty" ("What is Brewing in the Witch's Cauldron: Neo-Pagan Cults Have Gained Strength in Ukraine"), *Argumenty i fakty* (*Arguments and Facts*), 25 October 2022, https://aif.ru/society/religion/chto_varyat_v_vedminom_kotle_na_ukraine_nabrali_silu_neoyazycheskie_kulty [accessed: 23.07.2024].

Pelevin, Viktor, "Zombifikatsiia sovetskogo cheloveka" ("The Zombification of the Soviet Person"), *Novyi Zhurnal* (*New Journal*) 179, 1990, 324–338.

Proshina, Elena, "SMI rasskazali o 'zombie-atakakh' boicov VSU" ("The Media Reported about the 'Zombie-Attacks' by the Soldiers of the Armed Forces of Ukraine"), *Rambler*, 31 October 2022, https://news.rambler.ru/army/49607507-smi-rasskazali-o-zombi-atakah-boytsov-vsu/ [accessed: 23.07.2024].

Putin, Vladimir, "Obrashchenie prezidenta Rossiiskoi Federacii 'O provedenii spetsialnoi voyennoi operatsii'" ("The Address of the President of the Russian Federation 'On Conducting a Special Military Operation'"), *Prezident Rossii* (*The President of Russia*), 24 February 2022, http://kremlin.ru/events/president/news/67843 [accessed 23.07.2024].

Radio Svoboda (Radio Freedom) interview with Oleksandr Iabchanka, "'Ia takoho ne bachyv! Khiba shcho v filmach pro zombi-apokalipsys' – Oleksandr Iabchanka pro Bakhmut" ("I Have Never Seen Anything Like This! Except in Films about the Zombie Apocalypse' – Oleksander Iabchanka about Bakhmut"), 11 April 2023, https://www.radiosvoboda.org/a/oleksandr-yabchanka-bahmut/32358371.html [accessed: 23.07.2024].

Rafeyenko, Vladimir, *Dolgota dnei: Gorodskaya ballada* (*The Length of the Days: An Urban Ballad*), Kharkiv: Fabula, 2017.

Risch, William Jay, "Prelude to War?", in: David. R. Marples (ed.), *The War in Ukraine's Donbas: Origins, Contexts, and the Future*, Budapest: Central European University Press, 7–28.

Saprykin, Iurii, "Reviziya zla: Kak russkaya literature postsovetskogo perioda razbiralas, gde svet, a gde tma, i ne razobralas" ("Revision of Evil: How Russian Literature of the Post-Soviet Period Sorted Out Where the Light Is, Where the Darkness Is, and Failed to Do So"), *Kommersant* (*Merchant*), 16 December 2022, https://www.kommersant.ru/doc/5721611 [accessed: 23.07.2024].

Shkandrij, Myroslav, "Living with Ambiguities: Meanings of Nationalism in the Russian–Ukrainian War", in: Olga Bertelsen (ed.): *Revolution and War in Contemporary Ukraine: The Challenge of Change*, Stuttgart: Ibidem, 2016, 121–138.

Snyder, Timothy, "Fascism, Russia, and Ukraine", *The New York Review of Books*, 20 March 2014, https://www.nybooks.com/articles/2014/03/20/fascism-russia-and-ukraine/ [accessed 23.07.2024].

Sproede, Alfred, "'Mazepinstvo' and Other Ukrainian Vexations Featured in Russian Conspiracy Theories (from Poltava 1709 to the Maidan Revolt and After)", *Philologie im Netz* (*Philology Online*) 93, 2022, 83–112.

Vassilieva, Nataliia, and Nataliia Nekrasova, *Chernaya kniga Ardy* (*The Black Book of Arda*), Saint Petersburg: Acta Diurna, 2022.

Vihalemm, Triin, and Jānis Juzefovičs, "'They say we are all zombies': Rethinking the role of audiences in a mediatized international conflict", *Global Media and Communication* 19/1, 2023, 3–28.

Werber, Niels, "Geo- and Biopolitics of Middle-Earth: A German Reading of Tolkien's *The Lord of the Rings*", *New Literary History* 36/2, 2005, 227–246.

Wiggins, Bradley E., "Crimea River: Directionality in Memes from the Russia–Ukraine Conflict", *International Journal of Communication* 10, 2016, 451–485.

Yampolskii, Mikhail, "Rezhim imperskoi paranoi: voina v epokhu pustosloviia" ("The Regime of Imperial Paranoia: War in the Age of Empty Words"), *Re: Russia*, 26 December 2022, https://re-russia.net/expertise/043/ [accessed: 23.07.2024].

Yekelchyk, Serhy, "Naming the war: Russian aggression in Ukrainian official discourse and mass culture", *Canadian Slavonic Papers* 64/2–3, 2022, 232–246.

Zhurzhenko, Tatiana, "Russia's Never-ending War Against 'Fascism': Memory Politics in the Russian–Ukrainian Conflict", *Eurozine*, 08 May 2015, https://www.eurozine.com/russias-never-ending-war-against-fascism/ [accessed 23.07.2024].

The Russo-Ukrainian War as a Challenge to the Identity and Memory of Ukrainian Writers

Tetiana Shestopalova

The full-scale war began with a Russian attack that forced Ukraine out of its protracted 'transit state'[1] and into the formation of its postcolonial and post-totalitarian society. A sign of internal changes in the public life of Ukrainians is their realisation of the fundamental importance of national culture and the state language as a tool for representing a consolidated nation and a vital barrier between them and the Russians.[2] The Ukrainian language has become an absolutely necessary and natural expression of the inclusive identity of the Ukrainian political nation, which is composed of various ethnonational segments, as Ukraine is home to many ethnonational groups. Writer and journalist Tamriko Sholi, a Russified Georgian Ukrainian who grew up in Luhansk and spoke and wrote books in Russian before the war, attributed her transition to Ukrainian to a sense of responsibility for Ukraine and its key cultural codes. "In the new Ukrainian history that we are building right now, language is a very important element", she writes.[3]

It is well known that literature processes and verbalises the characteristics of national identity in different ways, strengthening or undermining people's perceptions of themselves and their past, present, and prospects. The purpose of this article is to reveal the nature of the linguistic and cultural identity of modern Eastern Ukrainian writers and to show how this nature determines their work with the individual and historical memory of Ukrainians against the background of the experi-

1 Tamara Hundorova characterised the "transit state" as a transitional period "after totalitarianism and colonialism". Tamara Hundorova, *Tranzytna kultura. Symptomy postkolonialnoi travmy: esei* (*Transit Culture: Symptoms of Postcolonial Trauma, Essays*), Kyiv: Hrani-T, 2012, 7 [author's trans.].

2 For more, see: Volodymyr Kulyk, "Mova ta identychnist v Ukraini na kinets 2022" ("Language and Identity in Ukraine at the End of 2022"), *Zbruč*, 01 January 2023, https://zbruc.eu/node/114247 [accessed: 08.06.2023].

3 Olena Iurchenko, "Nam mova bolyt: iak obiednaty ukraintsiv navkolo ukrainskoii movy?" ("Our Language Hurts Us: How to Unite Ukrainians Around the Ukrainian Language?"), *Osvitoriia* (*Education*), https://osvitoria.media/experience/nam-mova-bolyt-yak-ob-yednaty-ukrayintsiv-navkolo-ukrayinskoyi-movy/ [accessed: 31.07.2024] [author's trans.].

ence of the Russo–Ukrainian War. This article is based on speeches and literary texts by the Eastern Ukrainian writers Olena Stiazhkina, Volodymyr Rafeyenko, and Iya Kiva, for whom the war became a personal challenge from 2014 on, when Russia occupied the industrial parts of the Luhansk and Donetsk Oblasts, commonly known as the Donbas. The theoretical basis for this article is the work of Agneshka Matusiak and Tamara Hundorova, who examine the relationship between identity, memory, and style.[4]

Russia's full-scale war against Ukraine has exacerbated the issue of 'Russian–Ukrainian bilingualism' to the maximum extent possible.[5] After 24 February 2022, Ukrainian society began to perceive this issue through the prism of colonial and totalitarian trauma for the first time. This led to a fundamental revision of processes of national, civic, and cultural identity and collective memory of Ukrainians. Thus, before the full-scale invasion, the phenomenon of Russian-speaking Ukrainian writers was a relatively neutral subject of cultural reflection and self-reflection by the writers themselves. For example, Kiva, a well-known poet who lived in Donetsk until 2014, said in August 2021:

> [F]or a writer, language is not everyday life and not a realm where nothing much changes when you switch from one language to another. For a writer, losing a language is actually losing oneself, the ability to speak [...] [M]y main, or rather significant linguistic and poetic identity is connected with the Russian language, although it is connected with the Ukrainian reality.[6]

Iryna Starovoit, a philologist and cultural critic from Lviv, took a similar position. A little more than two weeks before Russia's full-scale invasion of Ukraine, she charac-

4 Agnieshka Matusiak, *Vyity z movchannia: Dekolonialni zmahannia ukrainskoi kultury ta literatury XXI stolittia z posttotalitarnoiu travmoiu* (*Breaking Out of Silence: Decolonial Struggles of Ukrainian Culture and Literature of the Twenty-First Century with Post-Totalitarian Trauma*), Lviv: LA "Piramida", 2020; and Hundorova, *Tranzytna kultura*.

5 Referring to the results of sociological surveys in Ukraine between 2014 and 2022, Volodymyr Kulyk stated: "Ukraine, despite a certain amount of use [...] of at least a dozen different languages, is generally a bilingual country, because only Ukrainian and Russian are used to some extent in all areas and in all regions". Volodymyr Kulyk, *Movna polityka v bahatomovnykh krainah: zakordonnyi dosvid ta ioho prydatnist dlia Ukrainy* (*Language Policy in Multilingual Countries: Foreign Experience and Its Applicability to Ukraine*), Kyiv: Dukh I Litera, 2021, 248–249 [author's trans.].

6 Oleh Kotsarev, "Iya Kiva: 'Ni u formi viiny, ni u myrnoho protestu vykhid z teplykh imperskyh "bratskyh" obiimiv ne bude lehkym'" ("Iya Kiva: 'Neither in the Form of War Nor in the Form of Peaceful Protest Will it Be Easy to Get out of the Warm Imperial "Brotherly" Embrace'"), *LB.ua*, 22 September 2021, https://lb.ua/culture/2021/08/22/491968_iya_kiva_ni_formi_viyni_ni_formi.html [accessed: 08.06.2023] [author's trans.].

terised the presence of Russian-speaking writers in the Ukrainian literary process as a specificity of national culture that requires understanding and attention:

> I extremely appreciate people who have made their ethical choice in favour of the Ukrainian language over the past eight years, but we must understand that it is much more difficult for a creative person to switch from another language to Ukrainian. And if we think about it, these are rare cases in world culture when a person has realised themselves equally well in two languages. And I would like to emphasise once again that this is not a problem in Poland, the Czech Republic, or Hungary. This is our specificity, and we have to treat it very responsibly.[7]

Russia's insidious attack on 24 February 2022 effectively pulled the rug of imperial culture and language out from under Ukrainians and caused radical changes in the self-identification of Ukrainian writers who, until that day, were Russian speakers. This became a point of no return for them. Kiva writes:

> In just one night, the shortest month of the year became the longest month of life. An immense, almost biblical day of creation. The river of war, which, despite the well-known proverb, had to be crossed for the second time, turned out to be a bottomless well of icy water. However, Ukrainians learned to swim there as well.[8]

While changing the language of creativity is a much more complex process than changing the language of communication, and requires time, psycho-emotional commitment, and purposeful intellectual efforts, the writers embarked on this path, emphasising their involvement in the decolonisation processes in Ukraine.

Kiva uses the concepts of ethical reconfiguration and psychophysiological reaction to the full-scale Russo–Ukrainian War to convey the depth of linguistic and cultural transformation, which involves the intersubjective (ethical) and intrasubjective (psychic and physiological) realms. Kiva is a poet, translator, journalist, and Ukrainian woman who was made a passive bilingual and an original Russian-language poet by the Russian language of the reality of her native Donetsk. She reclaimed Ukrainian as the language of her professional activity after the Russian occupation of Donetsk in 2014, realising that it was important for her to be part of

7 Bohdana Nebopak and Vadym Blonskii, "Iryna Starovoit: 'Ukraina staie liudynotsentrychnoiu'" ("Iryna Starovoit: 'Ukraine is Becoming Human-Centred'"), *The Ukrainians*, 07 February 2022, https://theukrainians.org/iryna-starovojt-pen/ [accessed: 31.07.2024] [author's trans.].

8 Iya Kiva, "Podali vid myru, blyzhche do peremohy" ("Away from Peace, Closer to Victory"), *Meridian Czernowitz*, 2023, https://www.meridiancz.com/blog/iia-kiva-podali-vid-myru-blyzhche-do-peremohy/ [accessed: 31.07.2024] [author's trans.].

the common Ukrainian-speaking space, to be present and involved in it.[9] "Through a few gestures of trust and faith in each other, which became our new language", she writes, is the way Ukrainians are reaching out to each other today to organise this space.[10] After 24 February 2022, Ukrainian became the language of Kiva's poetry. The poet takes her experience of returning to the Ukrainian language beyond the discourse of trauma. She emphasises that in her case, there is joy and freedom to be herself:

> But at some point, you feel it as if your vertebrae, which were hurting, finally fell into place and you can straighten your shoulders. I will still be thinking about working metaphors for all future explanations, but I want the choice of Ukrainian as a home (actually, when it is literally your home) to be articulated in this way, and not by the inertia of Russian discourse, which is often uncritically reproduced even by those who are fully in favour of Ukraine. Because sometimes all these language questions remind me of the need to explain why you are in love. Here, because I love it. There could be a simple explanation like this.[11]

Freedom can also begin where personal choice confronts the inertia and automatism of mass social life. It is based on a person's values and moral preferences. In this case, this choice takes place against the backdrop of deep internal dramas and crises. For example, Kiva admits that when she migrated to Kyiv in 2014, she took the "Ukrainian–Russian language" of Donetsk with her to save her mother's language from the "Russian world" and at the same time to emphasise the linguistic peculiarity of her true Ukrainian identity.[12] Russia's full-scale invasion in February 2022 shattered the poet's attempts to rehabilitate Russian as a language of life and culture. "Where there used to be Russian inside me, today I feel a dead animal that stinks and decomposes. I don't like pretentious statements, especially around the language, but now I feel that it will continue to be so", she writes.[13]

---

9 Kotsarev, "Iya Kiva".

10 Kiva, "Podali vid myru".

11 Iya Kiva, "Hotuiuchys do odnoho vystupu, znov bachu zapytannia pro..." ("When preparing for a speech, I see the question about..."), Facebook post, 09 May 2023, https://www.facebook.com/iya.kiva/posts/pfbid02zJ6ZiXSsoDrbHq5qZz6mUUhPJH1wHVdBan9WCNLhnytsMhgc7vZg3bfLBuUpBoBVl [accessed: 31.07.2024] [author's trans.].

12 Andrii Krasniashchykh, "Iya Kiva: 'Tam, de vseredyni mene ranishe bula rosiiska, siohodni ia vidchuvaiu mertvoho zvira'", ("Iya Kiva: 'Where There Used to Be Russian Inside Me, Today I Feel a Dead Animal'"), *Ukrainska Pravda* (*Ukrainian Truth*), 24 July 2022, https://www.pravda.com.ua/articles/2022/07/24/7359716/ [accessed: 31.07.2024] [author's trans.].

13 Ibid.

Rafeyenko also speaks of the "difficult and happy experience" of returning to the Ukrainian language of creativity: "The language is happiness, not a problem".[14] Rafeyenko has long been known as a successful Russian-language author and a winner of a number of literary awards (including Russian ones). After the occupation of Donetsk, he, like Kiva, moved to Kyiv, where he wrote his first Ukrainian-language work, the novel *Mondegreen*, with the genre subtitle "Songs of Death and Love".[15] The result is a story filled with mysticism and fairy tales, where he and the world around him undergo amazing transformations thanks to language: "It turns out that inside another language you have lived a completely different life. And who are you? The character goes through this path of gathering himself, as in a Christian prayer: 'God, gather me in yourself and bind me together'".[16]

The novel, which Rafeyenko wrote in the wake of his actual "growing into the language",[17] embodies, among other things, the phenomenon of the existential self-construction of the individual through language. As the Ukrainian writer Serhiy Zhadan, a volunteer and performer who is well known outside of Ukraine, said: "You can't switch to a language with the whole trolleybus".[18] While after 2014, Rafeyenko planned to write texts in Russian and Ukrainian alternately, in 2022, he stressed a complete break with the Russian language: "I will not do anything in Russian anymore. I don't want to have anything to do with this language. I don't want to and I can't. For me, a sense of home is Ukrainianness".[19]

---

14 Volodymyr Rafeyenko, "Iak mova vyznachaie pamiat" ("How Language Determines Memory"), *Zbruč*, 19 August 2019, https://zbruc.eu/node/91540 [accessed: 31.07.2024] [author's trans.].

15 Serhiy Zhadan states that "a well-made, important novel [...] has traditionally been missed by our [Ukrainian] criticism". Serhiy Zhadan, "Kilka sliv pro nerozuminnia..." ("A few words about misunderstanding..."), Facebook post, 24 October 2019, https://www.facebook.com/100044170792676/posts/2436920353022885/ [accessed: 31.07.2024] [author's trans.].

16 Rafeyenko, "Iak mova vyznachaie pamiat".

17 Ibid.

18 This phrase is Zhadan's answer to Iuriy Andrukhovych's question about whether there was an internal moment of conscious transition to the Ukrainian language in Kharkiv: "Zhadan: – Yes. I'm not going to switch to Russian with the [trolleybus] controller. Let me speak Ukrainian, even if she looks at me sideways. There was a thing that [...] many people don't understand when they talk about speaking Russian and the Russian language among Ukrainians in the East. Because you can't switch to the language with the whole trolleybus. Everyone switches personally". Iuriy Andrukhovych, "Serhii Zhadan – Iuriiu Andrukhovychu: 'V mene zminylosia vidchuttia, pro koho ia pyshu, chyim holosom hovoriu'" ("Serhiy Zhadan – Iuriy Andrukhovych: 'I Have a New Sense of Who I Am Writing About and in Whose Voice I Am Speaking'"), *Craft Magazine*, 21 March 2022, https://craftmagazine.net/sergiy-zhadan-yuri-andruhovychu/# [accessed: 31.07.2024] [author's trans.].

19 Stanislav Vrublevskyi, "'Rosiiskoiu bilshe nichoho ne budu robyty. Ne khochu maty zhodnoho stosunku do tsiiei movy' – pysmennyk Volodymyr Rafeyenko" ("'I Will Not Do Any-

A former resident of Donetsk, the academic historian and writer Stiazhkina also settled in Kyiv after the occupation of Donetsk by Russia, becoming one of the thousands of newly displaced persons. Revealing the bilingualism of her novel, *Cecil the Lion Had to Die*, Stiazhkina noted that she was unable to write in Russian when she approached the events of the occupation of Donetsk in 2014:

> If we want to win, we have to be Ukrainians and speak Ukrainian. And if we don't, we find ourselves somewhere in between, between worlds. This does not mean that we are there forever or that there is no way out. But there are not many ways out. Either you go to Moscow or you are a Ukrainian. It is both simple and very difficult.[20]

A look at the change of the language of creativity through the prism of the concept of identity allows us to emphasise the temporally and spatially unfinished and open process of the writer's creative realisation – a realisation that occurs in the consciously chosen Ukrainian language, since identity in today's dynamic world is often associated with more than one language and culture. In particular, the Ukrainian "home of being" is "almost always more than one language".[21] Thus, the issue of Ukraine's multilingualism, with a sharp bias towards Russian–Ukrainian bilingualism, did not disappear in the second year of the war. But for the first time, the Ukrainian language has marked a common inclusive space of national freedom and memory within a country from which the 'Russian antiworld'[22] is being squeezed out, albeit with difficulty, by rethinking the consequences of Ukraine's inoculation with the Russian language and Russian culture.

Writers who chose Ukrainian not only for daily communication but also for creative self-realisation during the war embody the fundamental disconnection of Ukrainian society from the colonial (19th-century) and totalitarian (20th-century) heritage that threatens the new political identity of Ukrainians. At the same time,

---

thing in Russian Anymore. I Don't Want to Have Anything to Do with This Language' – Writer Volodymyr Rafeyenko"), *Suspilne Kultura* (*Public Culture*), 31 May 2022, https://suspilne.media/245037-rosijskou-bilse-nicogo-ne-budu-robiti-ne-hocu-mati-zodnogo-stosunku-do-ciei-movi-pismennik-volodimir-rafeenko/ [accessed: 31.07.2024] [author's trans.].

20 *Vydavnytso Staroho Leva* (*The Old Lion Publishing House*), "Olena Stiazhkina: Knyha maie pokazaty shcho kozhen iz nas mozhe zminytysia" ("Olena Stiazhkina: A Book Should Show That Each of Us Can Change"), 25 June 2021, https://starylev.com.ua/news/olena-styazhkina-knyga-maye-pokazaty-shcho-kozhen-iz-nas-mozhe-zminytysya [accessed: 31.07.2024] [author's trans.].

21 Nebopak and Blonskii, "Iryna Starovoit".

22 This is a concept from Mikhail Epshtein. Mikhail Epshtein, *Russkii antimir: Politika na grani apokalipsisa* (*Russian Antiworld: Politics on the Brink of Apocalypse*), New York: Franc-Tireur USA, 2023.

the existential aspect of the linguistic and cultural transformation of the creative personality and the internal conflicts of changing one's identity are still poorly understood. Such questions require attention because the answers to them will testify to the depth and reliability of the new nation-centred project of Ukrainian identity, which has been intensified by the war. A healthy incorporation of representatives of different cultural environments and national communities into this project requires joint efforts and honesty. After all, as Kiva says, "[i]t is not at all a given fact that we can understand each other quickly, without sticking open wounds to each other. Honesty is tiring, but it is the only possible form of existence".[23]

Memory is a cultural phenomenon that ensures the strength of national identity. The prospect of the restoration of Ukrainian authority in the Donbas after the war poses the task of verbalising the common space of the historical memory of Ukraine and the Ukrainian Donbas. Turning to the mentioned novels of Stiazhkina and Rafeyenko, who consider the Donbas a small homeland within Ukraine, gives an artistic self-reflection of the Ukrainian space of the Donbas, with its inherent historical dramas, failures in collective memory, and identity quests.

In fact, Stiazhkina and Rafeyenko tell microstories of people on the frontier, which is the Donbas, appealing to the history of Ukraine as a 'politicised ethnicity'. This concept "opens up wide opportunities for establishing the relationship between national identity and historical memory, and most importantly, it fully justifies the naturalness of nations' desire to find their own roots in the ethnic past", as Iuliia Zernii writes.[24]

At the same time, the Soviet myth, which, according to historians Valerii Smolii and Larysa Yakubova,[25] underlies the identity of the Donbas and the historical memory of its inhabitants nowadays, blurred and hid the dramatic problems of the multiethnic past of the Donbas under the manipulative slogan of the formation of a new, progressive community of people – the so-called 'Soviet people'. Stiazhkina, in *Cecil the Lion Had to Die*, and Rafeyenko, in *Mondegreen*, play with the stereotypical idea of the Donbas's 'nomad' mentality against the background of endless migration and displacement, which define the entire modern history of Ukraine. At the same time,

---

23 Iya Kiva, "Podruha spytala mene, iak ia pochuvaiusia u Lvovi..." ("My friend asked me how I felt in Lviv..."), Facebook post, 30 January 2023, https://www.facebook.com/iya.kiva/posts/pfbid02ytzdtz4mrChBAHbJVh9TicbcF5y6rxEd9PyYQdLDWGqzepEFEuDY4eD2aznFXddcl [accessed: 31.07.2024] [author's trans.].

24 Iuliia Zernii, "Vzaiemozviazok istorychnoi pamiati ta natsionalnoi identychnosti" ("The Relationship Between Historical Memory and National Identity"), *politychnyi menedzhment* (*political management*) 5, 2008, 104–115, here 107 [author's trans.].

25 Valerii Smolii and Larysa Yakubova, *Donechchyna i Luhanshchyna: mistse v modernomu ukrainskomu natsionalnomu proekti, Analitychna dopovid* (*The Donetsk and Luhansk Oblasts: Place in the Modern Ukrainian National Project, An Analytical Report*), Valerii Smolii (ed.), Kyiv: Institute of History of Ukraine of the National Academy of Sciences of Ukraine, 2015, 26.

they draw attention to the phenomenon of the irrational connection of the inhabitants of this region with the Soviet past as the only roots of their history and the frame of the future.

For example, Stiazhkina depicted several Ukrainians, Russians, and Germans whose ancestors found themselves in the Donbas because of socioeconomic and geopolitical processes in the 19th and 20th centuries. Her work evokes the formation of a civil society in Ukraine out of a kaleidoscopic, heterogeneous mass of people in terms of ethnicity and worldview. Thus, some of the novel's characters overcome the trauma of silence and the ignorance of their history and consciously choose an inclusive Ukrainian national identity, while others experience Soviet and post-Soviet resentment, remaining in the field of the illusion of Donbas exclusivity and hoping for the return of the USSR.

Both authors use the motif of memory affected by historical amnesia and ignorance in the microstories of their main characters. This motif marks the unspoken trauma of ethnic communities and entire nations in the Soviet Union, forced to remain silent about the crimes of the totalitarian regime against them. The protagonist of Rafeyenko's *Mondegreen*, the Russified Ukrainian Haba Habinsky, overcomes 'historical amnesia' through his transition from the Russian to the Ukrainian language. He perceives Russian as the language of forgetting, ignorance, censorship, and silence – an instrument of the Soviet regime that prohibited the protagonist from knowing his family history and the language of his uprooting in general. As Rafeyenko writes in the novel,

> The catechism of blessed ignorance emerged slowly in his [Habinsky's] life. During childhood, you had to not know everything that you knew about those people who surrounded you. Because, firstly, they each had their own *Canon of Not-knowing* and, secondly, they were good people who knew not what they were doing. You had to not know about your country and city, about your male and female friends, about women and men, about their kids and desires, about light and darkness, mom and dad, brothers and sisters, about grandmother, grandfather and granduncle, about their past, and about your own future.
>
> The fate of your grandfather and his brother on your mother's side of the family – that is something that in Soviet times, and, honestly after those times, too, needed not to be known. The father and mother of his grandfather – Oleksii Iehorovych, and, respectively, of his granduncle – Ivan Iehorovych, were shot to death in the beginning of the 1920s by the Bolsheviks in front of their children when the older child had just turned six.[26]

---

26 Volodymyr Rafeyenko, *Mondegreen: Songs about Death and Love*, trans. Mark Andryczyk, Cambridge, MA: Harvard University Press, 2022, 77–78.

Unawareness, forgetting, and ignorance due to the lack of a claim to knowledge characterise an 'average' carrier of the Soviet myth, who is deprived of will and doomed to repeat the traumatic situation.[27] In Rafeyenko's novel, the epithet 'simple' is a marker of Habinsky's unconscious existence in a circle of ignorance and silence imposed by the language of the totalitarian regime. After migration from occupied Donetsk to Kyiv, for a long time Habinsky calls himself a "displaced person"[28] and a "simple refugee",[29] one that belongs to the sub-category "Simple Person Refugee",[30] and "a person that is intelligent, educated, simple, and a refugee".[31] This sarcastically emphasises Habinky's objectivity, not subjectivity.

In the finale of the novel, Habinsky ruptures the mythological cycle of his existence as a 'simple migrant' through painful and adventurous efforts to regain the Ukrainian language of communication and an understanding of the history of his family. This is a tool for therapeutically living through the trauma of his family, caused by the Bolsheviks' brutal massacre of his maternal ancestors, wealthy Ukrainians. Habinsky's fantastic meeting with his long-dead relatives in the novel's finale indicates that the character dared to leave the vicious circle of ignorance and got a chance to come "face to face with being":[32]

> Habinsky went up to the door. He felt that, if he would open it, he would never be able to fall asleep again. And if he didn't open it, he would never awaken. He took a breath and closed his eyes. He opened the door – and almost broke into tears. At the doorway stood five tiny children (sleep, little Jesus, sleep).[33]

According to the plot of *Mondegreen*, these children represent the awakened memory of Habinsky, a conscious knowledge of the tragedy of his Ukrainian ancestors caused by the Soviet regime. The rejection of ignorance as a way of life in Soviet and (by inertia) post-Soviet times requires the personal and special efforts of a person who has embodied the tradition of generational ignorance in the language of a totalitarian regime since birth.

In Stiazhkina's novel *Cecil the Lion Had to Die*, silence correlates with concealment, ignorance, and forgetting, and memory resembles a palimpsest. Most of her fictional characters are not sure of their own origins. Figuratively speaking, they are

---

27 Agnieshka Matusiak, *Vyity z movchannia*, 16.

28 Rafeyenko, *Mondegreen*, 52.

29 Ibid., 107, 126, 138.

30 Ibid., 126.

31 Ibid.

32 Ibid., 21.

33 Ibid., 145.

strangers to themselves. The work depicts the key character, Heinrich Fink, a descendant of German Mennonites, as a Donetsk resident at the novel's beginning. He recalls that his mother was afraid to remember the exact place of their German roots because of the Soviet repressions that their family suffered before World War II due to their German origin and the humiliation they faced during and after this war. She said that their family might have come from Baden or Prussia. However, for some reason, Fink's memory holds hints of Bavaria. The same problem of a lack of knowledge or even a void of memory about the fate of earlier generations in the USSR is characteristic of the novel's other protagonists, who are also Donetsk residents. The meeting and interaction of the characters on the pages of this novel are an artistic reflection on the consequences of Stalin's policy of deporting various ethnic groups.

Today, there are villages in the Donetsk and Luhansk Oblasts whose names changed depending on which ethnic group was deported to the village in place of another group deported to another region during the years of the Soviet Union. Boykivske, a village located in the Donetsk Oblast currently occupied by Russia, is an example of this.[34] Stiazhkina writes of the history of the names of this village in the novel. Over time, Boykivske was inhabited by Germans, Russians, and Boykos.[35] Accordingly, the names of this village are Ostheim, Velykokrasnoshchokove, Telmanove, and Boykivske:

> In Ostheim, which was later named Velykokrasnoshchokove, Telmanove, and now Boikivske... In Ostheim, from which the Germans were expelled, and red cheeks were removed, where poor Boikos were brought from the Polish border, and where Thaelmann was forgotten. And later, to complete the picture, Thaelmann was remembered, and it was occupied just like Prague, by the Russian tanks.[36]

---

34 *Wikipedia* "Boykivske", Ukrainian-language article, https://uk.wikipedia.org/wiki/%D0%91%D0%BE%D0%B9%D0%BA%D1%96%D0%B2%D1%81%D1%8C%D0%BA%D0%B5 [accessed: 31.07.2024].

35 As N. V. Karpovets writes in the *Encyclopedia of Modern Ukraine*, "[t]he Boykos are a distinctive ethnographic group of Ukrainians who inhabit the central and western parts of the Ukrainian Carpathians. They have a separate area of settlement, Boykivshchyna, which is based on ethnographic, linguistic, and dialectal data". N. V. Karpovets, "Boykos", *Encyclopedia of Modern Ukraine*, vol. 3, 2004, https://esu.com.ua/article-36041 [accessed: 31.07.2024] [author's trans.].

36 Olena Stiazhkina, *Smert leva Sesila mala sens* (*Cecil the Lion Had to Die*), Lviv: "VSL", 2021, 28 [translated for this essay by Viktoria Marinesco]. The English translation of this novel, *Cecil the Lion Had to Die*, will be published in August 2024. See: Harvard University Press, "Cecil the Lion Had to Die", https://www.hup.harvard.edu/catalog.php?isbn=9780674291669 [accessed: 31.07.2024].

In 2016, the Russian occupation regime abolished the name Boykivske and restored the name Telmanove (as Stiazhkina writes above, "Thaelmann was remembered"[37]). The Ukrainian Boykivske vis-à-vis Telmanove in the Russian-occupied Donbas is a defocused image of a place that a person comes from. It is a place that emphasises the dispersion of people's history and can serve not only as a metonymy of the 'Donbas rift'[38] at the level of topography but also as a marker of Russian/Soviet totalitarian practices in Ukraine and abroad. The memory of these practices borders on oblivion and amnesia and is reproduced and forgotten selectively and simultaneously.

In their work, Stiazhkina and Rafeyenko emphasise that the historical fate of the people of the Donbas goes far beyond the borders of this region. The characters' fates bear the imprint of the processes that shaped the life in the Donbas and other regions of Soviet Ukraine, such as forced displacement, repressions, the Holodomor, and World War II. Therefore, the concept of the so-called 'separateness of the Donbas', with its own borders of memory and identity, needs a rethinking, and writers can create specific incentives.

Describing the frontier zone of the Donbas, the writers suggest that the historical memory of its inhabitants is deformed and truncated by the Soviet demographic experiment to form the so-called Soviet people from a heterogeneous mass of many generations of migrants who came to live in the Donbas mainly under the pressure of harsh circumstances, and not voluntarily. This experiment significantly slowed down the processes of national identity formation in this region. However, the Russian occupation of the Ukrainian Donbas in 2014 gave an impetus to a part of the population to realise their Ukrainian identity and, at the same time, their rootedness in this region.

In Stiazhkina's novel, the image of the tree of life drawn by Fink's adopted granddaughter, Dina, is a marker of the Donbas's very damaged but still living Ukrainian national potential: "The tree has a lot of problems. There are too many holes, blocked and forgotten sprouts, too much uprooting in the root system".[39] But the common history of the characters who embody the identity of the Ukrainian Donbas and chose to fight for this identity began here; thin and invisible thread-roots stretch from Donetsk to their deeply dramatic stories, prerequisites of the settlement of the Donbas.

Thus, the Donbas does not only reflect the course and consequences of long-term hybrid processes and hybrid war in the 21st century. It is also integrated into the processes of the self-affirmation of the Ukrainian nation, for which the war is a tragic

37 Ibid.

38 I borrow the concept 'Donbas rift' from Smolii and Yakubova. Smolii and Yakubova, *Donechchyna i Luhanshchyna*, 26.

39 Stiazhkina, *Smert leva Sesila mala sens*, 234.

catalyst, but a catalyst nonetheless. The works of Kiva, Rafeyenko, and Stiazhkina, who bear the imprint of the experience of an internally displaced person, confirm this reasoning. For these three writers, 'displacement' is not just about social status but a personal focus on the correlation of the past and the present in the symbolic parameters of eradication and rooting.[40]

In the essay "People of the Donbas", Kiva also reflects on the ambivalent meaning of the image of the tree for former residents of the Donbas now occupied by Russia. She speaks of war as a boundary of existential experience that someone else can only understand through empathy: "You can only grow a great tree of love from tears".[41] In the poem "Faina" (from the poetic cycle *People of the Donbas*), the poet uses the metaphor of "empty nests of roots",[42] which unfolds into a semantically complex picture of the interplay of anthropic, spiritual, symbolic, and natural beginnings as the basis of human space after the catastrophe of war. For her, a tree symbolises rooting in a place one can call their own, where they can start all over again:

> we leave lists of traces like snow in the margins
> stained with blood of freedom from textuality
> they will someday return home with our traces, the trees.[43]

In this regard, the themes of home and the lost home as a familiar lifeworld filled with stable values and meanings acquire a characteristic aesthetic manifestation. Kiva defines the phenomenon of exile and refugees in the case of Ukraine as "the loss of home within oneself".[44] This figurative formula points to the displaced person's persecution by the painful doubt that home, as the pivot and guarantee of a stable and worthwhile life, ever existed. The title of the anthology of poems by Kiva from 2015 to 2018, *Far from Paradise*, correlates with this theme, raising the question of what paradise really was and whether home was paradise. A home under occupation needs protection and help itself, like an unattended child or a raped woman.[45]

---

40 Simona Veil, *Ukorinennia. Lyst do kliryka* (*Rooting: A Letter to a Cleric*), trans. Mykola Riabchuk et al., Kyiv: D.L., 1998, 36.

41 Iya Kiva, "Ia ne vmiiu nenavydity i ne vmiiu udavaty nenavyst..." ("I don't know how to hate and I don't know how to pretend to hate..."), Facebook post, 09 May 2023, https://www.facebook.com/iya.kiva/posts/pfbidoiqoHm6xxRtnNTdxRD89nrFfCcVoSAiBvLZnF19pbfu9AP5Q5LSSAGmCagQ8EXKqDl [accessed: 31.07.2024].

42 Iya Kiva, "People of the Donbas", trans. Maru Mushtrieva and Eugene Ostashevsky, *Common knowledge* 28/3, 2022, 352–356, here 355, https://doi.org/10.1215/0961754X-10046446.

43 Ibid.

44 Kotsarev, "Iya Kiva".

45 Iya Kiva, "The Dead Flowers of Forgetting", trans. Stephen Komarnyckyj, *Poetry School*, https://poetryschool.com/articles/stanzas-for-ukraine-16/ [accessed: 31.07.2024].

The use of the Ukrainian language clearly influences the authors' styles, which can be described as a search for and justification of a new 'home of being'. The use of two languages, the play on local Donetsk idioms, and the Ukrainian-language discourse of the mythological Baba in Stiazhkina's novel reproduce and, at the same time, problematise the traditionally Russian-speaking landscape of this urban centre in Eastern Ukraine.

In *Mondegreen*, the protagonist's 'entry' into the Ukrainian language turns on the 'mechanism' of self-awareness through a return *ad fontes* of childhood, as indicated by the mythological motifs and elements of fairy-tale children's horror inherent in the novel. The reidentification of the protagonist is accompanied by the split of his consciousness, fantastic transformations, a play with words and sounds, and intertextual passages. However, the novel's architecture, which is "built on the Gospels",[46] reflects the complexity and unprecedented seriousness of constructing a new character's identity based on mastering the Ukrainian language.

Kiva also expresses the depth and importance of the problem of the language of creativity as the basis of the author's personality: "[W]riters do not use a ready-made language; they create a new one. Therefore, they cannot move anywhere but only make the language they will move into".[47] Following this thesis, we can say that the creative processes of all three authors are based on their internal search for a new linguistic and poetic identity in the Ukrainian language and Ukrainian culture. Literary scholarly interest in the collisions of this search is not well developed, with specialists' attention mostly focused on works on military subjects. However, it can only grow, as it is linked to an understanding of the depth and scope of decolonisation processes in Ukraine as a multiethnic and multicultural environment.

Bibliography

Andrukhovych, Iuriy, "Serhii Zhadan – Iuriiu Andrukhovychu: 'V mene zminylosia vidchuttia, pro koho ia pyshu, chyim holosom hovoriu'" ("Serhiy Zhadan – Iuriy Andrukhovych: 'I Have a New Sense of Who I Am Writing About and in Whose Voice I Am Speaking'"), *Craft Magazine*, 21 March 2022, https://craftmagazine.net/sergiy-zhadan-yuri-andruhovychu/# [accessed: 23.07.2024].

Harvard University Press, "Cecil the Lion Had to Die", https://www.hup.harvard.edu/catalog.php?isbn=9780674291669 [accessed: 23.07.2024].

Hundorova, Tamara, *Tranzytna kultura. Symptomy postkolonialnoi travmy: esei* (*Transit Culture: Symptoms of Postcolonial Trauma, Essays*), Kyiv: Hrani-T, 2012.

46 Rafeyenko, "Iak mova vyznachaie pamiat".

47 Kotsarev, "Iya Kiva".

Iurchenko, Olena, "Nam mova bolyt: iak obiednaty ukraintsiv navkolo ukrainskoii movy?" ("Our Language Hurts Us: How to Unite Ukrainians Around the Ukrainian Language?"), *Osvitoriia* (*Education*), https://osvitoria.media/experience/nam-mova-bolyt-yak-ob-yednaty-ukrayintsiv-navkolo-ukrayinskoyi-movy/ [accessed: 23.07.2024].

Karpovets, N. V., "Boykos", *Encyclopedia of Modern Ukraine*, vol. 3, 2004, https://esu.com.ua/article-36041 [accessed: 23.07.2024].

Kiva, Iya, "Hotuiuchys do odnoho vystupu, znov bachu zapytannia pro..." ("When preparing for a speech, I see the question about..."), Facebook post, 09 May 2023, https://www.facebook.com/iya.kiva/posts/pfbid02zJ6ZiXSsoDrbHq5qZz6mUUhPJH1wHVdBan9WCNLhnytsMhgc7vZg3bfLBuUpBoBVl [accessed: 23.07.2024].

Kiva, Iya, "Ia ne vmiiu nenavydity i ne vmiiu udavaty nenavyst..." ("I don't know how to hate and I don't know how to pretend to hate..."), Facebook post, 09 May 2023, https://www.facebook.com/iya.kiva/posts/pfbid0iqoHm6xxRtnNTdxRD89nrFfCcVoSAiBvLZnF19pbfu9AP5Q5LSSAGmCagQ8EXKqDl [accessed: 23.07.2024].

Kiva, Iya, "Podruha spytala mene, iak ia pochuvaiusia u Lvovi..." ("My friend asked me how I felt in Lviv..."), Facebook post, 30 January 2023, https://www.facebook.com/iya.kiva/posts/pfbid02ytzdtz4mrChBAHbJVh9TicbcF5y6rxEd9PyYQdLDWGqzepEFEuDY4eD2aznFXddcl [accessed: 23.07.2024].

Kiva, Iya, "The Dead Flowers of Forgetting", trans. Stephen Komarnyckyj, Poetry School, 2023, https://poetryschool.com/articles/stanzas-for-ukraine-16/ [accessed: 23.07.2024].

Kiva, Iya, "People of the Donbas", trans. Maru Mushtrieva and Eugene Ostashevsky, *Common knowledge* 28/3, 2022, 352–356.

Kiva, Iya, "Podali vid myru, blyzhche do peremohy" ("Away from Peace, Closer to Victory"), *Meridian Czernowitz*, 2023, https://www.meridiancz.com/blog/iia-kiva-podali-vid-myru-blyzhche-do-peremohy/ [accessed: 23.07.2024].

Kotsarev, Oleh, "Iya Kiva: 'Ni u formi viiny, ni u myrnoho protestu vykhid z teplykh imperskyh "bratskyh" obiimiv ne bude lehkym'" ("Iya Kiva: 'Neither in the Form of War Nor in the Form of Peaceful Protest Will it Be Easy to Get out of the Warm Imperial "Brotherly" Embrace'"), *LB.ua*, 22 September 2021, https://lb.ua/culture/2021/08/22/491968_iya_kiva_ni_formi_viyni_ni_formi.html [accessed: 23.07.2024].

Krasniashchykh, Andrii, "Iya Kiva: 'Tam, de vseredyni mene ranishe bula rosiiska, siohodni ia vidchuvaiu mertvoho zvira'", ("Iya Kiva: 'Where There Used to Be Russian Inside Me, Today I Feel a Dead Animal'"), *Ukrainska Pravda* (*Ukrainian Truth*), 24 July 2022, https://www.pravda.com.ua/articles/2022/07/24/7359716/ [accessed: 23.07.2024].

Kulyk, Volodymyr, "Mova ta identychnist v Ukraini na kinets 2022" ("Language and Identity in Ukraine at the End of 2022"), *Zbruč*, 01 January 2023, https://zbruc.eu/node/114247 [accessed: 23.07.2024].

Kulyk, Volodymyr, *Movna polityka v bahatomovnykh krainah: zakordonnyi dosvid ta ioho prydatnist dlia Ukrainy* (*Language Policy in Multilingual Countries: Foreign Experience and Its Applicability to Ukraine*), Kyiv: Dukh i Litera, 2021.

Matusiak, Agnieshka, *Vyity z movchannia: Dekolonialni zmahannia ukrainskoi kultury ta literatury XXI stolittia z posttotalitarnoiu travmoiu* (*Breaking Out of Silence: Decolonial Struggles of Ukrainian Culture and Literature of the Twenty-First Century with Post-Totalitarian Trauma*), Lviv: LA "Piramida", 2020.

Nebopak, Bohdana, and Vadym Blonskii, "Iryna Starovoit: 'Ukraina staie liudynotsentrychnoiu'" ("Iryna Starovoit: 'Ukraine is Becoming Human-Centred'"), *The Ukrainians*, 07 February 2022, https://theukrainians.org/iryna-starovojt-pen/ [accessed: 23.07.2024].

Rafeyenko, Volodymyr, *Mondegreen: Songs about Death and Love,* trans. Mark Andryczyk, Cambridge, MA: Harvard University Press, 2022.

Rafeyenko, Volodymyr, "Iak mova vyznachaie pamiat" ("How Language Determines Memory"), Zbruč, 19 August 2019, https://zbruc.eu/node/91540 [accessed: 23.07.2024].

Smolii, Valerii, and Larysa Yakubova, *Donechchyna i Luhanshchyna: mistse v modernomu ukrainskomu natsionalnomu proekti, Analitychna dopovid* (*The Donetsk and Luhansk Oblasts: Place in the Modern Ukrainian National Project, An Analytical Report*), Valerii Smolii (ed.), Kyiv: Institute of History of Ukraine of the National Academy of Sciences of Ukraine, 2015.

Stiazhkina, Olena, *Smert leva Sesila mala sens* (*Cecil the Lion Had to Die*), Lviv: "VSL", 2021.

Veil, Simona, *Ukorinennia. Lyst do kliryka* (*Rooting: A Letter to a Cleric*), trans. Mykola Riabchuk et al., Kyiv: D.L., 1998.

Vrublevskyi, Stanislav, "'Rosiiskoiu bilshe nichoho ne budu robyty. Ne khochu maty zhodnoho stosunku do tsiiei movy' – pysmennyk Volodymyr Rafeyenko" ("'I Will Not Do Anything in Russian Anymore. I Don't Want to Have Anything to Do with This Language' – Writer Volodymyr Rafeyenko"), *Suspilne Kultura* (*Public Culture*), 31 May 2022, https://suspilne.media/245037-rosijskou-bilse-nicogo-ne-budu-robiti-ne-hocu-mati-zodnogo-stosunku-do-ciei-movi-pismennik-volodimir-rafeenko/ [accessed: 23.07.2024].

Vydavnytso Staroho Leva (The Old Lion Publishing House), "Olena Stiazhkina: Knyha maie pokazaty shcho kozhen iz nas mozhe zminytysia" ("Olena Stiazhkina: A Book Should Show That Each of Us Can Change"), 25 June 2021, https://starylev.com.ua/news/olena-styazhkina-knyga-maye-pokazaty-shcho-kozhen-iz-nas-mozhe-zminytysya [accessed: 23.07.2024].

Wikipedia, "Boykivske", Ukrainian-language article, https://uk.wikipedia.org/wiki/%D0%91%D0%BE%D0%B9%D0%BA%D1%96%D0%B2%D1%81%D1%8C%D0%BA%D0%B5 [accessed: 23.07.2024].

Zernii, Iuliia, "Vzaiemozviazok istorychnoi pamiati ta natsionalnoi identychnosti" ("The Relationship Between Historical Memory and National Identity"), politychnyi menedzhment (political management) 5, 2008, 104–115.

Zhadan, Serhiy, "Kilka sliv pro nerozuminnia..." ("A few words about misunderstanding..."), Facebook post, 24 October 2019, https://www.facebook.com/100044170792676/posts/2436920353022885/ [accessed: 23.07.2024].

The Beginning of the Occupation

The City of Mariupol in Media Reports (Spring 2022)

Yuliia Soroka

The city of Mariupol has been occupied by Russian troops since 20 May 2022 and remains the largest occupied city of the Russo–Ukrainian War. Yet, when this territory of Ukraine will be liberated and de-occupied, how will Ukrainian society greet the citizens of Mariupol, who are currently under occupation? And how do these occupied people appear to those outside of the city during the war? The media holds the decisive role in predefining the answers to these questions. The military conditions and their consequences in Mariupol limit information access for those both in and outside of the city and result in a lack of communication, information isolation, propaganda distortions, and information restrictions by the military state. Thereby, an understanding of the events in Mariupol and their participants can mainly form based on media reports. Accordingly, the messages of these reports will be the basis for the postwar reintegration of Ukrainian society.

So as not to get lost in the many information narratives currently present, I isolated specific periods when the attention paid to the occupation of Mariupol was at its highest. I made this selection using the Google Trends web application, which shows the frequency of a particular search term compared to other search queries. Periods when the level of this indicator reached its maximum value are significant. This suggests that an audience's attention was highest at this time, and the presented media interpretations of events were the most widespread. Additionally, the events mentioned at these points were the most important, and their participants received the most attention.

A search of data over several years (starting in 2004) suggests that the leading indicators connected to Mariupol were in March 2022. I carried out this investigation in Ukrainian, Russian, and English. Although the dynamics of the popularity of search terms in the different languages vary, in March and April 2022, all three languages reached their highest level. Searching over the last 12 months gave me a more detailed and differentiated picture. The maximum index of the Ukrainian-language search appeared in the week of 13–20 March, the Russian-language search a week earlier, on 6–13 March, and the English-language search on 10–17 April. I carried out this data fixation through Google Trends on 3 November 2022, using the following Google Trends search options: all over the world, in the last 12 months, all categories, and internet search.

The following paper is an overview of media reports in Ukrainian, Russian, and English published during the above-mentioned periods and still available online through Google search. The reviewed reports give three perspectives of the events: two from countries that are direct participants in the war and one from 'external' observers. To focus on these perspectives, I excluded from this analysis translations of reports from, for example, Ukrainian mass media into English, Russian into English, Ukrainian into Russian, or English into Ukrainian or Russian. In the text, I name the three perspectives as Ukrainian-speaking, Russian-speaking, and English-speaking, corresponding to the data that I analysed. Each language is separated into its own section of the text. Stylistically, these sections function as collages made from the main news stories. I have provided quotes or information from the news sources in the text, while writing the details of the sources in the footnotes.

I associate the Ukrainian-speaking and Russian-speaking perspectives with public discourses on the war in the respective countries, although the definitive argumentation of such a connection requires further research. Linking English-language messages to specific official or ideological discourses also requires more research. This study of the three language-based perspectives is relevant when considering the average media consumer. Lacking the capacity for multilingual communication and access to independent analyses of information, many consumers of internet news, and those using Google in particular, fall into the space of a certain language, where the 'political', the 'ideological', and the 'sociocultural' exist as part of an indistinguishable naturalised whole.[1] The English-language perspective, for instance, has changed during the war. Or, more specifically, the official positions of European countries have shifted. It is, however, essential to record what these positions were initially. That is, which events news stories paid attention to and which actors they highlighted in the said stories.

The focus of such stories in my research is Mariupol. Located on the northern coast of the Sea of Azov, before the war it was the tenth most populous city in Ukraine (with about 440,000 inhabitants). It is known primarily for its metallurgical and machine-building industries (e.g., the Ilyich, Azovstal, and Azovmash plants) and the seaport, which played a significant role in Ukrainian exports of industrial and agricultural products. In the 16th century, Zaporizhian Cossacks founded a settlement at the mouth of the Kalmius River on the territory of present-day Mariupol (starting with the Domakha Fortress) as a stopping point on their trading route running

1 For more on the concept of naturalisation as a cultural mechanism of power, see: Yuliia Soroka, "Denaturalisation of Collective Identities within pro-Euromaidan Discourse (on field of Facebook Representation)", *Władza Sądzenia (Judicial Power)* 8, 2016, 42–54.

from the Dnipro River to the Black Sea. The settlements around the fortress focused on agriculture, crafts, and trade. Through these industries and the Russian imperial policy of settling the northern Azov region (in particular, the resettlement of Orthodox Greeks from Crimea) at the end of the 18th century, the county town of Mariupol appeared, officially founded in 1778.[2] In the contemporary inhabitants' imagination, the commercial and industrial achievements of the city (e.g., the Azovstal Metallurgical Plant, a flagship of Soviet industrialisation) often overshadow Mariupol's cultural distinctiveness and ethnic diversity. The city has also always been in the shadow of Donetsk, the oblast's centre, while simultaneously having a competitive advantage over it – namely, a seacoast with beaches within the city's limits and connected to nearby villages. In 1948, the city was renamed Zhdanov, in honour of Joseph Stalin's associate, Andriy Zhdanov, who was born there. In 1989, a civil movement pushed for the return of the city's historical name.[3] This movement can be seen as a part of the larger sociopolitical tectonic shifts that preceded the declaration of independent Ukraine.

Siege, Shelling and Bombing, and Humanitarian Hell: Ukrainian-Language Sources

On 13–20 March 2022, Mariupol was already under siege by the Russian Army and the so-called Donetsk People's Republic (DNR). This section details the situation in Mariupol based on the Ukrainian-language sources I consulted for this period. On 13 March 2022, *Word and Deed* (*Slovo i dilo*) and *The Voice of Ukraine* (*Holos Ukrainy*) wrote, respectively:

2 D. Ya. Telegin, M. Lillie, I. D. Potekhina, and M. M. Kovaliukh, "Settlement and economy in Neolithic Ukraine: a new chronology", *Antiquity* 77/297, 2003, 456–470, https://doi.org/10.1017/S0003598X00092528; V. O. Pirko, *Zaselennia i hospodarske osvoennia Stepovoi Ukrainy v XVI-XVIII st.* (*Settlement and Economic Development of the Ukrainian Steppe in the 16th–18th Centuries*), Donetsk: Skhidnyi Publishing House, 2004; A. Z. Didova (ed.), *Nashchadky kozakiv u Donbasi: kozatskomu rodu nema perevodu* (*Descendants of the Cossacks in the Donbas: There is No Substitute for the Cossack Family*), Donetsk: Donbass, 2005; and Roman Adrian Cybriwsky, "Mariupol: Seaside City", in: *The Ukrainian Panorama: Dispatches from the Road about People, Places, Progress, and Problems*, Kyiv: Dnipro-Podil Books, 2019, 311–318.

3 Yuliia Soroka, "Vid Zhdanova do Mariupolia: pytannia pereimenuvannia mista u publikatsiiakh mistsevoi presy" ("From Zhdanov to Mariupol: The Issue of Renaming the City in the Local Press"), in: O. K. Mikheevoi (ed.), 2010, *Sotsiolohiia mista* (*Sociology of the City*), Donetsk: Knowledge Publishing House, 329–353.

> Since Russia's invasion of Ukraine began, about 100 aerial bombs have been dropped on Mariupol, and 2,187 civilians have already died. This was reported by the press service of the Mariupol City Council on Sunday, 13 March.[4]
>
> Russian troops took this fortress of the Ukrainian south by storm. They artificially created a humanitarian disaster there: they blocked the "green corridors" to the city, prevented the evacuation of the population, prevented the passage of humanitarian goods, and robbed them. Every day, the blocked city is "ironed" from the air by Russian "liberators".[5]

In an address on 13 March 2022, the President of Ukraine, Volodymyr Zelenskyy, referred to 100 tonnes of humanitarian cargo accompanied by Orthodox priests, which the Russian occupiers did not allow to enter.[6] Meanwhile, there was no information about diplomatic actions taken to organise humanitarian corridors.

The Telegram channel of the Mariupol City Council became a vital information source for the media. Quoting it, as done below, the media reported on airstrikes and casualties:

> The occupiers cynically and purposefully hit residential buildings and crowds of people, destroyed children's hospitals, and destroyed the city's infrastructure. Each bombardment brings terrible destruction and claims the most important thing – the lives of peaceful Mariupol residents.[7]

At the same time, the General Staff of the Armed Forces of Ukraine emphasised that the city was heroically defending itself and that the Russian occupiers violated international humanitarian laws.[8]

---

4 *Slovo i dilo* (*Word and Deed*), "Zelenskyy rozrakhovue na dostavku humdopomohy do Mariupolia" ("Zelenskyy Expects Humanitarian Aid to Be Delivered to Mariupol"), 13 March 2022, https://www.slovoidilo.ua/2022/03/13/novyna/polityka/zelenskyj-rozraxovuye-dostavku-humdopomohy-mariupolya [accessed: 23.07.2023] [author's trans.].

5 Olha Baulina, "Mariupol stav mistom-muchenykom liutoi viyny, iaka spustoshue Ukrainu" ("Mariupol Has Become a Martyr-City of the Fierce War That Is Devastating Ukraine"), Holos Ukrainy (The Voice of Ukraine), 13 March 2022, http://www.golos.com.ua/article/357153 [accessed: 31.07.2024] [author's trans.].

6 Slovo i dilo, "Zelenskyy rozrakhovue na".

7 Novynarnia (Newsroom), "Trahediia Mariupolia: rosiiany vbyly vzhe maizhe 2200 tsyvilnykh" ("The Tragedy of Mariupol: Russians Have Already Killed Almost 2200 Civilians"), 13 March 2022, https://novynarnia.com/2022/03/13/tragediya-mariupolya-rosiyany-vbyly-vzhe-majzhe-2200-czyvilnyh/ [accessed: 31.07.2024] [author's trans.].

8 Violetta Orlova, "Sproby okupantiv zakhopyty Mariupol zalyshaiutsia bezuspishnymy – Henshtab ZSU" ("The Attempts of the Occupants to Capture Mariupol Remain Unsuccessful – The General Staff of the Armed Forces of Ukraine"), UNIAN, 14 March 2022, https://www.unian.ua/war/viyna-z-rosiyeyu-sprobi-okupantiv-zahopiti-mari

In the city, 80 percent of the housing stock was destroyed. Following damage to civilian infrastructure, there was no access to electricity, drinking water, and gas, and people hid from airstrikes wherever they could.[9] From 50 to 100 aerial bombs were dropped on the city per day. The mayor of Mariupol reported that the registered number of civilian casualties, whose bodies were found in the streets and buried, was 2,358.[10] Doctors and patients of the regional intensive care hospital, who were hiding in its undamaged basement, were held by the occupiers and could not leave.[11]

The media reported three more events on 16 March 2022. An airstrike destroyed the Neptune Pool, which served as a shelter for residents around the Ilyich Steel and Iron Works. Pregnant women, women in labour, and children from a nearby maternity hospital were killed in the pool building.[12] In the centre of the city, an aerial bomb was dropped on a theatre. People from the surrounding areas and those who remained in the city centre after the evacuation attempts on 5 March 2022 were hiding in its basement and on its other floors.[13] "Around 3:30 p.m., the Russian occupiers fired at a convoy of civilians evacuating from Mariupol to Zaporizhzhia with a BM-21 Grad MLRS".[14]

According to various sources (the Mariupol City Council, the Azov Regiment, and the former head of the Donetsk Oblast State Administration, Serhiy Taruta), there

---

upol-zalishayutsya-bezuspishnimi-novini-vtorgnennya-rosiji-v-ukrajinu-11742391.html [accessed: 31.07.2024].

9 Radio Svoboda (Radio Freedom), "Radnyk mera Mariupolia: kilkist zahyblykh u misti mozhe nablyzhatysia do 20 tysiach" ("The Advisor to the Mariupol Mayor: The Death Toll in the City Could Be Approaching 20 Thousand"), 15 March 2022, https://www.radiosvoboda.org/a/news-mariupol-zahybli/31752967.html [accessed: 31.07.2024].

10 Kateryna Shapoval, "'Liudei khovaiut v bratskykh mohylakh, deiakykh – u svoikh dvorakh': Interviu zastupnyka mera Mariupolia pro katastrofu v misti" ("'People Are Buried in Mass Graves, Some in Their Own Yards': Interview with the Deputy Mayor of Mariupol About the Disaster in the City"), Forbes, 16 March 2022, https://forbes.ua/inside/intervyu-mariupol-16032022-4685 [accessed: 23.07.2024].

11 Tetiana Kotenko, "Rashysty u Mariupoli vzialy u zaruchnyky likariv ta patsientiv" ("Ruscists in Mariupol Take Doctors and Patients Hostage"), Hlavkom, 15 March 2022, https://glavcom.ua/country/criminal/rashisti-u-mariupoli-vzyali-u-zaruchniki-likariv-ta-pacijentiv-830022.html [accessed: 23.07.2024].

12 Suspilne (Society), "Rosiiki viiskovi z 'Hradiv' obstrilialy kolonu avtivok, iaki ikhaly z Mariupolia – shtab ZSU" ("Russian Servicemen Fired at a Convoy of Vehicles Travelling from Mariupol with Grad Multiple Rocket Launchers – Ukrainian Armed Forces HQ"), 16 March 2022, https://suspilne.media/218279-rosijki-vijskovi-z-gradiv-obstrilali-kolonu-avtivok-aki-ihali-z-mariupola-stab-zsu/ [accessed: 23.07.2024].

13 Roman Petrenko, "Rosiiany skynuly nadpotuzhnu bombu na dramteatr Mariupolia, de khovaiutsia sotni liudei" ("Russians Drop a High-Powered Bomb on Mariupol Drama Theatre Where Hundreds of People Are Hiding"), Pravda (Truth) 16 March 2023, https://www.pravda.com.ua/news/2022/03/16/7331956/ [accessed: 23.07.2024].

14 Suspilne, "Rosiiki viiskovi z 'Hradiv'" [author's trans.].

were between 600 and 1,200 people in the drama theatre before the explosion; after the explosion, about 130 people survived. About 100 people – that is, everyone in the field kitchen outside the theatre during the shelling – died. Later, a bomb was dropped on an art school in the Left Bank District of the city.[15] A day earlier, representatives of the Red Cross left the city. On the way out, locals also trying to leave saw their cars.[16]

We also learn about events in the city from the eyewitness testimonies of Mariupol residents. Occasionally, people got internet access and sent a message or made a phone call. These stories then made their way to journalists from people's friends or relatives. Reporters also managed to talk to people who were able to leave the city and save themselves. On 14 March 2022, an agreement was reached to create a corridor for citizens to leave Mariupol, although, "they [the Russians] did not allow humanitarian aid [to enter]".[17] Further witness testimonies are below.

After the city had been blockaded for one week, Anna, a resident of Mariupol, was miraculously able to make a call, and an audio recording was shared with a newsroom. She said:

> Everything is terrible and hard for us today. [...] We're trembling. The floors are all shaking from the [explosive] wave. [...] They're just shooting wherever they can. It flies into the yard. [...] There will be a natural disaster. Everything is on fire. The corpses lie [around]. They bury them in the park. Just bury them. There is no glass [in the windows]. [...] There is no water. [...] 3,000 people are sitting in basements. I don't know what will happen next. But it can't get any worse. [...] There is nothing to hit here anymore. There are just residential buildings. The military isn't particularly visible here. I don't know why they're shooting![18]

---

15 Khmarochos (Skyscraper), "Mariupol: bomby na shkolu mystetstv, nasylne vyvezennia do RF, holodomor u susidnikh selakh" ("Mariupol: Bombs Hit an Art School, Forced Deportation to Russia, Famine in Neighbouring Villages"), 20 March 2022, https://hmarochos.kiev.ua/2022/03/20/mariupol-bomby-na-shkolu-mystecztv-nasylne-vyvezennya-do-rf-golodomor-u-susidnih-selah/ [accessed: 23.07.2024].

16 0629.com, "Chervonyi Khrest zalyshyv Mariupol. A yak zhe poraneni?" ("The Red Cross Has Left Mariupol. What About the Wounded?"), 16 March 2022, https://www.0629.com.ua/news/3351323/cervonij-hrest-zalisiv-mariupol-a-ak-ze-poraneni [accessed: 23.07.2024].

17 Iurii Bratiuk, "Arestovych poiasnyv, chomu zaraz ne mozhna vriatuvaty Mariupol viiskovym shliakhom" ("Arestovych Explains Why Mariupol Cannot Be Saved by Military Means Now"), zaxid.net, 18 March 2022, https://zaxid.net/arestovich_poyasniv_chomu_zaraz_ne_mozhna_vryatuvati_mariupol_viyskovim_shlyahom_n1538838 [accessed: 23.07.2024] [author's trans.].

18 Anastasiia Fedchenko, "'Trupy lezhat na vulytsiakh. Ikh zakopuiut tam zhe na shtyklopatu'. Monoloh zhytelky Mariupolia" ("'Corpses Are Lying in the Streets. They Are Buried There with Bayonets and Shovels': A Monologue by a Resident of Mariupol"), Novynarnia

Anna Murlykina, a journalist from Mariupol, also wrote about her acquaintances:

> The family has very little gas left. They keep it as the most valuable treasure. Because these 20 litres of fuel are their last hope for survival. The last hope to make it to the humanitarian corridor, get into an old car, and escape from this hell that Russia has created.[19]

Oksana, a 46-year-old local woman who managed to leave on 4 March 2022, told a journalist that there was "an air raid every twenty minutes. Bombs destroy everything indiscriminately. Residential high-rise buildings. Schools. Hospitals. Administrative buildings".[20] She does not provide her last name out of fear for her husband and parents, who stayed behind in a basement without water or food. The same article has a statement from 28-year-old Diana Palkina from Kyiv, who has close relatives in Mariupol: "It's simply a genocide. They are being starved to death, freezing to death. Plus, the airstrikes that kill hundreds of innocent people. No words can describe what is happening – it is beyond human morality".[21]

A resident of Kyiv shared messages from her brother in Mariupol with journalists. His SMS messages, starting at the beginning of the invasion and lasting until 14 March 2022, became a diary of the siege:

> Houses are burning, many people with children are in basements, we have about 30 people [here]. There are dead people, they're being gathered in a nearby store. [...] There is no government, people are abandoned. There are no police, firefighters, or others. Deaths from hypothermia, malnutrition, disease, and the inability to move will soon begin.[22]

(Newsroom), 11 March 2022, https://novynarnia.com/2022/03/11/trupy-lezhat-na-vulyczyah-mariupol/ [accessed: 23.07.2024] [author's trans.].

19 Anna Murlykina, "'Donechko, shcho vidbuvaetsia?' Yak vyzhyvaiut mariupoltsi v pekli shchodennoho znyshchennia" ("'My Daughter, What's Going On?' How Mariupol Residents Survive in the Hell of Daily Destruction"), Texty (Texts), 13 March 2023, https://texty.org.ua/articles/105960/donechka-sho-vidbuvayetsya-yak-vyzhyvayut-mariupolci-v-pekli-shodennoho-znyshennya/ [accessed: 23.07.2024] [author's trans.].

20 Maksim Butchenko, "Misto u vohni. Tila na vulytsiakh, vidsutnist vody ta izhi ta postiinyi vohon po zhytlovykh masyvakh – rozpovidi mariupoltsiv" ("The City Is on Fire. Bodies on the Streets, a Lack of Water and Food, and the Constant Shelling of Residential Areas – Stories from Mariupol Residents"), New Voice, 14 March 2022, https://nv.ua/ukr/ukraine/events/mariupol-zhive-pid-postiynimi-obstrilami-bez-vodi-ta-jizhi-50224909.html [accessed: 23.07.2024] [author's trans.].

21 Ibid.

22 Viktoriia Prysedska, "'Zahyblykh skladaiut u susidnomu mahazyni'. Shchodennyk z blokadnoho Mariupolia" ("'The Dead Are Being Buried in a Nearby Shop': A Diary from Blockaded Mariupol"), BBC, 15 March 2022, https://www.bbc.com/ukrainian/features-60750253 [accessed: 23.07.2024] [author's trans.].

In an interview, a woman explained how she decided to leave, choosing between the mortal danger of staying and the mortal danger of going: "I understood that we might not make it, that we might be shot, hit a mine, or come under shelling, but I also understood that we would die in Mariupol. And we had to take the risk".[23] In another interview, Yulia, a 30-year-old woman, talked about the lack of contact with those who remained: "On the one hand, you are happy that you were able to leave, and on the other hand, you want to cry because there are loved ones who are still in danger, you don't know what happened to them, where they are".[24] A local journalist reported that there was

> [c]onstant shelling, rockets, bombs. Piles that no one can sort out. Fires that no one can put out. Human bodies that no one hides. Not a single hospital, not a single safe house remains. People are surviving in basements, collecting water from puddles, starving and praying to be saved.[25]

In these messages, people who were left alone under tragic circumstances with numerous threats to their lives retell their experiences. Some of them managed to escape with relatives, acquaintances, colleagues, or the help of volunteers, who were from the territories controlled by Ukraine. Some were saved thanks to their own desperate efforts. Dmytro from Mariupol, for example, swam in the Sea of Azov for three hours until he was able to get to the shore of a seaside village, from which he reached

23 Televiziinoi sluzhby novyn (TSN) (Television news service), "'U Mariupoli my zahynemo, treba ryzykuvaty': istoriia zhinky, iaka zmohla vyrvatysia z otochenoho okupantamy mista" ("'We Will Die in Mariupol, We Have to Take a Risk': The Story of a Woman Who Managed to Escape from the City Surrounded by the Occupiers"), 15 March 2022, https://tsn.ua/ato/u-mariupoli-mi-zaginemo-treba-rizikuvati-istoriya-zhinki-yaka-zmogla-virvatisya-z-otochenogo-okupantami-mista-2009971.html [accessed: 23.07.2024] [author's trans.].

24 Ksiusha Savoskina, "'Shchodnia my liahaly spaty i ne znaly, chy prokynemos'. Istoriia zhytelky Mariupolia, iakii vdalosia vybratysia z mista" ("'Every Day We Went to Bed and Did Not Know Whether We Would Wake Up': The Story of a Mariupol Resident Who Managed to Get Out of the City"), hromadske (mass), 16 March 2022, https://hromadske.ua/posts/shodnya-mi-lyagali-spati-i-ne-znali-chi-prokinemos-istoriya-zhitelki-mariupolya-yakij-vdalosya-vibratisya-z-mista [accessed: 23.07.2024] [author's trans.].

25 Kateryna Rodak, "'U susidnomu budynku zhinku rozirvalo, ii khovaly na podviri': Ruskii mir v Mariupoli" ("'In the Neighbouring House, a Woman Was Torn to Pieces, and She Was Buried in the Yard': The Russian World in Mariupol"), zahid.net, 18 March 2022, https://zaxid.net/v_susidnomu_budinku_zhinku_rozirvalo_yiyi_hovali_na_podviryi_n1538736 [accessed: 23.07.2024] [author's trans.].

Zaporizhzhia.[26] Some people remained, and it is unclear whether they survived. And some were taken to the territory of the Russian Federation.[27]

During the considered period, Ukrainian media also reprinted material that featured Mariupol in a broader cultural and historical context:

> The Greeks of Nadazov remember each of their homelands: from the valleys of the Peloponnese and Anatolia to the slopes of the Crimean Mountains. This memory allows them to reproduce an almost erased image of themselves every time. Despite past hardships, deportations, and executions. Despite the current division by Russian aggression (first published in 2020).[28]

Such stories also mentioned the Cossack outpost of Domakha, which was the centre of the Kalmius palanquin of the Zaporizhian Cossacks, a place of the development of industries and trade, and a border fortress. This historical reference concluded by saying that, "in the middle of the 17th century, the expansion from the east stopped in Mariupol" (first published in 2014 in the newspaper United Ukraine, Ukraina yedyna).[29]

Alongside the history, the memory of the 2014 events in Mariupol was also updated:

> [Mariupol, a]n outpost of Ukrainian independence. Here, they've known well since 2014 what the "Russian world" is. [...] At that time, the people of Mariupol were under the control of the militants of the self-proclaimed DNR for a month and even survived a pseudo-referendum. Despite the ambiguous situation, they still managed to expel the separatists and Russian occupiers from the city and the government. [...] Even before the beginning of the invasion, the people of Mariupol publicly declared that they were ready to go to demonstrations every day, proving that Mariupol is Ukraine and Russia is the aggressor country. And Mariupol has no flowers for them.[30]

---

26 Nastoiashchee Vremia. Ciuzhety (The Present Tense: Stories), "Pobeh yz Maryupolia vplav" ("Escaped Mariupol by Swimming"), YouTube video, 15 April 2022, 3:53, https://www.youtube.com/watch?v=lg_Olq6li-Q [accessed: 23.07.2024].

27 Khmarochos, "Mariupol".

28 Mykhailo Drapak, "Mariupol ta hreky: zberehty svii dim" ("Mariupol and the Greeks: Saving Your Home"), Lokalna Istoraiia (Local History), 17 March 2022, https://localhistory.org.ua/texts/reportazhi/mariupol-tse-ukrayina/ [accessed: 23.07.2024] [author's trans.].

29 Maksim Maiorov, "Mariupol zupynyv navalu zi skhodu" ("Mariupol Stops an Invasion from the East"), istorychna pravda (historical truth), 18 March 2022, https://www.istpravda.com.ua/columns/2022/03/18/161082/ [accessed: 23.07.2024] [author's trans.].

30 Instytut Prosvity (Institute of Enlightenment), "Mariupol: zhyva rana Ukrainy ta druhyi Niurnberh dlia tsyvilizovanoho suspilstva" ("Mariupol: Ukraine's Open Wound and a Second Nuremberg for Civilised Society"), 18 March 2022, https://iprosvita.com/ma

By 19 March 2022, the defenders of Mariupol – the Azov Regiment, the soldiers of the marines, and the National Guard – were surrounded, yet "continue[d] to defend the city and wait for help".[31] The same article states that,

> [f]or the defence of Mariupol, the defenders of the city – the commander of the Azov Regiment, Denis Prokopenko "Redis", and the commander of the 36th Marine Brigade, Volodymyr Baraniuk – received the title of Hero of Ukraine.[32]

The Liberation of the Territory of the DNR by the National Militia under the Cover of Russian Troops: Russian-Language Sources

In Russian-language media from 6–13 March 2022, Mariupol appears as "the hottest spot after Volnovakha was liberated".[33] These stories represent a different perspective from those given above. Here, the Russian Federation calls itself a liberator. Despite my impulse to deny and refute the invader's claims, I give these Russian-language narratives to show how they present the events and residents of Mariupol.

In the Russian-language publication regnum, these texts were published as part of the recurring thematic broadcast on the 'special military operation' (spetsialnaia voiennaia operatsiia). The theme was titled "The History of this Issue" and started with Vladimir Putin's speech from 24 February 2022. In the speech, Putin explains that the operation was to be a "protection against the actions of the nationalist junta" in Kyiv, which the West supports, and the "demilitarisation and denazification" of the territories of Ukraine. Another text that was part of this broadcast mentioned that "earlier, the heads of the DNR and LNR [the Luhansk People's Republic] asked Vladimir Putin to help repel the aggression of the Kyiv regime to avoid casualties among the peaceful population and a humanitarian disaster in the Donbas".[34]

In Russian-language reports, the leading actors in events connected to Mariupol were the 'military units of the Donbas republics' and the 'People's Militia of the DNR', which, "with the support of the Russian Armed Forces, are liberating their territory

---

riupol-zhyva-rana-ukrainy-ta-druhyj-niurnberh-dlia-tsyvilizovanoho-suspilstva/ [accessed: 23.07.2024] [author's trans.].

31 Viktor Kruk, "Ukrainski '300 spartantsiv': zakhysnyky Mariupolia vidtiahnuly na sebe 10% armii okupantiv" ("The Ukrainian '300 Spartans': The Defenders of Mariupol Repelled 10% of the Occupiers' Army"), Telehraf (Telegraph), 19 March 2022, https://www.telegraf.in.ua/kremenchug/10104272-ukrajinski-300-spartanciv-zahisniki-mariupolja-vidtjagnula-na-sebe-10-armiji-okupantiv.html [accessed: 23.07.2024] [author's trans.].

32 Ibid.

33 regnum, "Pushilin: Mariupol – samaya goryachaya tochka posle Volnovakhi" ("Pushilin: Mariupol is the Hottest Point after Volnovakha"), 12 March 2022, https://regnum.ru/news/3531173 [accessed: 27.01.2024] [author's trans.].

34 Ibid.

from Ukrainian occupation".[35] The same article reported that these military units approached the Azovstal plant.[36]

The Ministry of Defence of the Russian Federation reported that "armed forces strike only at military infrastructure and Ukrainian troops".[37] These sources also blamed the Ukrainian authorities and the military for the difficult humanitarian situation "in this city [Mariupol], like in many others".[38] Lastly, according to such sources, Ukrainians "reject the majority of Russian initiatives to evacuate civilians from combat areas [and] prohibit civilians from leaving the city on their own".[39] These Russian-language articles described military actions with emotionally neutral military expressions (e.g., "tighten the ring",[40] "squeeze the enemy",[41] "strike",[42] "ensure a safe exit",[43] etc.).

Other sources reported on the consequences of the actions of the Russian troops, and that the Russian Ministry of Defence denied them. For instance, following the airstrike on the maternity hospital on 9 March 2022, Russian representatives accused Ukraine of "staged provocation".[44] Among other things, statements from a local resident named Ihor, who was evacuated to the village of Bezymenne, served as

---

35 EurAsia Daily, "V Mariupole voiska DNR vyshli k zavodu 'Azovstal' – Minoborony" ("In Mariupol, DNR Troops Reached the Azovstal Plant – Defence Ministry"), 10 March 2022, https://eadaily.com/ru/news/2022/03/10/v-mariupole-voyska-dnr-vyshli-k-zavodu-azovstal-minoborony [accessed: 23.07.2024] [author's trans.].

36 Ibid.

37 Krasnaia Vesna (Red Spring), "Zhiteli Mariupolya vyrazili zhelanie, chtoby natsionalisty ubralis iz goroda" ("Mariupol Residents Expressed Their Desire for Nationalists to Get Out of the City"), 08 March 2022, https://rossaprimavera.ru/news/bb28287a [accessed: 23.07.2024] [author's trans.].

38 Roman Kretsul and Bogdan Stepovoi, "V gorodskoi cherte: podrazdeleniya Donbassa prodolzhayut osvobozhdat Mariupol" ("Within the City Limits: Donbas Units Continue to Liberate Mariupol"), Izvestia (News), 11 March 2022, https://iz.ru/1303439/roman-kretcul-bogdan-stepovoi/v-gorodskoi-cherte-podrazdeleniia-donbassa-prodolzhaiut-osvobozhdat-mariupol [accessed: 23.07.2023] [author's trans.].

39 Ibid.

40 Krasnaia Vesna, "Zhiteli Mariupolya".

41 Kretsul and Stepovoi, "V gorodskoi cherte".

42 Krasnaia Vesna, "Zhiteli Mariupolya".

43 Violetta Khaneneva, "V DNR soobshchili o rasstrele natsionalistami mirnykh grazhdan, pokidavshikh Mariupol" ("The DNR Reported that Nationalists Shot Civilians Fleeing Mariupol"), gazeta.ru (newspaper.ru), 06 March 2022, https://www.gazeta.ru/army/news/2022/03/06/17389471.shtml?updated [accessed: 23.07.2024] [author's trans.]; and Moskva24, "Mariupol zablokirovan, vse mosty i podstupy k gorodu razrusheny – Minoborony RF" ("Mariupol Blocked, All Bridges and Entrances to the City Destroyed – the Russian Defence Ministry"), 11 March 2022, https://www.m24.ru/news/politika/11032022/439609 [accessed: 23.07.2024] [author's trans.].

44 RIA Novosti (RIA News), "V Minoborony nazvali 'aviaudar' po Mariupolyu srezhissirovannoy provokatsiei" ("The Defence Ministry Called the 'Airstrike' on Mariupol an Orches-

the basis for this explanation. Ihor, whose mother was an employee of the maternity hospital, said that "the [Ukrainian] military broke all the locks, dispersed the staff of the maternity hospital, and set up firing points in the building".[45]

Russian news called Ukrainian participants in the events in Mariupol nationalists. Articles claimed that these Ukrainians shot at a humanitarian convoy and mined the city's main roads.[46] When articles mentioned the Azov Regiment, instead of calling them by just a generalisation (e.g., 'nationalists'), they always indicated that this is an "extremist organisation prohibited in the Russian Federation".[47]

According to these sources, residents evacuated from Mariupol "express their desire for the nationalists to leave the city",[48] gratefully accept Russian humanitarian and medical aid, and agree to the conditions of their stays in the temporary accommodation points.[49] At the same time, representatives of the DNR police were suspicious of residents of the 'liberated' village of Talakovka: "It is important to understand that the locals are favourable to us at first glance. They smile at you, wave, but could just as well stick a knife in your back".[50]

Mariupol is a Strategic Goal of the Russian Federation and Revenge for Their Defeat Near Kyiv: English-Language Sources

In English-language reports from 10–17 April 2022, Mariupol is completely surrounded and the site of the "fiercest urban warfare" since the beginning of the invasion.[51] Such articles called Mariupol a southern port of Ukraine, whose population before the war was about 400,000 inhabitants. Six weeks of fighting, shelling, and bombing destroyed a large part of the city, as confirmed by satellite

---

trated Provocation"), 10 March 2022, https://ria.ru/20220310/provokatsiya-1777547947.html [accessed: 23.07.2024] [author's trans.].

45 Dmitrii Plotnikov, "'Bolshe nedeli im ne proderzhatsya'. Zhiteli Mariupolya – o gumanitarnoi katastrofe, kotoraya razvorachivaetsya u nikh na glazakh" ("'They Won't Last More Than a Week': Mariupol Residents on the Humanitarian Catastrophe Unfolding Before Their Eyes"), lenta.ru, 08 March 2022, https://lenta.ru/articles/2022/03/08/mariupol/ [accessed: 23.07.2024] [author's trans.].

46 Khaneneva, "V DNR soobshchili"; and Moskva24, "Mariupol zablokirovan".

47 Kretsul and Stepovoi, "V gorodskoi cherte".

48 Krasnaya Vesna, "Zhiteli Mariupolya".

49 Plotnikov, "'Bolshe nedeli im ne proderzhatsya'".

50 Dmitrii Grigoriev, "Kak bliz Mariupolya nachalas denatsifikatsiya Ukrainy" ("How the Denazification of Ukraine Began near Mariupol"), URA.RU, 11 March 2022, https://ura.news/articles/1036284140 [accessed: 23.07.2024] [author's trans.].

51 Emma Brown and Taylor Umlauf, "After More Than a Month of Fighting, Much of Mariupol Lies in Ruins", The Wall Street Journal, 17 April 2022, https://www.wsj.com/articles/mariupol-in-ruins-11650132943 [accessed: 23.07.2024].

image analysis. The number of deaths among the population was not known. Residents remained without electricity, water, and communication, and many could not evacuate. The media referenced President Zelenskyy, who reported that tens of thousands of Mariupol residents were killed,[52] and quoted Foreign Minister Dmytro Kuleba, who apocalyptically stated that "[t]he city doesn't exist anymore".[53]

English-language media consistently pointed to the uncertainty of reporting war events, particularly when referring to the claims of the Russian Federation. One article, for example, stated that "Russia said on Wednesday [that] more than 1,000 Ukrainian marines, among the last defenders holed up in the Azovstal industrial district, had surrendered, though Ukraine did not confirm that".[54] These sources referenced both the Russian claims that they were gaining control over the city and the Ukrainian claims that the fighting was continuing: "Ukraine Says Mariupol Has Not Fallen" (headline).[55] Ukraine's statements about the use of chemical weapons on the city's territory remained unconfirmed: "Ukrainian authorities are investigating a report by troops in the port city of Mariupol that they came under a Russian chemical-weapons attack on Monday".[56] Ukraine also claimed that tens of thousands were killed in Mariupol and accused Russian troops of torture and executions; Reuters, for instance, "confirmed widespread destruction in Mariupol but could not verify the alleged crimes".[57]

These media sources marked the dramatic culmination of the military confrontation by announcing the deadline for surrender that the Russian command set for the Ukrainian military in Mariupol. Media reports on this topic gestured to their

---

52 BBC, "Mariupol: Battle for key port city continues, Ukraine says", 11 April 2022, https://www.bbc.com/news/world-europe-61068650 [accessed: 23.07.2024].

53 CBS News, "Transcript: Ukrainian Foreign Minister Dmytro Kuleba on 'Face the Nation'", 17 April 2022 https://www.cbsnews.com/news/dmytro-kuleba-transcript-face-the-nation-04-17-2022 [accessed: 23.07.2024].

54 Pavel Polityuk and Natalia Zinets, "Explainer: Mariupol: ruins of port could become Russia's first big prize in Ukraine", Reuters, 13 April 2022, https://www.reuters.com/world/europe/mariupol-strategic-prize-russia-symbol-resistance-ukraine-2022-03-30/ [accessed: 23.07.2024].

55 VOA News, "Ukraine Says Mariupol Has Not Fallen", 17 April 2022, https://www.voanews.com/a/ukraine-says-mariupol-has-not-fallen-/6533156.html [accessed: 23.07.2024].

56 The Wall Street Journal, "What Is Happening in the Besieged Port City of Mariupol", 12 April 2022, https://www.wsj.com/livecoverage/russia-ukraine-latest-news-2022-04-12/card/what-is-happening-in-the-besieged-port-city-of-mariupol-vE3kfFl6BocQpGKclhkN [accessed: 23.07.2024].

57 Pavel Polityuk, "Ukraine says tens of thousands killed in Mariupol, accuses Russia of abuses", Reuters, 12 April 2022, https://www.reuters.com/world/europe/ukraine-says-tens-thousands-killed-mariupol-accuses-russia-slowing-evacuations-2022-04-11/ [accessed: 23.07.2024].

sympathies for one of the parties, quoting either Russian or Ukrainian officials, and emphasising the motives of humanity or dignity:

> Russia's defence ministry has told the Ukrainian forces still fighting in the besieged southern port of Mariupol to lay down their arms starting at 6 a.m. Moscow time (03:00 GMT) on Sunday (17 April) to save their lives.[58]

> Ukrainian forces besieged in Mariupol have rejected Russia's demands to surrender and are still resisting an unrelenting assault on the southeastern port city, top Ukrainian officials said on Sunday.[59]

> "Mariupol in final siege; Ukrainian forces 'will fight till the end'" (headline).[60]

English-language media emphasised the strategic position of Mariupol. This position, according to them, explained the current situation of the war, the reasons for the extreme intensity of military operations, the force and means used, the number of victims, the level of destruction, and the ravaging of the city:

> Mariupol is a strategic objective for Moscow. Taking the city would create an overland corridor from Russia across the northern lip of the Azov Sea to the Russia-annexed Crimean Peninsula.[61]

> Russia attempts to solidify its grip on an area that provides strategically important access points to the Black Sea and beyond.[62]

> [A s]trategic city, which lies between Russian-annexed Crimea and eastern areas of Ukraine held by Russian-backed separatists.[63]

---

58 Euractiv.com with Reuters, "Russia sets deadline for Ukraine troops in Mariupol to surrender", Euractiv.com, 17 April 2022, https://www.euractiv.com/section/global-europe/news/russia-sets-deadline-for-ukraine-troops-in-mariupol-to-surrender/ [accessed: 23.07.2024].

59 Jessie Yeung et al., "Ukraine rejects deadline to surrender in Mariupol as Russia threatens to eliminate resistance", CNN, 17 April 2022, https://edition.cnn.com/2022/04/17/europe/ukraine-mariupol-russia-assault-intl-hnk/index.html [accessed: 23.07.2024].

60 Fenit Nirappil et al., "Mariupol in final siege; Ukrainian forces 'will fight till the end'", The Washington Post, 17 April 2022, https://www.washingtonpost.com/national-security/2022/04/17/ukraine-russia-mariupol/ [accessed: 23.07.2024].

61 Brown and Umlauf, "After More Than a Month".

62 Nirappil et al., "Mariupol in final siege".

63 Polityuk, "Ukraine says tens of thousands".

> The city is in a strategic location just south of the Donbas area of Ukraine and has an excellent port on the Sea of Azov – an arm of the Black Sea. Mariupol would provide the Russians "unfettered and unhindered land access between the Donbas and Crimea".[64]

English-language media also often explained the attacks on Mariupol through the broader context of the Russo–Ukrainian War. Judging by the labelling and tagging that such media used, they mainly perceived these events in this context. This explanation linked the situation in Mariupol with Kyiv: "The Kremlin hopes an attack in the east could reverse the battlefield fortunes for Russia after a humiliating failure to quickly storm the capital, Kyiv".[65] In this way, the destruction and killing in Mariupol were revenge for the Russian defeat around Kyiv: Mariupol "could become the first big city captured by Russia since its invasion".[66] Noting the frank emotion of this interpretation, many other media sources reprinted or referred to a Reuters quote,[67] which read, "ruins of port could become Russia's first big prize in Ukraine".[68]

Lastly, English-language reports allowed for a heroic interpretation of the losses in Mariupol. In these interpretations, the city was a symbol of Ukrainian resistance: "Mariupol holds out against Russia's siege, a symbol of Ukrainian resistance"[69] and the city shows a "resistance that has thwarted the Kremlin's invasion plans".[70]

---

64 Jim Garamone, "Russian Forces, Ukrainians Vie for Mariupol", U.S. Department of Defense, 12 April 2022, https://www.defense.gov/News/News-Stories/Article/Article/2997624 [accessed: 23.07.2024].

65 Yuras Karmanau, "Ukraine's port of Mariupol holding out against all odds", AP, 15 April 2022. https://apnews.com/article/russia-ukraine-kyiv-business-europe-moscow-f5b814ca711f0679cf362016cd46cd47 [accessed: 23.07.2024].

66 Polityuk and Zinets, "Explainer", Reuters.

67 See, for example: Derek Saul, "Ukraine Effectively Surrenders Mariupol – Here's Why The City Is Such A Prized Target For Russia", Forbes, 17 May 2022, https://www.forbes.com/sites/dereksaul/2022/05/17/ukraine-effectively-surrenders-mariupol-heres-why-the-city-is-such-a-prized-target-for-russia/ [accessed: 23.07.2024]; Pavel Polityuk and Natalia Zinets, "EXPLAINER-Mariupol: ruins of port could become Russia's first big prize in Ukraine", Mail Online, 13 April 2022, https://www.dailymail.co.uk/wires/reuters/article-10715165/EXPLAINER-Mariupol-ruins-port-Russias-big-prize-Ukraine.html [accessed: 23.07.2024]; and Pavel Polityuk and Natalia Zinets, "Explainer-Mariupol: ruins of port could become Russia's first big prize in Ukraine", The Star, 13 April 2022, https://www.thestar.com.my/news/world/2022/04/13/explainer-mariupol-ruins-of-port-could-become-russia039s-first-big-prize-in-ukraine [accessed: 23.07.2024].

68 Polityuk and Zinets, "Explainer", Reuters.

69 Yuras Karmanau, "Mariupol holds out against Russia's siege, a symbol of Ukrainian resistance", PBS, 15 April 2022, https://www.pbs.org/newshour/world/mariupol-holds-out-against-russias-siege-a-symbol-of-ukrainian-resistance [accessed: 23.07.2024].

70 Karmanau, "Ukraine's port of Mariupol".

Conclusions

The media reports that I analysed in this article have a common object of focus: the city of Mariupol, its territory and infrastructure, and its residents. These articles all appeared within a short time of each other and described the course of military operations in Mariupol and nearby areas. At times, the reports in different languages referred to the same sources (e.g., representatives of the Mariupol City Council, the Ukrainian Ministry of Defence, the Russian Ministry of Defence, etc.) and used the same photo and video materials.

The articles, however, differ in their perspectives on and perceptions of the events. The Ukrainian-language sources spoke from the perspective of the attacked country and region and the people resisting this aggression. Meanwhile, the perspective of the Russian-language sources focused on the DNR and the 'liberation' of its territory from 'nationalists' – which is also the official narrative of the Russian Federation. Lastly, the perspective of English-language sources was oriented around war strategies and security issues.

Mariupol was presented with different interpretations for audiences using one of the three languages for Google searches. In these sources, Mariupol was a victim of the aggression of a neighbouring country, the object of liberation from nationalists, and a means and key point for the realisation of another military goal. It is unlikely that the average user would read all three versions at the same time. This is hindered not only by the information limitations of wartime but, above all, by a commitment to a particular picture of reality. Knowledge of such narratives, however, helps to understand the behaviour of people who hold a particular perspective, including how they form communication strategies.

Returning to the questions I posed at the beginning – how those outside of Mariupol will greet the occupied citizens after the war and what beliefs about their current situation different societies have – I can formulate some conclusions based on my study of the media representations of Mariupol. In the English-language sources, a focus on the strategic goals of the military operations prioritises military troops and institutions. Everyone else in this context is called a 'civilian', whose condition is determined by the rules of warfare. During military operations inside the city, those with 'civilian' status can potentially become 'civilian casualties', or victims of the war. In fact, the English-language sources explain and justify (i.e., legitimise) the losses of the civilian population in the context of the strategic aims of the Russian authorities. The Ukrainian-language perspective tends to victimise the people under occupation, placing the responsibility for the casualties and the destruction on the Russian authorities, which invaded the territory of a sovereign neighbouring state unprovoked. The Ukrainian perspective, however, avoids any justifications for such losses. Russian-language sources label Mariupol residents as 'rescued' and in need of external guidance and control. These same sources, however, also present such people as unreliable, treacherous, and dangerous for their 'saviours'.

As I argue in this text, the Ukrainian-language, Russian-language, and English-language sources offer different messages in terms of their content, the context given with the explanations and arguments, and their emotional colouring. The narratives and discourses to which these three perspectives belong influence the perceptions of the studied categories of people and urgently require further research.

Bibliography

0629.com, "Chervonyi Khrest zalyshyv Mariupol. A yak zhe poraneni?" ("The Red Cross Has Left Mariupol. What About the Wounded?"), 16 March 2022, https://www.0629.com.ua/news/3351323/cervonij-hrest-zalisiv-mariupol-a-ak-ze-poraneni [accessed: 23.07.2024].

Baulina, Olha, "Mariupol stav mistom-muchenykom liutoi viyny, iaka spustoshue Ukrainu" ("Mariupol Has Become a Martyr-City of the Fierce War That Is Devastating Ukraine"), *Holos Ukrainy (The Voice of Ukraine)*, 13 March 2022, http://www.golos.com.ua/article/357153 [accessed: 23.07.2024].

BBC, "Mariupol: Battle for key port city continues, Ukraine says", 11 April 2022, https://www.bbc.com/news/world-europe-61068650 [accessed: 23.07.2024].

Bratiuk, Iurii, "Arestovych poiasnyv, chomu zaraz ne mozhna vriatuvaty Mariupol viiskovym shliakhom" ("Arestovych Explains Why Mariupol Cannot Be Saved by Military Means Now"), *zaxid.net*, 18 March 2022, https://zaxid.net/arestovich_poyasniv_chomu_zaraz_ne_mozhna_vryatuvati_mariupol_viyskovim_shlyahom_n1538838 [accessed: 23.07.2024].

Brown, Emma, and Taylor Umlauf, "After More Than a Month of Fighting, Much of Mariupol Lies in Ruins", *The Wall Street Journal*, 17 April 2022, https://www.wsj.com/articles/mariupol-in-ruins-11650132943 [accessed: 23.07.2024].

Butchenko, Maksim, "Misto u vohni. Tila na vulytsiakh, vidsutnist vody ta izhi ta postiinyi vohon po zhytlovykh masyvakh – rozpovidi mariupoltsiv" ("The City Is on Fire. Bodies on the Streets, a Lack of Water and Food, and the Constant Shelling of Residential Areas – Stories from Mariupol Residents"), *New Voice*, 14 March 2022, https://nv.ua/ukr/ukraine/events/mariupol-zhive-pid-postiynimi-obstrilami-bez-vodi-ta-jizhi-50224909.html [accessed: 23.07.2024].

CBS News, "Transcript: Ukrainian Foreign Minister Dmytro Kuleba on 'Face the Nation'", 17 April 2022 https://www.cbsnews.com/news/dmytro-kuleba-transcript-face-the-nation-04-17-2022 [accessed: 23.07.2024].

Cybriwsky, Roman Adrian, “Mariupol: Seaside City”, in: *The Ukrainian Panorama: Dispatches from the Road about People, Places, Progress, and Problems*, Kyiv: Dnipro-Podil Books, 2019, 311–318.

Didova, A. Z. (ed.), *Nashchadky kozakiv u Donbasi: kozatskomu rodu nema perevodu* (*Descendants of the Cossacks in the Donbas: There is No Substitute for the Cossack Family*), Donetsk: Donbass, 2005.

Drapak, Mykhailo, “Mariupol ta hreky: zberehty svii dim” (“Mariupol and the Greeks: Saving Your Home”), *Lokalna Istoraiia (Local History)*, 17 March 2022, https://localhistory.org.ua/texts/reportazhi/mariupol-tse-ukrayina/ [accessed: 23.07.2024].

Euractiv.com with Reuters, “Russia sets deadline for Ukraine troops in Mariupol to surrender”, *Euractiv.com*, 17 April 2022, https://www.euractiv.com/section/global-europe/news/russia-sets-deadline-for-ukraine-troops-in-mariupol-to-surrender/ [accessed: 23.07.2024].

EurAsia Daily, “V Mariupole voiska DNR vyshli k zavodu ‘Azovstal’ – Minoborony” (“In Mariupol, DNR Troops Reached the Azovstal Plant – Defence Ministry”), 10 March 2022, https://eadaily.com/ru/news/2022/03/10/v-mariupole-voyska-dnr-vyshli-k-zavodu-azovstal-minoborony [accessed: 23.07.2024].

Fedchenko, Anastasiia, “‘Trupy lezhat na vulytsiakh. Ikh zakopuiut tam zhe na shtyk-lopatu’. Monoloh zhytelky Mariupolia” (“‘Corpses Are Lying in the Streets. They Are Buried There with Bayonets and Shovels’: A Monologue by a Resident of Mariupol”), *Novynarnia (Newsroom)*, 11 March 2022, https://novynarnia.com/2022/03/11/trupy-lezhat-na-vulyczyah-mariupol/ [accessed: 23.07.2024].

Garamone, Jim, “Russian Forces, Ukrainians Vie for Mariupol”, U.S. Department of Defense, 12 April 2022, https://www.defense.gov/News/News-Stories/Article/Article/2997624/ [accessed: 23.07.2023].

Grigoriev, Dmitrii, “Kak bliz Mariupolya nachalas denatsifikatsiya Ukrainy” (“How the Denazification of Ukraine Began near Mariupol”), *URA.RU*, 11 March 2022, https://ura.news/articles/1036284140 [accessed: 23.07.2024].

Instytut Prosvity (Institute of Enlightenment), “Mariupol: zhyva rana Ukrainy ta druhyi Niurnberh dlia tsyvilizovanoho suspilstva” (“Mariupol: Ukraine’s Open Wound and a Second Nuremberg for Civilised Society”), 18 March 2022, https://iprosvita.com/mariupol-zhyva-rana-ukrainy-ta-druhyj-niurnberh-dlia-tsyvilizovanoho-suspilstva/ [accessed: 23.07.2024].

Karmanau, Yuras, “Mariupol holds out against Russia’s siege, a symbol of Ukrainian resistance”, PBS, 15 April 2022, https://www.pbs.org/newshour/world/mariupol-holds-out-against-russias-siege-a-symbol-of-ukrainian-resistance [accessed: 23.07.2024].

Karmanau, Yuras, “Ukraine’s port of Mariupol holding out against all odds”, AP, 15 April 2022. https://apnews.com/article/russia-ukraine-kyiv-business-europe-moscow-f5b814ca711f0679cf362016cd46cd47 [accessed: 23.07.2024].

Khaneneva, Violetta, "V DNR soobshchili o rasstrele natsionalistami mirnykh grazhdan, pokidavshikh Mariupol" ("The DNR Reported that Nationalists Shot Civilians Fleeing Mariupol"), *gazeta.ru* (newspaper.ru), 06 March 2022, https://www.gazeta.ru/army/news/2022/03/06/17389471.shtml?updated [accessed: 23.07.2024].

Khmarochos (Skyscraper), "Mariupol: bomby na shkolu mystetstv, nasylne vyvezennia do RF, holodomor u susidnikh selakh" ("Mariupol: Bombs Hit an Art School, Forced Deportation to Russia, Famine in Neighbouring Villages"), 20 March 2022, https://hmarochos.kiev.ua/2022/03/20/mariupol-bomby-na-shkolu-mystecztv-nasylne-vyvezennya-do-rf-golodomor-u-susidnih-selah/ [accessed: 25.07.2024].

Kotenko, Tetiana, "Rashysty u Mariupoli vzialy u zaruchnyky likariv ta patsientiv" ("Ruscists in Mariupol Take Doctors and Patients Hostage"), Hlavkom, 15 March 2022, https://glavcom.ua/country/criminal/rashisti-u-mariupoli-vzyali-u-zaruchniki-likariv-ta-pacijentiv-830022.html [accessed: 25.07.2024].

Krasnaia Vesna (Red Spring), "Zhiteli Mariupolya vyrazili zhelanie, chtoby natsionalisty ubralis iz goroda" ("Mariupol Residents Expressed Their Desire for Nationalists to Get Out of the City"), 08 March 2022, https://rossaprimavera.ru/news/bb28287a [accessed: 26.07.2024].

Kretsul, Roman, and Bogdan Stepovoi, "V gorodskoi cherte: podrazdeleniya Donbassa prodolzhayut osvobozhdat Mariupol" ("Within the City Limits: Donbas Units Continue to Liberate Mariupol"), *Izvestia (News)*, 11 March 2022, https://iz.ru/1303439/roman-kretcul-bogdan-stepovoi/v-gorodskoi-cherte-podrazdeleniia-donbassa-prodolzhaiut-osvobozhdat-mariupol [accessed: 25.07.2024].

Kruk, Viktor, "Ukrainski '300 spartantsiv': zakhysnyky Mariupolia vidtiahnuly na sebe 10% armii okupantiv" ("The Ukrainian '300 Spartans': The Defenders of Mariupol Repelled 10% of the Occupiers' Army"), *Telehraf (Telegraph)*, 19 March 2022, https://www.telegraf.in.ua/kremenchug/10104272-ukrajinski-300-spartanciv-zahisniki-mariupolja-vidtjagnula-na-sebe-10-armiji-okupantiv.html [accessed: 25.07.2024].

Maiorov, Maksim, "Mariupol zupynyv navalu zi skhodu" ("Mariupol Stops an Invasion from the East"), *istorychna pravda (historical truth)*, 18 March 2022, https://www.istpravda.com.ua/columns/2022/03/18/161082/ [accessed: 25.07.2024].

Moskva24, "Mariupol zablokirovan, vse mosty i podstupy k gorodu razrusheny – Minoborony RF" ("Mariupol Blocked, All Bridges and Entrances to the City Destroyed – the Russian Defence Ministry"), 11 March 2022, https://www.m24.ru/news/politika/11032022/439609 [accessed: 23.07.2024].

Murlykina, Anna, "'Donechko, shcho vidbuvaetsia?' Yak vyzhyvaiut mariupoltsi v pekli shchodennoho znyshchennia" ("'My Daughter, What's Going On?' How Mariupol Residents Survive in the Hell of Daily Destruction"), *Texty (Texts)*, 13 March 2023, https://texty.org.ua/articles/105960/donechka-sho-vidbuvaye

tsya-yak-vyzhyvayut-mariupolci-v-pekli-shodennoho-znyshennya/ [accessed: 23.07.2024].

Nastoiashchee Vremia. Ciuzhety (The Present Tense: Stories), "Pobeh yz Maryupolia vplav" ("Escaped Mariupol by Swimming"), YouTube video, 15 April 2022, 3:53, h ttps://www.youtube.com/watch?v=lg_Olq6Ii-Q [accessed: 23.07.2024].

Nirappil, Fenit, et al., "Mariupol in final siege; Ukrainian forces 'will fight till the end'", *The Washington Post*, 17 April 2022, https://www.washingtonpost.com/nat ional-security/2022/04/17/ukraine-russia-mariupol/ [accessed: 23.07.2024].

Novynarnia (Newsroom), "Trahediia Mariupolia: rosiiany vbyly vzhe maizhe 2200 tsyvilnykh" ("The Tragedy of Mariupol: Russians Have Already Killed Almost 2200 Civilians"), 13 March 2022, https://novynarnia.com/2022/03/13/tragediya-mariu polya-rosiyany-vbyly-vzhe-majzhe-2200-czyvilnyh/ [accessed: 23.07.2024].

Orlova, Violetta, "Sproby okupantiv zakhopyty Mariupol zalyshaiutsia bezuspishnymy – Henshtab ZSU" ("The Attempts of the Occupants to Capture Mariupol Remain Unsuccessful – The General Staff of the Armed Forces of Ukraine"), *UNIAN*, 14 March 2022, https://www.unian.ua/war/viyna-z-rosiyeyu-sprobi-o kupantiv-zahopiti-mariupol-zalishayutsya-bezuspishnimi-novini-vtorgnenny a-rosiji-v-ukrajinu-11742391.html [accessed: 23.07.2024].

Petrenko, Roman, "Rosiiany skynuly nadpotuzhnu bombu na dramteatr Mariupolia, de khovaiutsia sotni liudei" ("Russians Drop a High-Powered Bomb on Mariupol Drama Theatre Where Hundreds of People Are Hiding"), *Pravda (Truth)* 16 March 2023, https://www.pravda.com.ua/news/2022/03/16/7331956/ [accessed: 23.07.2024].

Pirko, O., *Zaselennia i hospodarske osvoennia Stepovoi Ukrainy v XVI-XVIII st. (Settlement and Economic Development of the Ukrainian Steppe in the 16th–18th Centuries)*, Donetsk: Skhidnyi Publishing House, 2004.

Plotnikov, Dmitrii, "'Bolshe nedeli im ne proderzhatsya'. Zhiteli Mariupolya – o gumanitarnoi katastrofe, kotoraya razvorachivaetsya u nikh na glazakh" ("'They Won't Last More Than a Week': Mariupol Residents on the Humanitarian Catastrophe Unfolding Before Their Eyes"), *lenta.ru*, 08 March 2022, https://lenta.ru/ articles/2022/03/08/mariupol/ [accessed: 23.07.2024].

Polityuk, Pavel, "Ukraine says tens of thousands killed in Mariupol, accuses Russia of abuses", *Reuters*, 12 April 2022, https://www.reuters.com/world/europe/ukra ine-says-tens-thousands-killed-mariupol-accuses-russia-slowing-evacuations -2022-04-11/ [accessed: 23.07.2024].

Polityuk, Pavel, and Natalia Zinets, "Explainer: Mariupol: ruins of port could become Russia's first big prize in Ukraine", *Reuters*, 13 April 2022, https://www.r euters.com/world/europe/mariupol-strategic-prize-russia-symbol-resistance -ukraine-2022-03-30/ [accessed: 23.07.2024].

Polityuk, Pavel, and Natalia Zinets, "EXPLAINER-Mariupol: ruins of port could become Russia's first big prize in Ukraine", *Mail Online*, 13 April 2022, https://w

ww.dailymail.co.uk/wires/reuters/article-10715165/EXPLAINER-Mariupol-ruins-port-Russias-big-prize-Ukraine.html [accessed: 23.07.2024].

Polityuk, Pavel, and Natalia Zinets, "Explainer-Mariupol: ruins of port could become Russia's first big prize in Ukraine", *The Star*, 13 April 2022, https://www.thestar.com.my/news/world/2022/04/13/explainer-mariupol-ruins-of-port-could-become-russia039s-first-big-prize-in-ukraine [accessed: 23.07.2024].

Prysedska, Viktoriia, "'Zahyblykh skladaiut u susidnomu mahazyni'. Shchodennyk z blokadnoho Mariupolia" ("'The Dead Are Being Buried in a Nearby Shop': A Diary from Blockaded Mariupol"), BBC, 15 March 2022, https://www.bbc.com/ukrainian/features-60750253 [accessed: 23.07.2024].

Radio Svoboda (Radio Freedom), "Radnyk mera Mariupolia: kilkist zahyblykh u misti mozhe nablyzhatysia do 20 tysiach" ("The Advisor to the Mariupol Mayor: The Death Toll in the City Could Be Approaching 20 Thousand"), 15 March 2022, https://www.radiosvoboda.org/a/news-mariupol-zahybli/31752967.html [accessed: 23.07.24].

regnum, "Pushilin: Mariupol – samaya goryachaya tochka posle Volnovakhi" ("Pushilin: Mariupol is the Hottest Point after Volnovakha"), 12 March 2022, https://regnum.ru/news/3531173 [accessed: 25.07.2024].

RIA Novosti (RIA News), "V Minoborony nazvali 'aviaudar' po Mariupolyu srezhissirovannoy provokatsiei" ("The Defence Ministry Called the 'Airstrike' on Mariupol an Orchestrated Provocation"), 10 March 2022, https://ria.ru/20220310/provokatsiya-1777547947.html [accessed: 25.07.2024].

Rodak, Kateryna, "'U susidnomu budynku zhinku rozirvalo, ii khovaly na podviri': Ruskii mir v Mariupoli" ("'In the Neighbouring House, a Woman Was Torn to Pieces, and She Was Buried in the Yard': The Russian World in Mariupol"), *zahid.net*, 18 March 2022, https://zaxid.net/v_susidnomu_budinku_zhinku_rozirvalo_yiyi_hovali_na_podviryi_n1538736 [accessed: 23.07.2024].

Saul, Derek, "Ukraine Effectively Surrenders Mariupol – Here's Why The City Is Such A Prized Target For Russia", *Forbes*, 17 May 2022, https://www.forbes.com/sites/dereksaul/2022/05/17/ukraine-effectively-surrenders-mariupol-heres-why-the-city-is-such-a-prized-target-for-russia/ [accessed: 23.07.2024].

Savoskina, Ksiusha, "'Shchodnia my liahaly spaty i ne znaly, chy prokynemos'. Istoriia zhytelky Mariupolia, iakii vdalosia vybratysia z mista" ("'Every Day We Went to Bed and Did Not Know Whether We Would Wake Up': The Story of a Mariupol Resident Who Managed to Get Out of the City"), *hromadske (mass)*, 16 March 2022, https://hromadske.ua/posts/shodnya-mi-lyagali-spati-i-ne-znali-chi-prokinemos-istoriya-zhitelki-mariupolya-yakij-vdalosya-vibratisya-z-mista [accessed: 23.07.2024].

Shapoval, Kateryna, "'Liudei khovaiut v bratskykh mohylakh, deiakykh – u svoikh dvorakh': Interviu zastupnyka mera Mariupolia pro katastrofu v misti" ("'People Are Buried in Mass Graves, Some in Their Own Yards': Interview with the Deputy

Mayor of Mariupol About the Disaster in the City"), *Forbes*, 16 March 2022, https ://forbes.ua/inside/intervyu-mariupol-16032022-4685 [accessed: 23.07.2024].

Slovo i dilo (Word and Deed), "Zelenskyy rozrakhovue na dostavku humdopomohy do Mariupolia" ("Zelenskyy Expects Humanitarian Aid to Be Delivered to Mariupol"), 13 March 2022, https://www.slovoidilo.ua/2022/03/13/novyna/po lityka/zelenskyj-rozraxovuye-dostavku-humdopomohy-mariupolya [accessed: 23.07.2024].

Soroka, Yuliia, "Denaturalisation of Collective Identities within pro-Euromaidan Discourse (on field of Facebook Representation)", *Władza Sądzenia (Judicial Power)* 8, 2016, 42–54.

Soroka, Yuliia, "Vid Zhdanova do Mariupolia: pytannia pereimenuvannia mista u publikatsiiakh mistsevoi presy" ("From Zhdanov to Mariupol: The Issue of Renaming the City in the Local Press"), in: O. K. Mikheevoi (ed.), *Sotsiolohiia mista (Sociology of the City)*, Donetsk: Knowledge Publishing House, 2010, 329–353.

Suspilne (Society), "Rosiiki viiskovi z 'Hradiv' obstrilialy kolonu avtivok, iaki ikhaly z Mariupolia – shtab ZSU" ("Russian Servicemen Fired at a Convoy of Vehicles Travelling from Mariupol with Grad Multiple Rocket Launchers – Ukrainian Armed Forces HQ"), 16 March 2022, https://suspilne.media/218279-rosijki-vi jskovi-z-gradiv-obstrilali-kolonu-avtivok-aki-ihali-z-mariupola-stab-zsu/ [accessed: 23.07.2024].

Telegin, D. Ya., M. Lillie, I. D. Potekhina, and M. M. Kovaliukh, "Settlement and economy in Neolithic Ukraine: a new chronology", *Antiquity* 77/297, 2003, 456–470, https://doi.org/10.1017/S0003598X00092528.

The Wall Street Journal, "What Is Happening in the Besieged Port City of Mariupol", 12 April 2022, https://www.wsj.com/livecoverage/russia-ukraine-latest-news-2022-04-12/card/what-is-happening-in-the-besieged-port-city-of-mariupol-v E3kfFl6BocQpGKclhkN [accessed: 23.07.2024].

Televiziinoi sluzhby novyn (TSN) (Television news service), "'U Mariupoli my zahynemo, treba ryzykuvaty': istoriia zhinky, iaka zmohla vyrvatysia z otochenoho okupantamy mista" ("'We Will Die in Mariupol, We Have to Take a Risk': The Story of a Woman Who Managed to Escape from the City Surrounded by the Occupiers"), 15 March 2022, https://tsn.ua/ato/u-mariupoli-mi-zaginemo-treb a-rizikuvati-istoriya-zhinki-yaka-zmogla-virvatisya-z-otochenogo-okupanta mi-mista-2009971.html [accessed: 23.07.2024].

VOA News, "Ukraine Says Mariupol Has Not Fallen", 17 April 2022, https://www.v oanews.com/a/ukraine-says-mariupol-has-not-fallen-/6533156.html [accessed: 23.07.2024].

Yeung, Jessie, et al., "Ukraine rejects deadline to surrender in Mariupol as Russia threatens to eliminate resistance", *CNN*, 17 April 2022, https://edition.cnn.com /2022/04/17/europe/ukraine-mariupol-russia-assault-intl-hnk/index.html [accessed: 23.07.2024].

Experiences of Displacement

The Politics of Distorted Data

How Many War-Displaced Ukrainian Citizens Are in Russia?

Lidia Kuzemska

"War turns people into numbers", said Oleksandra Matviichuk, the Head of the Ukrainian Nobel Peace Prize-winning Centre for Civil Liberties, during her Speech to Europe in Vienna in May 2023.[1] But what if the numbers are turned into people? The infamous 'fog of war' spreads not only to the actual battlefields with unknown war casualties on both sides but also reaches civilian – yet highly political and emotionally charged – matters. This text focuses on one such issue – the attempt to calculate how many Ukrainian citizens have been forcefully displaced to Russia since the start of the full-scale invasion on 24 February 2022 and how many might remain there. We need to understand where the publicly circulating numbers, which range from 1.3 to 5.4 million, come from, so that the real people behind them remain on the political agenda of Ukraine and its international partners during the war and afterwards.[2] When the time comes, decisions about Ukrainian citizens in Russia should be included in post-war negotiations. Like Ukrainians displaced in Europe and elsewhere, Ukrainians in Russia should have the opportunity to decide on their future settlement and return options. Better estimates on how many displaced Ukrainians remain in Russia can help us plan the necessary steps for their support.

I argue that in the case of the forced displacement of Ukrainians to Russia, the inflated and unverified number of border crossings between Ukraine and Russia – provided, moreover, only by the Russian side – wrongfully transformed into the number of supposedly real individual Ukrainians fleeing the Russian invasion in the

---

1 Oleksandra Matviichuk, "A Speech to Europe by Oleksandra Matviichuk", *Documenting Ukraine Blog*, https://www.iwm.at/documenting-ukraine/blog/a-speech-to-europe-2023-by-oleksandra-matviichuk [accessed: 25.07.2024].

2 For instance, point 4 of President Volodymyr Zelenskyy's peace formula states: "Release of all prisoners and deportees, including war prisoners and children deported to Russia". See: *Reuters*, "Explainer: What is Zelenskiy's 10-point peace plan?", 28 December 2022, https://www.reuters.com/world/europe/what-is-zelenskiys-10-point-peace-plan-2022-12-28/ [accessed: 25.07.2024].

direction of the aggressor state. To analyse the politics behind these distorted numbers, I look closer at the available, albeit limited, data we have in the public domain on the forced migration flow of Ukrainians to and through Russia in 2022 and 2023. I conclude that a more realistic estimate of the number of Ukrainian citizens displaced to Russia after the invasion is up to a maximum of 1 million people and that, moreover, this number is probably decreasing as people are transiting through Russia to elsewhere.

Why Focus on the Numbers?

First, it is important to note that we do not know what the exact number of people residing in the territories of the temporarily occupied Zaporizhzhia, Kherson, Donetsk, and Luhansk Oblasts (see Figure 12) was before the start of the full-scale invasion because the last Ukrainian census took place in 2001. At that time, the combined population of these four oblasts amounted to about 10 million people.[3] Since then, Crimea was annexed by Russia in March 2014, and some parts of the Donetsk and Luhansk Oblasts (ORDLO) were occupied by Russia in April/May 2014 and have been governed through the self-proclaimed 'republics' (marked by the red line in Figure 1). In addition to the natural process of demographic decline that all Ukrainian regions experience, hundreds of thousands of people left the occupied territories between 2014 and 2021, moving either to other areas in Ukraine (there are a registered 1.4 million Internally Displaced Persons (IDPs) as of December 2021[4]), to Russia (estimated to be as high as 1 million people[5]), or somewhere abroad (no estimates available).

---

3 Derzhavnyi komitet statystyky Ukrainy (State Statistics Committee of Ukraine), "Vseukrainskyi perepys naselennia 2001" ("All-Ukrainian Population Census"), http://2001.ukrcensus.go v.ua/publications/#p1 [accessed: 25.07.2024].

4 National Social Service of Ukraine, "Sotsialnyi zakhyst vnutrishno peremishchenykh osib" ("Social Protection of Internally Displaced Persons"), https://nssu.gov.ua/vpo [accessed: 25.07.2024].

5 Irina Kuznetsova, "To Help 'Brotherly People'? Russian Policy Towards Ukrainian Refugees", *Europe–Asia Studies* 72/3, 2020, 505–527. For more information on the processes of the depopulation of the occupied territories from 2014 to 2021, and on the most current developments, see: Tetyana Malyarenko and Borys Kormych, "New Wild Fields: How the Russian War Leads to the Demodernization of Ukraine's Occupied Territories", *Nationalities Papers*, 2023, 1–19, h ttps://doi.org/10.1017/nps.2023.33; Tetyana Malyarenko and Borys Kormych, "Russian Policy towards the Economy of Occupied Ukrainian Territories: Crawling de-Modernization", *Eurasian Geography and Economics* 64/2, 2023, 1–18, https://doi.org/10.1080/15387216.2023.2167097 ; and Tatiana Zhurzhenko, "Terror, Collaboration and Resistance: Russian Rule in the Newly Occupied Territories of Ukraine", *Eurozine*, 17 January 2023, https://www.eurozine.com/terro r-collaboration-and-resistance/ [accessed: 25.07.2024].

Figure 12: Map of the Russian-occupied territories of Ukraine (as of 11 August 2023)

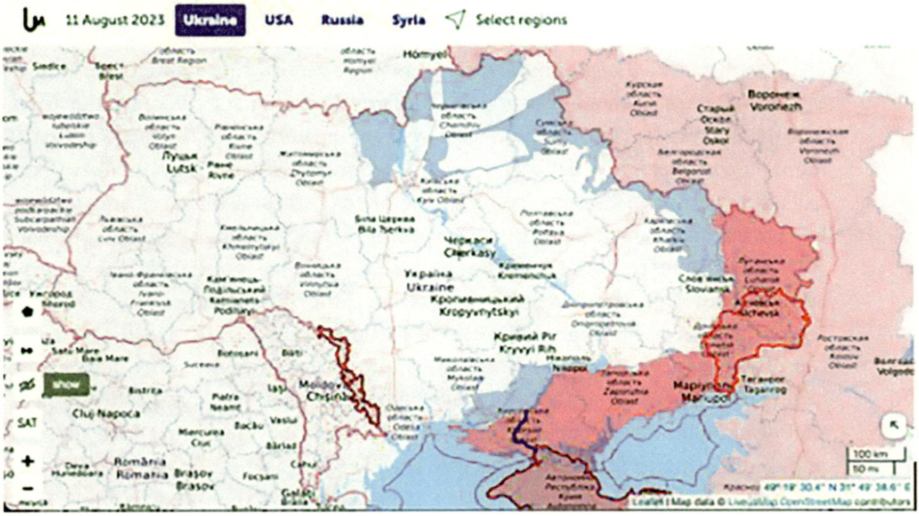

Image from Liveuamap, 11 August 2023, https://liveuamap.com [accessed: 11.08.2023]

After the beginning of the full-scale Russian invasion in February 2022, parts of Northern, Eastern, and Southern Ukraine were occupied. Some of them were soon liberated by the Ukrainian Armed Forces (marked grey in Figure 1), whereas others remained under occupation. Russian forces often prevented the civilian population of these regions from evacuating to Ukrainian-controlled territory. Some civilians were taken hostage and transferred to Russian territory, while others endured military actions, repressions, and ecological and humanitarian challenges but had to remain under occupation. This was especially true for those with reduced mobility or other obligations. We do not know how many people temporarily left the occupied territories in the direction of Russia and then returned to their homes because they could not find accommodation or work in Russia, left its territory to other countries, or had to visit the occupied territories for other reasons.[6]

The lack of reliable demographic data leaves room for speculation about the number of people fleeing the military actions, and this is especially so considering the absence of independent oversight and verification about how the data have been produced, by whom, and for what purposes. Recognising the sources and agendas of data-producing and data-circulating actors can help us be more critical towards

6 International Organization for Migration (IOM) UN Migration, *LATVIA. On the Way Back to Ukraine: Surveys with Refugees on Destinations, Length of Stay & Assistance*, report, April–June 2023, https://dtm.iom.int/sites/g/files/tmzbdl1461/files/reports/DTM_2023_LVA_Crossing_back_survey_Ukraine_Q2.pdf [accessed: 25.07.2024].

the numbers and mitigate the potential negative effects of such circulations. These numbers do not exist in a vacuum; they have concrete political effects and shape and legitimise policies, primarily towards the (un)counted people themselves.[7]

War-displaced Ukrainians in Russia remain largely outside of international protection schemes and without support from the Ukrainian state because the diplomatic ties between Ukraine and Russia were cut in February 2022. Russia closed all humanitarian corridors between the occupied territories and the Ukrainian-controlled territories of Ukraine in the spring of 2022. Most civilians fleeing the war had little choice about their route of escape from active warzones, and many are considered deportees by the Ukrainian government and some international observers.[8] Some civilians were transported by the Russian authorities, but the majority escaped the war on their own in the only available direction of Russia. All had to undergo a 'filtration' procedure: a mandatory screening process that involved a document check, having their fingerprints and photo taken, phone inspections, body searches, questioning, and, for some people, (often) arbitrary detention and torture.[9] The international community has rightly focused on the forcible transfer of Ukrainian children from the occupied territories to Russia and has noted that these may be qualified as genocidal deportations.[10]

---

7 Peter Andreas and Kelly M. Greenhill, "Introduction: The Politics of Numbers", in: Peter Andreas and Kelly M. Greenhill (eds.), *Sex, Drugs, and Body Counts: The Politics of Numbers in Global Crime and Conflict*, Ithaca, NY: Cornell University Press, 2010, 1–18.

8 5:00 AM Coalition, *Deportation of Ukrainian citizens from the territory of active military operations or from the temporarily occupied territory of Ukraine to the territory of the Russian Federation and the Republic of Belarus*, report, https://zmina.ua/wp-content/uploads/sites/2/2023/01/deportation_eng.pdf [accessed: 25.07.2024]; and Human Rights Centre ZMINA, *Deportation of Ukrainian Citizens to the Territory of the Russian Federation: Signs and Context*, report, April 2023, https://zmina.ua/wp-content/uploads/sites/2/2023/05/deport_people_eng_web.pdf, [accessed: 25.07.2024].

9 Amnesty International, *"Like A Prison Convoy": Russia's Unlawful Transfer And Abuse of Civilians In Ukraine During 'Filtration'*, report, 10 November 2022, https://www.amnesty.org/en/documents/eur50/6136/2022/en/ [accessed: 12.08.2023]; Yale School of Public Health Humanitarian Research Lab, *System of Filtration: Mapping Russia's Detention Operations in Donetsk Oblast*, report, 25 August 2022, https://hub.conflictobservatory.org/portal/sharing/rest/content/items/7d1c90eb89d3446f9e708b87b69ad0d8/data [accessed: 25.07.2024]; and Daria Getmanova and Svitlana Matviyenko, "Producing the Subject of Deportation: Filtration Processes during the Russia–Ukraine War", *Sociologica* 16/2, 2022, 239–252.

10 Oksana Dudko, "A Conceptual Limbo of Genocide: Russian Rhetoric, Mass Atrocities in Ukraine, and the Current Definition's Limits", *Canadian Slavonic Papers* 64/2–3, 2022, 133–145; Kristina Hook, *The Russian Federation's Escalating Commission of Genocide in Ukraine: A Legal Analysis*, report, July 2023, https://newlinesinstitute.org/wp-content/uploads/20230726-Genocide-Ukraine-Report-NISLAP_.pdf [accessed: 25.07.2024]; Victoria Colvin and Phil Orchard, "Forced Deportations and the Ukraine War: Russian Culpability in Atrocity Crimes", *Violence: An International Journal* 3/2, 2023, 1–20; Parliamentary Assembly Council

Unsurprisingly, since the full-scale invasion, the Russian authorities have published even more limited migration statistics[11] that do not explicitly separate Ukrainians displaced due to the Russian invasion from other cross-border travellers. They also do not publish the number of transit international travellers (including Ukrainians fleeing the invasion) who left the territory of the Russian Federation.

Nonetheless, it is regrettable to see how Ukrainian officials repeat and amplify Russian falsifications. For instance, in a report published in August 2023, Russian Presidential Children's Ombudswoman Maria Lvova-Belova (who was issued an arrest warrant by the International Criminal Court (ICJ) in March 2023 for crimes against Ukrainian children) stated: "From February 2022, the Russian Federation accepted [prinyala, Russian] 4.8 million residents from Ukraine and the republics of the Donbas, among them are more 700 thousand children".[12] Ukrainian Ombudsman Dmytro Lubinets quickly reacted to this report, stating, "in 2022, Russia transferred [vyvezla, Ukrainian] more than 700,000 children from Ukraine",[13] and said that this is yet further proof of the deportation of Ukrainian children. Other

of Europe, "Deportations and Forcible Transfers of Ukrainian Children and Other Civilians to Russian Federation or to Ukrainian Territories Temporarily Occupied", Resolution 2495, 2023, https://pace.coe.int/en/files/31776/html [accessed: 25.07.2024]; Veronika Bilkova, Cecilie Hellestveit, and Elina Steinerte, *Report on Violations and Abuses of International Humanitarian and Human Rights Law, War Crimes and Crimes against Humanity, Related to the Forcible Transfer and/or Deportation of Ukrainian Children to the Russian Federation*, Organization for Security and Co-operation in Europe, Office for Democratic Institutions and Human Rights, report, 2023, https://www.osce.org/files/f/documents/7/7/542751_1.pdf [accessed: 12.08.2023]; Yulia Ioffe, "Forcibly Transferring Ukrainian Children to the Russian Federation: A Genocide?", *Journal of Genocide Research* (Forthcoming), 2022, https://papers.ssrn.com/sol3/papers.cfm?abstract_id=4236369 [accessed: 25.07.2024]; Anti-Discrimination Centre Memorial Brussels, *Violation of the Rights of Children Taken from Ukraine to Russia and Belarus as a Result of Russian Military Aggression*, report, 12 June 2023, https://adcmemorial.org/en/publications/violation-of-the-rights-of-children-taken-from-ukraine-to-russia-and-belarus-as-a-result-of-russian-military-aggression/ [accessed: 25.07.2024]; and Kidmapping map, https://mapping.kids [accessed: 25.07.2024].

11 Anastasija Kokourova, "17 organov vlasti zasekretili statistiku s fevralya proshlogo goda" ("17 Governmental Institutions Made Statistics Secret as of February of Last Year"), *Esli byt tochnym* (*To Be Precise*), 18 May 2023, https://tochno.st/materials/zasekretili-statistiku-s-fevralya-proshlogo-goda [accessed: 25.07.2024].

12 Maria Lvova-Belova, *Doklad o deyatelnosti Upolnomochennogo pri Prezidente Rossiiskoi Federatsii po pravam rebenka v 2022 godu* (*Report on the Activity of the Russian Federation's Presidential Children's Rights Ombudsman in 2022*), report, 2023, p.117, http://deti.gov.ru/detigray/upload/documents/July2023/7JkHUTqLIsZL45JDp4XI.pdf [accessed: 12.08.2023] [author's trans.].

13 Ombudsman Lubinets Dmytro, "Deportatsiia ditei – ne 'dobra sprava', a zlochyn!" ("The Deportation of Children is Not a 'Good Deed', but a Crime"), Telegram post, 31 July 2023, https://t.me/dmytro_lubinetzs/3194 [accessed: 25.07.2024] [author's trans.].

officials doubt the number of 700,000, for example, Deputy Prime Minister Iryna Vereshchuk, who often comments on the issue of the forced transfer of children.[14] Nonetheless, Lubinets's statement illustrates that the Ukrainian side has limited sources of information about the number of Ukrainian citizens displaced to Russia, yet it uses Russia's falsified numbers to highlight the scale of its war crimes. To compare the range of discrepancies, as of 12 August 2023, the official Ukrainian number of documented children forcibly transferred to Russia was 19,546, of whom 386 were returned to Ukraine.[15] Where does this discrepancy in numbers come from?

In trying to provide answers, I first briefly discuss the concept of the 'politics of numbers' and its relevance for my analysis in this case study. Second, I compare data on the forced displacement of Ukrainians to Russia provided by the United Nations High Commissioner for Refugees (UNHCR), official Ukrainian sources, and official Russian sources, noting discrepancies, inconsistencies, and gaps. Third, I focus on the available – albeit limited and scrutiny-requiring – migration statistics of the Russian Ministry of Internal Affairs to demonstrate that even based on official Russian sources, we can conclude that the publicly stated numbers of Ukrainians in Russia are inflated and do not match the records of the Russian institutions responsible for migration statistics. Finally, I conclude with a reflection on why these purposefully distorted numbers continue to circulate in the official narratives of not only Russia but also Ukraine, and why international agencies and Ukrainian officials should be more critical in repeating these falsified numbers.

The Politics of Numbers

Statistics on the number of the displaced are used for a variety of purposes: to justify the allocation of resources, anticipate the social and economic impacts of displacement, envisage potential security challenges, and ensure that the displaced are taken into consideration when policies are being formulated.[16] For these reasons,

14 Anastaiia Poia, "Do Ukrainy povernuly shchonaimenshe 380 ukrainskykh ditei, yaki buly deportovani do RF – Vereshchuk" ("At Least 380 Ukrainian Children Deported to the Russian Federation Were Returned to Ukraine"), *Ukrainska Pravda (Ukrainian Truth)*, 10 August 2023, https://life.pravda.com.ua/society/2023/08/10/255831/ [accessed: 25.07.2024].

15 See updated data on the Children of War portal: Dity viiny (Children of War), https://childrenofwar.gov.ua [accessed: 25.07.2024]. Civic initiatives, such as Save Ukraine, Helping to Leave, SOS Ukraine, and The Ark help with evacuating children and adults from the temporarily occupied territories and from Russia to Ukraine or European countries.

16 Jeff Crisp, "'Who Has Counted the Refugees?' UNHCR and the Politics of Numbers", *New Issues in Refugee Research*, June 1999, https://www.refworld.org/pdfid/4ff58e4b2.pdf [accessed: 25.07.2024].

it is important to know not only the overall number of the displaced but also their composition (e.g., gender, age), education levels, skills, occupations, and other dynamically changing needs. Reliable, comprehensive, and up-to-date data is thus essential for state policies. However, the 'politics of numbers', that is "intentional efforts by individuals or institutions [to lower or inflate numbers] to pursue their own interests and to influence the behaviour of others"[17], interfere with this equation. Reliable data is difficult to obtain in a situation of war with unclear realities on the ground. Discrepancies, omissions, and errors in the numbers collected can occur for a multitude of reasons: poor training, a lack of technological infrastructure and local knowledge, human error, a lack of access to certain areas, the urgency of intervention, and the breakdown of institutions. But, as Joël Glasman and Brendan Lawson argue, this "can also be due to manipulation. A whole series of studies shows that states often have an interest in disguising humanitarian statistic".[18] The number of casualties, the displaced, and people particular in need or vulnerable situations carry not only humanitarian or technical value but also political and moral weight, often used to highlight the scale of man-made inequalities and injustices.[19]

The scales of displacement and return have symbolic meanings for state actors, either of political failure (a massive outflow of the population) or political success (a high number of returns). Hosting displaced people or returnees is also a political gesture to show a country's humanitarian effort and an argument for obtaining international aid. Countries often use an exaggerated number of incoming displaced people to embarrass the country of origin and point out its human rights violations or other reasons that forced people to flee.[20] Lowering the number might mean the opposite – minimising and legitimising the actions of those who provoked the displacement or denying the scale of the problem.

Gabriel Cardona-Fox argues that the collection of data is inherently political, especially in such countries as Russia, which are often 'blind spots' for international statistical bodies.[21] Both exaggerating and lowering the numbers may serve operational, conceptual, and political purposes to heighten or hide certain social, economic, or demographic phenomena. In this regard, Caress Schenk's analysis of migration statistics in Russia demonstrates gaps due to corruption and informality

---

17 Ibid., 17.

18 Joël Glasman and Brendan Lawson, "Ten Things We Know about Humanitarian Numbers", *Journal of Humanitarian Affairs* 5/1, 2023, 1–10, here 2.

19 Ibid., 2–4.

20 Ibid., 17.

21 Gabriel Cardona-Fox, "The Politics of IDP Data", *Refugee Survey Quarterly* 39/4, 2020, 620–633.

within the responsible institutions, frequent changes in migration policies and data collection regulations, as well as the arbitrariness of data collection on the ground.[22]

When we look at the exaggerated Russian number of persons displaced from Ukraine to its territory (about 5.4 million), the reasoning for such distortion seems to be threefold. First, this is to embarrass the Ukrainian state that supposedly failed to prevent the war and to protect and evacuate its citizens and, as a result, now experiences a large-scale outflow of the population and faces long-term demographic problems.[23] Second, a clear intention is to portray Russia as the biggest 'humanitarian' host of displaced Ukrainians since 2014 – as a country that is 'evacuating' civilians from the combat zone and opening its borders to people fleeing the 'anti-Russian hostile regime' and willing to 'find refuge' in Russia, which provides them with all kinds of support [sic].[24] Third, an inflated number of displaced Ukrainians in Russia questions the mandates and effectiveness of the UNHCR and other UN institutions that accept their de facto powerlessness to even count the displaced, not to even raise the issue of protection and the rights of the displaced in a country that caused their displacement and dispossession in the first place.

UNHCR Data

The last available UNHCR Ukraine Data Portal number of border crossings from Ukraine to Russia since the start of the full-scale invasion on 24 February 2022 amounts to 2.85 million (see Figure 13).[25] It is dated 3 October 2022, two days before the Russian Federation annexed the four occupied oblasts of Ukraine (Donetsk, Luhansk, Zaporizhzhia, and Kherson) and declared their residents Russian cit-

---

22 Caress Schenk, "Counting Migrants in Russia: The Human Dimension of Administrative Data Production", *International Migration Review*, 2023, 1–28, https://doi.org/10.1177/01979183231154565; Caress Schenk, "The Kremlin Has Another Weapon in Its Arsenal: Migration Policy", *The Washington Post*, 11 April 2022, https://www.washingtonpost.com/politics/2022/04/11/russia-ukraine-weaponized-migration/ [accessed: 12.08.2023].

23 For instance, already in March 2022, the Head of the Russian National Centre for Defence, Command General Mikhail Mezetsev, announced that the Ukrainian government is using civilians as 'human shields' and that they have a list of 2.7 million people willing to be relocated to Russia. See: *RIA Novosti* (*RIA News*), "Minoborony: bolee 2,7 milliona ukraintsev hotyat evakuirovatsya v Rossiyu" ("The Ministry of Defence: More than 2.7 Million Ukrainians Want to Evacuate to Russia"), 19 March 2022, https://ria.ru/20220319/evakuatsiya-1779069058.html [accessed: 31.07.2024].

24 Kuznetsova, "To Help 'Brotherly People'?", 509, 520.

25 United Nations High Commissioner for Refugees (UNHCR) Operational Data Portal, "Ukraine Refugee Situation", https://data.unhcr.org/en/situations/ukraine/location [accessed: 31.07.2024].

izens.[26] Since then, we have seen no UNHCR updates on the number of border crossings between Ukraine and Russia. I assume this is due to the Russian position that residents in the occupied territories are now 'Russian' citizens moving within 'Russian' (in fact occupied) territory and, hence, should no longer be considered as cross-border 'refugees'. The UNHCR's history of involvement in handling post-Soviet displacements was limited and not particularly successful, according to its own evaluation,[27] and it looks like they reverted to their usual approach when divergent statistics emerged: "UNHCR staff … see no value risking the confrontation with the host government […]".[28] As Irina Mützelburg notes, the UNHCR often compiles numbers measuring different facts from different countries (border crossings, estimates of the displaced, the number of registered people) into one number of 'refugees from Ukraine' to demonstrate the extent of the crisis.[29]

There is no doubt that counting the displaced is a complicated task, especially amidst the ongoing war. This task involves establishing criteria and a methodology for who is counted, the capacity (or lack thereof) to organise the process, accounting for the natural processes of birth, death, and onward or return movement among the displaced, and political considerations.[30] Nonetheless, the UNHCR does not provide information about any independent monitoring mechanism to verify (or at least review the initial sources) the data it makes publicly available under its logo on the UNHCR portal, side-by-side with data coming from other countries. Moreover, the lags in updates and discrepancies in numbers are also unexplained, leaving open questions about the reliability and comprehensiveness of UNHCR-branded data.

---

26 Ofitsialnoe opublikovanie pravovykh aktov (Official Publication of Legal Acts), Federal Laws the Russian Federation from 04 October 2022, no. 372-F3, no. 373-F3, no. 374-F3, and no. 375-F3, http://publication.pravo.gov.ru/search?pageSize=30&index=1&DocumentTypes=82a8bf1c-3bc7-47ed-827f-7affd43a7f27&PublishDateSearchType=1&PublishDate=05.10.2022&NumberSearchType=0&DocumentDateSearchType=0&JdRegSearchType=0&SortedBy=6&SortDestination=1 [accessed: 31.07.2024].

27 United Nations High Commissioner for Refugees (UNHCR), "Displacement in the former Soviet region", in: *The State of the World's Refugees 2000: Fifty Years of Humanitarian Action*, report, 2000, 185–209, https://www.unhcr.org/media/state-worlds-refugees-2000-fifty-years-humanitarian-action-chapter-8-displacement-former [accessed: 31.07.2024].

28 Crisp, "'Who Has Counted the Refugees?'", 16.

29 Brendan Lawson and Irina Mützelburg, "Humanitarian Numbers in the Russian–Ukrainian War: An Interview with Irina Mützelburg (October 2022)", *Journal of Humanitarian Affairs* 5/1, 2023, 52–61, here 54.

30 Jeff Crisp, "Who Is Counting the Refugees? Displacement Data, Its Limitations, and Potential for Misuse", *Refugee History*, 04 August 2022, https://refugeehistory.org/blog/2022/8/4/who-is-counting-refugees-displacement-data-its-limitations-and-potential-for-misuse [accessed: 31.07.2024].

Figure 13: UNHCR data on the number of "refugees and displaced persons from Donetsk, Luhansk, and other oblasts of Ukraine who arrived in Russia from 24 February to 4 October 2022"[31]

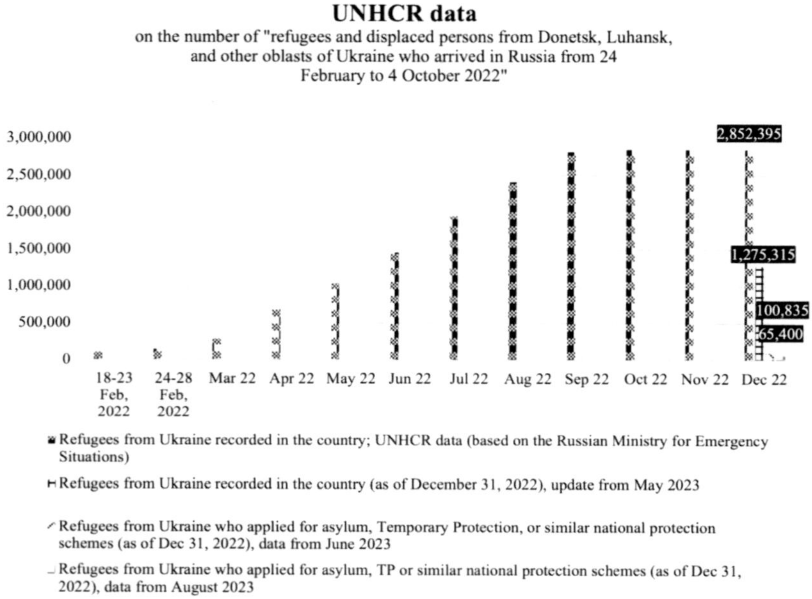

All Figures are based on the sources/numbers in Figure 23 (see the Appendix).

War-displaced Ukrainian citizens in Russia cannot rely on the large-scale help of international organisations that usually operate in situations of mass refugee influx, such as the UNHCR or the International Committee of the Red Cross (ICRC). The ICRC's activities in Russia have been severely criticised in Ukraine for their ineffectiveness in the search for the missing and their lack of meaningful impact on the lives of captured civilians and military personnel.[32] Even though the UNHCR office

31 This is a definition used by the UNHCR Russia in its monthly digests. See: "*UNHCR Russia Monthly Digest, December 2022*", 1, https://www.unhcr.org/ru/wp-content/uploads/sites/73/2023/03/UNHCR_monthly_digest_Russia_December_2022_EN.pdf [accessed: 13.08.2023]. Here and throughout the text I put this definition in quotation marks because, in fact, forcibly displaced Ukrainians do not receive refugee status in Russia, nor do the majority of them receive any other national humanitarian protection status, as I explore in section *B. Migration Registration Data (from the Russian Ministry of Internal Affairs)*.

32 See, for instance, the report of the Central Tracing Agency of the ICRC on its activity during the Russo–Ukrainian War as of July 2023: International Committee of the Red Cross, *ICRC's Central Tracing Agency Bureau for the International Armed Conflict between the Rus-*

in Russia exists and provides general information about the entry and condition of the reception of displaced Ukrainians, it does not work with them directly (or rather, it is not allowed to by the Russian authoritarian regime). Rather, the UNHCR in Russia relies on its cooperation with local Russian organisations, such as the Civic Assistance Committee (*Grazhdanskoe sodeistvie*), the Russian Red Cross, the Health and Life Charitable Foundation (*Zdorovie i zhyzn*), and the Silsila Foundation for the Distribution of Humanitarian Aid.[33] The UNHCR depends on the data and access provided by the state, which is limited to occasional visits to the Temporary Accommodation Centres (TAPs) across the country accompanied by Russian officials and, in particular, the Ombudswoman's representatives. Noteworthily, the total number of displaced people residing in the 807 TAPs in 58 Russian regions reached only 40,680 people in October 2022, including 12,470 children.[34] This was less than half of the initially planned number of 95,909 displaced people who should have been mandatorily distributed and accommodated in 1,533 TAPs, as became apparent from the Russian government's quotas established in the early days of the full-scale invasion.[35] What then happened to the supposedly remaining 2.84 million not hosted in the TAPs? The UNHCR gives no answers.

Nonetheless, looking at Figure 13, we see that up until June 2023, the number of 2.85 million border crossings was mistakenly equated to the actual number of individuals who were displaced to Russia. However, when we look at the recently published data on the UNHCR portal (Figure 13), the number of individuals recorded as "refugees from Ukraine [sic]"[36] as of December 2022 is significantly fewer than 2.85 million. In fact, it is only 1.27 million. Even more striking is the unexplained discrepancy between 1.27 million "refugees from Ukraine" and the number of individuals

sian Federation and Ukraine, report, 2023, https://t.me/mkkk_ru/596 [accessed: 12.08.2023]. Note the overall number of applications (more than 86,000) and the number of cases where information about the whereabouts of the missing person has been provided (6,000).

33 United Nations High Commissioner for Refugees (UNHCR) Russia, "Kuda mozhno obratitsya za pomoshchyu litsam, pribyvayushchim na territoriyu RF v svyazi s konfliktom v Ukraine?" ("Where Can People Arriving on the Territory of the Russian Federation in Connection with the Conflict in Ukraine Apply for Assistance?"), 2023, https://www.unhcr.org/ru/28617-helpforukrref.html [accessed: 31.07.2024].

34 RIA Novosti (RIA News), "Chislo PVR dlya bezhentsev v Rossii dostiglo 807" ("The Number of TAPs in Russia Reached 807"), 24 October 2022, https://ria.ru/20221024/bezhentsy-1826256366.html [accessed: 31.07.2024].

35 Ofitsialnoe opublikovanie pravovykh aktov (Official Publication of Legal Acts), Resolution of the Government of the Russian Federation from 12 March 2022, no. 349, http://www.publication.pravo.gov.ru/Document/View/0001202203120005?index=6 [accessed: 31.07.2024].

36 I discuss the legal statuses of forcibly displaced Ukrainian citizens later in the text.

who applied for any kind of legal status in Russia by the end of 2022. The latter number has also decreased from the 100,000 reported in June 2023 to 65,400 in August 2023.[37] How did 2.85 million transform into 65,000? Does the 65,000 include those residing in the TAPs? This is not clear.

Official Ukrainian Data

There is currently no mechanism for Ukrainians in Russia to declare their (involuntary) presence on Russian territory since the embassy and consulates of Ukraine do not function on the territory of the aggressor state. The familiar number of 2.85 million 'border crossings' has been circulating in Ukrainian and international official reports as the actual number of forcibly displaced Ukrainians in Russia. This was the only available estimate coming from the UN agency that Ukrainian officials could rely on, although this number was, in fact, initially coming from the Russian Ministry for Emergency Situations. As visible in Figure 14 and Figure 15, there is no consistency among Ukrainian officials on the number of Ukrainians who are considered forcibly displaced or deported to Russia. Sometimes the number is closer to the UNHCR estimates, sometimes to the numbers published by Russia, and sometimes there is no explanation provided as to where the numbers come from.

Looking at the timelines of the total number of the displaced and the number of displaced children, it is noticeable that since early 2023, Ukrainian officials have gradually moved to commenting only on the number of forcibly transferred/deported children and do not comment on the total number of Ukrainians who might be in Russia. This shift might be related to the fact that until recently there were no UNHCR updates (though the recent figures from the summer of 2023 have not been commented on by Ukrainian officials either) or because Ukrainian officials acknowledge that they cannot estimate the fluctuating number of people who move from the occupied territories to Russia and/or onwards.

Considering that the forcefully displaced Ukrainians are coming from an active warzone, they often do not have the necessary documents, or these might have been destroyed, lost during the journey, or taken away during the 'filtration' procedure, which makes daily life and further travel difficult for them. Children, and especially newborns, might not have any Ukrainian documents, while older people might only have birth certificates and not IDs or other documents necessary for daily lives abroad and travel. Furthermore, Ukrainian bank cards and SIM cards do not work in Russia. The displaced are also not allowed to exchange Ukrainian currency, so their actions in Russia are severely constrained. Registering with the Russian authorities

37 Please see all the details about the numbers and sources in Figure 23.

is thus necessary for Ukrainian citizens to cover their basic needs in Russia, but it also makes them part of the Russian 'politics of numbers'.

Figure 14: Ukrainian officials' estimates on the total number of forcefully displaced or deported Ukrainians (April 2022–August 2023)

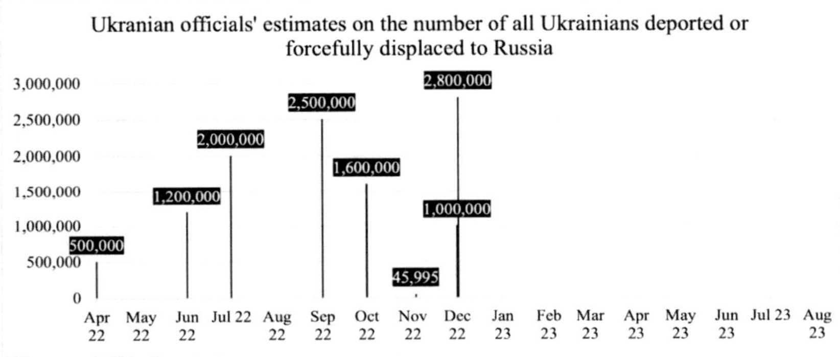

All Figures are based on the sources/numbers in Figure 23 (see the Appendix).

Figure 15: Ukrainian officials' estimates on the number of forcefully displaced or deported Ukrainian children (April 2022–August 2023)

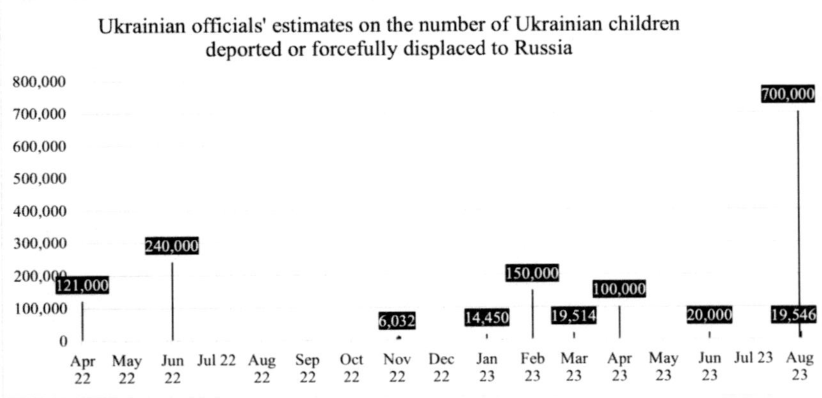

All Figures are based on the sources/numbers in Figure 23 (see the Appendix).

Once in Russia, forcefully displaced Ukrainians have limited choices for further actions that depend on their social ties, available resources, and sociodemographic category. Those who have relatives or friends in Russia, have sufficient financial means, or do not want to be under increased surveillance can try evading the governmental pathway of being mandatorily distributed across the Russian regions and settled into one of the TAPs (located in hostels, summer camps, sanatoria, or sports facilities). TAPs provide the displaced with free accommodation and meals, but they are usually in remote areas far from employment opportunities, education, and healthcare facilities.

Ukrainian citizens outside the government-run TAPs struggle to access any public services without first legalising their stay in Russia, which can take up to six months (see more in the following sections). Official employment and long-term renting require legal status too. Kindergarten and school places for war-displaced children are only available if they officially register as residing in the same district, which is not always possible due to landlords' unwillingness to register temporary dwellers, often with no income. While waiting for their documentation, many people take precarious informal jobs and live in extremely strenuous conditions. Often, displaced people earn just enough to cover expenses and necessities but cannot afford medical care or clothes. Nongovernmental organisations (NGOs) report that it takes months to receive the one-off cash payment of 10,000 RUB (about 100 EUR) promised by the Russian government. Until then, people remain without financial help and rely on volunteer donations of food, clothes, non-food items, toiletries, basic furniture, and second-hand gadgets to study and work online.[38]

People with disabilities and/or chronic illnesses, the elderly, orphaned children, or those under state care are dependent on the decisions taken on their behalf by the Russian authorities who organised the so-called 'evacuations' from the occupied territories.[39] These groups are the most vulnerable and have little say about where they

38 See, for instance, reports of the House with a Lighthouse Foundation for Assistance to Refugees (which is donation funded), the Civic Assistance Committee (which is UNHCR and donation funded), the Russian Red Cross (which is state and donation funded), and the Russian Orthodox Church (which is state and donation funded): Fond pomoshchi bezhentsam "Dom s mayakom" (House with a Lighthouse Foundation for Assistance to Refugees), official website, https://mayak.fund [accessed: 31.07.2024]; Komitet "Grazhdanskoe sodeistvie" (Civic Assistance Committee), official website, https://refugee.ru [accessed: 31.07.2024]; Russian Red Cross, "Tsentr Rossiiskogo Krasnogo Kresta po voprosam migratsii" ("The Russian Red Cross Centre for Migration Issues"), https://www.redcross.ru/activity/migratsiya/ [accessed: 31.07.2024]; and the Russian Orthodox Church, "Tserkovnaya pomoshch bezhentsam i postradavshim mirnym zhitelyam" ("Church Aid to Refugees and Affected Civilians"), https://помочьвбеде.рф [accessed: 31.07.2024].

39 Human Rights Centre ZMINA, *Deportation of Custodial Settings from Occupied Territories of Ukraine*, report, 2023, https://zmina.ua/wp-content/uploads/sites/2/2023/07/deportation_f_eng_web.pdf [accessed: 31.07.2024].

will be evacuated to and which status they will receive. According to the Ukrainian delegation to the UN Committee on the Rights of Persons with Disabilities, "7700 persons with disabilities, including children, were in institutions in areas that had fallen under Russian occupation".[40] Some institutions have not been evacuated to Ukrainian-controlled territory due to rapidly advancing Russian forces, the lack of human and logistical resources for evacuation, and the medical needs of the patients. Some children from these institutions were later transferred to Russia by the occupying authorities for placement in 'foster care families', often without the consent of their parents or legal guardians in Ukraine.[41]

Figure 16: Ukrainian officials' estimates on the number of children under state care forcefully displaced or deported to Russia (April 2022–August 2023)

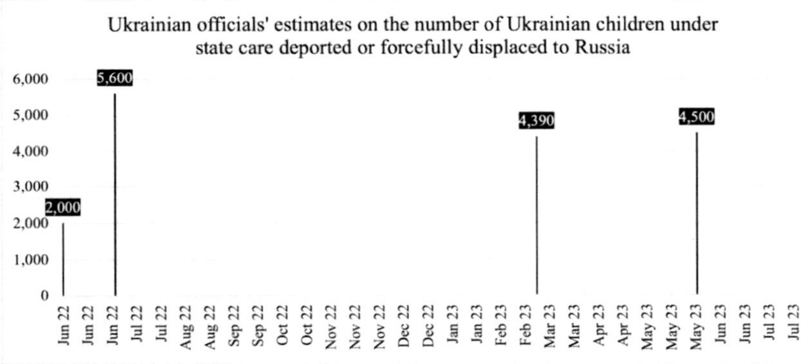

All Figures are based on the sources/numbers in Figure 23 (see the Appendix).

Looking at Figure 16, we see that Ukrainian officials have more consistently estimated the category of children under state care. It is, however, unclear whether the numbers announced by Ukrainian officials include children under state care from territories occupied since 2014. Russian Presidential Children's Ombudswoman Lvova-Belova acknowledged that up to 1,500 children from these territories have

40 Human Rights Watch, *"We Must Provide a Family, Not Rebuild Orphanages": The Consequences of Russia's Invasion of Ukraine for Children in Ukrainian Residential Institutions*, report, 13 March 2023, https://www.hrw.org/report/2023/03/13/we-must-provide-family-not-rebuild-orphanages/consequences-russias-invasion [accessed: 31.07.2024].

41 Georgette Mulheir et al., *Bridging the Gaps: Four Studies on the Situation of Ukrainian Children with Disabilities and Their Families since the War Began*, European Disability Forum, report, 15 February 2023, 43–45, 61–62, https://www.edf-feph.org/content/uploads/2023/02/221215-BRIDGING-THE-GAPS-extended-summary-FINAL.pdf [accessed: 12.07.2024].

been (at least temporarily) transferred to Russia since February 2022.[42] To note, many were born after the occupation of Crimea and parts of the Donetsk and Luhansk Oblasts in 2014 and have not been registered in Ukraine at all.

Overall, data circulated by Ukrainian officials about the number of Ukrainians forcefully displaced to Russia reflect the uncertainty and speculations about the potential scale of such displacement. Even though Ukrainian authorities are creating a database of verified and documented individual cases,[43] time and changing realities in the occupied territories (in 2014 and 2022) complicate tracing people, who gradually fall beyond the registers of living, missing, or deceased Ukrainian citizens. Those displaced to Russia, unfortunately, become part of the inflated number spread by the government-controlled Russian media.

Official Russian Data

In this section, I analyse three types of data coming from the Russian authorities: 1) data from the state media source TASS (and other outlets quoting TASS), which regularly reported on the dynamic of the overall number of displaced people from February 2022 to March 2023; 2) statistics on the migration registrations of Ukrainian citizens after their arrival to Russia; and 3) statistics on the number of Ukrainian nationals who received any kind of legal status in Russia in 2022/2023.

A. TASS Reporting from a Source in Russian Security Services

In March 2023, the official Russian press agency TASS reported a staggering number of people displaced from Ukraine to Russia: 5.4 million, including 744,000 children (see Figure 17 and Figure 18).[44] However, this independently unverified number is misleading. It most probably reflects the overall number of crossings between Russia and the occupied Ukrainian territories during 2022. For instance, according to a report by the Civic Assistance Committee – one of the few NGOs advocating for

42 Lvova-Belova, *Doklad o deyatelnosti*, 117.

43 See: Dity viiny, https://childrenofwar.gov.ua. Also, since May 2023, the Unified Database of Missing Persons has registered over 24,000 Ukrainian citizens (military and civilian) as missing due to war. Alona Mazurenko, "Do reestru znyklykh bezvisty vnesly informatsiiu pro ponad 24 tysiatchi osib – upovnovazhenei" ("More than 24,000 Persons Were Registered in the Database of Missing Persons"), *Ukrainska Pravda* (*Ukrainian Truth*), 12 July 2023, https://www.pravda.com.ua/news/2023/07/12/7410945/ [accessed: 31.07.2024].

44 TASS, "Chislo pribyvshikh v RF bezhentsev s territorii Ukrainy i Donbassa prevysilo 5,4 mln chelovek" ("The Number of Refugees Coming to Russia from the Territory of Ukraine and the Donbas Surpassed 5.4 Mil People"), 13 March 2023, https://tass.ru/obschestvo/17248303 [accessed: 31.07.2024].

refugee rights in Russia – this manipulation is covered using multiple, often contradictory, and mutually exclusive labels to describe who is moving and their motives and intentions.

Figure 17: The total number of "people coming from the Donbas and Ukraine to the territory of the Russian Federation" (the label most used by TASS[45])

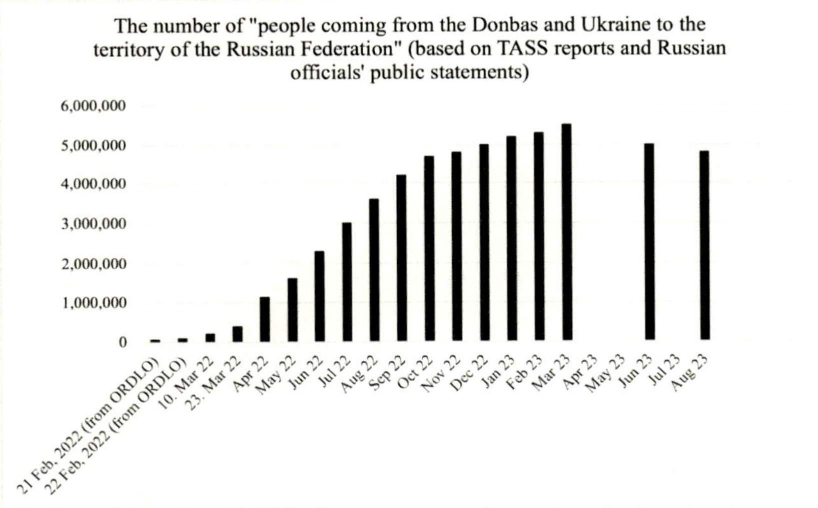

This Figure is based on the sources/numbers in Figure 23 (see the Appendix).

A range of labels has been used to categorise this migration flow, such as 'arriving people' (*pribyvshie*), 'refugees' (*bezhentsy*), 'people who crossed the border' (*peresekshyie granitsu*), 'people currently in the Russian Federation' (*nakhodyashchiesya v Rossiiskoi Federatsii*), 'people accepted by the Russian Federation' (*lyudi, kotorykh prinyala Rossiiskaya Federatsiya*), 'evacuees' (*evakuirovannye*), the '(self)-evacuated' (*evakuirovavshiesya*), and the 'forcibly resettled' (*vynuzhdennye pereselentsy*). The labels are also political. They signal a relationship of power and have consequences in terms of status as well as the aid and moral obligations the host state and society have towards them.[46] Noteworthy are the absence of any mention of the reason

45 See, for example: TASS, "Chislo pribyvshikh v RF bezhentsev s territorii Ukrainy i Donbassa prevysilo 5,4 mln chelovek" ("The Number of Refugees Coming to Russia from the Territory of Ukraine and the Donbas Surpassed 5.4 Mil People"), 13 March 2023, https://tass.ru/obschestvo/17248303 [accessed: 31.07.2024].

46 Rebecca Hamlin, *Crossing: How We Label and React to People on the Move*, Redwood City: Stanford University Press, 2021, 12–13.

why people were displaced as well as an emphasis on either the humanitarian (e.g., 'evacuees') or neutral (e.g., 'arriving', 'accepted') character of their migration. These labels and consequently their numbers presented by the authorities do not distinguish between Ukrainian nationals and other cross-border travellers (Russian or third-country nationals) or between those displaced by war and those travelling for other reasons; they also include people who transited through Russia and left its territory, as well as those who returned to live in the occupied territories.[47] Combining all these different categories of travellers and labelling them 'refugees from Ukraine in Russia' is thus misleading.

Figure 18: The number of children who are part of the "people coming from the Donbas and Ukraine to the territory of the Russian Federation" (the label most used by TASS[48])

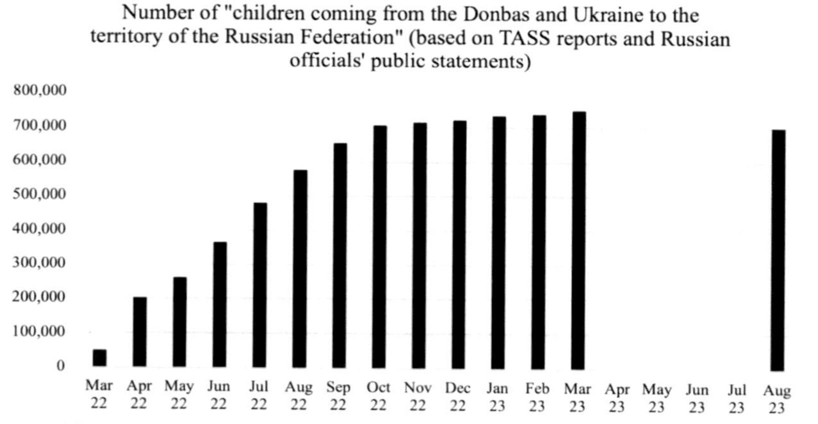

This Figure is based on the sources/numbers in Figure 23 (see the Appendix).

By the end of 2022, Georgia recorded 25,204 Ukrainian refugees, Azerbaijan almost 7,000, Armenia 360, and Kazakhstan around 7,000. As these countries do not share direct land borders with Ukraine, and considering that air travel has been suspended in Ukraine since the first day of the invasion, Ukrainian refugees reached

47 Konstantin Troitskii, Skolko bezhentsev s Ukrainy nakhoditsya v Rossiiskoi Federatsii? (How Many Refugees from Ukraine Are in the Russian Federation?), Komitet "Grazhdanskoe sodeistvie" (Civic Assistance Committee), report, 2023, https://refugee.ru/wp-content/uploads/2023/03/troiczkij-k.e.-skolko-bezhenczev-iz-ukrainy-v-rossijskoj-federaczii_-1-1.pdf [accessed: 31.07.2024].

48 See previous footnote.

these countries predominantly by transiting through Russia. The number of registered Ukrainian refugees in these countries does not account for those Ukrainian citizens who entered from Russia and transited onwards, so the overall number of exits from Russia is even higher than the number of registered refugees in these countries.[49] For example, a report by UNHCR and World Vision Georgia indicates that at least half of the Ukrainian refugees in the country entered from Russia and originated from the Donetsk and Kherson Oblasts.[50] Similarly, looking westward, in 2022, Estonia and Latvia respectively recorded (in addition to those Ukrainian refugees who stayed) 53,000 and 230,000 Ukrainian citizens entering from Russia or Belarus and transiting through their territories to reach other EU countries or Ukraine.[51] We can also assume that some Ukrainian nationals who were already holders of Russian citizenship left Russia in 2022 as part of the larger Russian anti-war and draft evasion emigration.[52]

We should also take into account that, according to TASS, in the first months of the full-scale invasion, the majority and later at least half of the crossings reported as part of the overall 5.4 million were done (in March–June 2022) by residents of the Donetsk and Luhansk Oblasts, which have been occupied since 2014.[53] This is significant, as many of these residents travelled using either their Russian passports or documents issued by the self-proclaimed 'republics'.[54] Technically, they did not cross

49 International Centre for Migration Policy Development (ICMPD), *ICMPD Migration Outlook: Eastern Europe and Central Asia, 2023*, report, 2023, 20, https://www.icmpd.org/file/download/59104/file/230215_ICMPD_Migration_Outlook_EasternEuropeCentralAsia_2023_final.pdf [accessed: 31.07.2024].

50 United Nations High Commissioner for Refugees (UNHCR) and World Vision Georgia, *Ukrainian refugees in Georgia: Profile, Intentions and Needs*, report, November 2022, 3, https://data.unhcr.org/en/documents/details/97675 [accessed: 31.07.2024].

51 United Nations High Commissioner for Refugees (UNHCR), *Ukraine Regional Refugee Response Plan (January–December 2023)*, report, 2023, 84, 120, https://data.unhcr.org/en/documents/details/97958 [accessed: 31.07.2024].

52 Emil Kamalov et al., *Russia's 2022 Anti-War Exodus: The Attitudes and Expectations of Russian Migrants*, PONARS Eurasia, report, September 2022, https://www.ponarseurasia.org/wp-content/uploads/2022/09/Pepm790_Kamalov-Kostenko-Sergeeva-Zavadskaya_Sept2022.pdf [accessed: 12.08.2023]; and Athina Anastasiadou, Artem Volgin, and Douglas R. Leasure, "War and Migration: Quantifying the Russian Exodus through Yandex Search Trends", SocArXiv Papers, 18 May 2023, 1–25, https://osf.io/preprints/socarxiv/92zam/ [accessed: 31.07.2024].

53 TASS, "Svyshe 2,3 mln bezhentsev pribyli v Rossiyu s Ukrainy, iz DNR i LNR" ("More than 2.3 Mil Refugees Arrived to Russia from Ukraine, from the DNR and the LNR"), 04 July 2022, https://tass.ru/armiya-i-opk/15112613 [accessed: 31.07.2024].

54 An estimated 1.44 million people received Russian citizenship on the occupied territories of the Donetsk and Luhansk Oblasts between 2014 and 2021. Komitet "Grazhdanskoe sodeistvie" (Civic Assistance Committee), *Ubezhyshche dlya 0,04% bezhentsev v mire: rossiiskaya migratsyonnajy statistika za 2021 god i ee analitika* (Asylum for 0.04 Per-

the Ukrainian–Russian border as Ukrainian nationals and did not have the obligation to undertake migration registration in Russia (see the following subsection). They could come and go as many times as they needed; however, we must note that the occupying administrations imposed a strict ban on men (ages 18–55) leaving the territories of the self-proclaimed republics due to forced conscription.[55]

On 22 February 2022, Russia recognised these occupied territories as the independent so-called Donetsk and Luhansk 'People's Republics' (the DNR and LNR). Therefore, the migration flow data between these territories and Russia is available for the period between the end of February and the beginning of October 2022, until their annexation by Russia. For instance, according to the information reported by the Russian *Mediazona* outlet, Russian Border Guards recorded a total of 1,129,441 crossings of Russian nationals to these territories in 2022.[56] Separately, 142,991 border crossings of Russian nationals to Ukraine (apart from those crossing to the so-called Donetsk and Luhansk 'People's Republics') in 2022 have been recorded since the start of the full-scale invasion on 24 February 2022.[57] Therefore, looking

---

cent of World Refugees: Russian Migration Statistics in 2021 and Their Analysis), report, 2022, 15, https://refugee.ru/wp-content/uploads/2022/06/migraczionnaya-statistika-za-2021-god-i-ee-kratkaya-analitika.docx.pdf [accessed: 31.07.2024].

55 5:00 AM Coalition, *Forced conscription of Ukrainian citizens in the occupied territory of Ukraine by the Russian Federation: facts and legal classification*, report, 2023, https://zmina.ua/wp-content/uploads/sites/2/2023/01/mobilization_eng.pdf [accessed: 31.07.2024].

56 Sergei Golubev, "Rossiyane postavili rekord po vyezdam v Tsentralnuyu Aziyu. Chto govoryat poslednie dannye o peresecheniyakh granitsy" ("Record Entry of Russians into Central Asia: What the Latest Data Says About Border Crossings"), *Mediazona* (*Mediazone*), 08 November 2022, https://zona.media/article/2022/11/08/exit [accessed: 31.07.2024].

57 This number comes from the following calculation: the total number of border crossings of Russian nationals from Russia into Ukraine reported in 2022 was 471,326. From this, we need to deduct the number recorded in the first quarter of 2022 (largely before the full-scale invasion), which was 328,435. Data source: *Mediazona* (*Mediazone*), "Kuda vyezzhali grazhdane Rossii" ("Where Russian Citizens Went"), graphic in a Telegram post, 03 February 2023, https://t.me/mediazzzona/10585 [accessed: 31.07.2024]. Having in mind that Ukraine introduced a visa regime with Russia in July 2022 and strictly controls the entry of nationals of the aggressor state, we can assume that this number of 142,991 may be an estimate of Ukrainian nationals receiving Russian passports and travelling back to Ukraine through available humanitarian corridors throughout the rest of 2022. However, this number does not match the 18,000 Ukrainians travelling back from Russia to Ukraine through humanitarian corridors in the Sumy and Volyn Oblasts from February 2022 to August 2023, which were recorded by the Ukrainian Border Guards. Data source: *Radio Svoboda* (*Radio Freedom*), "Cherez zakryti dilianky kordonu vid pochatku povnomasshtabnoho vtorhnennia povernulos ponad 18 tysiach ukraintsiv – DPSU" ("Over 18 Thousand Ukrainians Have Returned through Closed Border Sections since the Beginning of the Full-Scale Invasion – SBGS"), 08 September 2023, https://www.radiosvoboda.org/a/news-kordon-poverennya-ukrayintsi-rosiya-demchenko-viyna/32538868.html [accessed: 31.07.2024]. In any case, further research is necessary.

at the migration balance, we can assume at least 1.26 million border crossings from Russian to Ukrainian territory (both occupied and government-controlled) in 2022 based on the Russian Border Guard's data. Adding this to the available numbers of transit migration to other countries through Russian and Belarusian territory in 2022 (as indicated above, approximately 300,000 people), we end up with at least 1.56 million exit border crossings of Ukrainian nationals (or those with Ukrainian and Russian citizenships) from Russia.

Keeping in mind that people might have been travelling multiple times between the occupied territories and Russia, we can stress that it is incorrect 1) to equate the number of border crossings with the number of individuals; 2) to assume that all individuals travelled because of the war; 3) to frame all individuals as 'arriving' in Russia and not staying temporarily, returning, or travelling onwards; 4) to think that all travellers were only Ukrainian citizens; and 5) to ignore the fact that such large-scale, supposedly permanent displacement of 5.4 million people could not have been managed by such limited government resources as the state-provided TAP accommodations (which is used by 40,000 people – less than one percent of the supposed 5.4 million) and the onetime 10,000 RUB cash payments, which were distributed to a maximum of 1.4 million people based on government funding data.[58] What about the other millions of supposedly existing 'refugees'? This scale of displacement could not have been simply dispersed across the country.

B. Migration Registration Data (from the Russian Ministry of Internal Affairs)

As noted above, Ukrainian nationals entering Russia and staying at least temporarily must complete a migration registration (*vstat´ na migratsionnyi uchet*), indicating their personal information, place of residence, and reason for entering Russia. Migration registration is a necessary first step in their legalisation and a prerequisite for receiving any kind of social support, employment, or educational placement. In principle, after changing their place of residence, a person has to deregister in their current Russian region and reregister in the new one, or deregister completely if they intend to leave the Russian territory. These (de/re)registrations are not always done or not done on time, so this data is not an accurate reflection of the current situation on the ground but is mostly indicative of the dynamics of migration flow.

58 TASS, "Svyshe 14,1 mlrd rublei vyplatili bezhentsam pribyvshim v Rossiyu s Ukrainy i iz Donbassa" ("Over 14.1 Billion Roubles Paid to Refugees Arriving in Russia from Ukraine and the Donbas"), 05 May 2023, https://tass.ru/obschestvo/17683379 [accessed: 31.07.2024].

Figure 19: Russian migration statistics on Ukrainian nationals in 2022/2023 (based on information from the Russian Ministry of Internal Affairs).

	January–December 2022[59]	**January–June 2023**[60]
Total number refugees recorded in the country (UNHCR, as of 31 December 2022)	1,275,315	No updated number

59 This is based on the 2022 statistics of the Ministry of Internal Affairs of the Russian Federation and a Civic Assistance Committee report. See: Ministry of Internal Affairs of the Russian Federation, *Otdelnye pokazateli migratsionnoi situatsii v Rossiiskoi Federatsii za yanvar-dekabr 2022 goda s raspredeleniem po stranam i regionam (Selected Indicators of the Migration Situation in the Russian Federation for January–December 2022 with Distribution by Countries and Regions)*, report, 18 January 2023, https://мвд.рф/dejatelnost/statistics/migracionnaya/item/35074711/ [accessed: 31.07.2024], (please note that since March 2024 the migration statistics information is no longer publicly available; you can access the previously downloaded copy of this document here https://docs.google.com/spreadsheets/d/1aGhBCaO7V2-QIQ1LcQIPBzAofGE9P1kd/edit?usp=share_link&ouid=118041966722631615728&rtpof=true&sd=true); and Komitet "Grazhdanskoe sodeistvie" (Civic Assistance Committee), *Pasport RF stal "toksichnym aktivom". Statistika MVD za 2022 god: 277 oftssialnykh "bezhentsev", snizhenie interesa k grazhdanstvu (The Russian Passport Has Become a "Toxic Asset". Ministry of Internal Affairs Statistics for 2022: 277 Official "Refugees", Declining Interest in Citizenship)*, report, 23 February 2022, https://refugee.ru/dokladyi/stats-2022-toxic/ [accessed: 31.07.2024].

60 Based on the 2023 statistics of the Ministry of Internal Affairs of the Russian Federation and a Civic Assistance Committee report. See: Ministry of Internal Affairs of the Russian Federation, *Otdelnyje pokazateli migratsionnoi situatsiji v Rossijskoj Federatsiji za janvar-ijun 2023 goda s raspredelieniem po stranam I regionam (Selected Indicators of the Migration Situation in the Russian Federation for January-June 2023 with Distribution by Countries and Regions)*, report, n.d., https://мвд.рф/dejatelnost/statistics/migracionnaya/item/40034334/ [accessed: 31.07.2024] (please note that since March 2024 the migration statistics information is no longer publicly available; you can access the previously downloaded copy of this document here https://docs.google.com/spreadsheets/d/1tjUoXntl8asWmCtTVQyab5MCzM1FL96Y/edit?usp=share_link&ouid=118041966722631615728&rtpof=true&sd=true); and Komitet "Grazhdanskoe sodeistvie" (Civic Assistance Committee), *Statistika MVD: chislo ofitsialnykh "bezhentsev" upalo na tret za god, prodolzhaetsya padenie interesa k grazhdanstvu RF (Ministry of Internal Affairs Statistics: The Number of Official "Refugees" Fell by a Third over the Year, Interest in Russian Citizenship Continues to Fall)*, report, 28 July 2023, https://refugee.ru/dokladyi/stats-1q-2023/ [accessed: 31.07.2024].

MIGRATION REGISTRATIONS (*migratsionnyi uchet*)		
Migration registration (there can be multiple instances per person)	1,069,896	125,903
Migration deregistration (there can be multiple instances per person)	831,611	150,075
Migration registration balance in the given period	+238,285	-24,172
UKRAINIAN NATIONALS – LEGAL STATUS HOLDERS IN RUSSIA BY THE END OF THE PERIOD	**January–December 2022**	**January–June 2023**
Temporary asylum status (*vremennoe ubezhyshche, VU*)	65,374 status-holders by the end of Dec 2022 (97,591 persons received the status in 2022)[61]	51,549 status-holders by the end of March 2023 (2,050 persons received the status between January–March 2023)
Refugee status (*status bezhentsa*)	26 status-holders by the end of 2022 (5 persons received the status in 2022)	25 status-holder by the end of March 2023
Temporary residence permit (*razreshenie na vremennoe prozhivannie, RVP*)	35,603 permit-holders by the end of 2022 (29,389 persons received it in 2022)	25,418 status-holders by the end of June 2023 (356 persons received it during the six months of 2023)
Permanent residence permit (*vid na zhitelstvo, VNZh*)	71,258 permit-holders by the end of 2022 (25,489 persons received it in 2022)	57,351 permit-holders by the end of June 2023 (5,396 persons received it during the six months of 2023)
Citizenship acquisition (excluding passports issued in the occupied territories)	296,901 persons received it during 2022	39,053 persons received it during the six months of 2023
Total number of people with any kind of legal status by the end of 2022	**469,162**	

61 The lower overall number of temporary protection status-holders by the end of 2022 (65,374) compared to the total number of people who receive the status during 2022 (97,591) is explained by people changing their status to a more permanent one, receiving the Russian citizenship or leaving Russia altogether.

When we look closer at the migration registrations of Ukrainian nationals in Russia in 2022 and 2023 (Figure 19), we see that the UNHCR number of 'refugees recorded in the country' – 1.27 million people as of December 2022 – is closer to the number of all migration registrations than any other estimates of the number of displaced Ukrainians. The combined number of migration registrations (and there can be multiple instances per person) in 2022 was over 1 million, but the overall migration balance in that year is an addition of only 238,285, which means that people were registering and then either moving elsewhere in Russia or leaving the Russian territory altogether. The situation in the first six months of 2023 is even more telling, as the migration registration balance is negative (a subtraction of 24,172). Ukrainians either exiting Russia more than entering it or receiving Russian citizenship (which means the person must deregister as a Ukrainian national on Russian territory) might explain this dynamic.

In the entry goals that Ukrainian nationals indicated when doing migration registrations in 2022 and the first months of 2023 (Figure 20), 'private' matters – meaning visiting relatives or friends or temporary stays for other reasons – were indicated in two-thirds of all registrations (Figure 21). As the simplest reason (looking the 'safest' and requiring the least documented confirmation), this entry goal far exceeded 'humanitarian' reasons (totalling 9,029 in 2022 and 581 in the first six months of 2023), which presumably should have been the main entry goal in a situation of mass displacement and people looking for refuge.

We need qualitative data to explain why Ukrainian nationals prefer to indicate 'private' matters as their entry goal for migration registration in Russia, but we can assume that it implies fewer bureaucratic hurdles in the future and less questioning from the authorities. Moreover, to decrease the burden on the state, the authorities might only register those residents in the state-run TAP accommodations who enter for 'humanitarian' reasons. Since we do not have publicly available and detailed statistics according to region and district (*raion*) on the entry goals, we cannot verify this assumption.

Figure 20: Migration registration of Ukrainian nationals in Russia (2022–2023) by entry goals.

The number of migration registrations of Ukrainian citizens in Russia (January–December 2022) by entry goals.[62] Total number of registrations during the period: 1,069,896	
Private	759,110
Work	102,258
Tourism	25,656
Education	14,479
Humanitarian	9,029
Other	94,235

Figure 21: The migration registration of Ukrainian nationals in Russia (2022–2023) divided into entry goals.

The number of migration registrations of Ukrainian citizens in Russia (January–June 2023) by entry goals.[63] Total number of registrations during the period: 125,903	
Private	82,212
Work	11,258
Tourism	4,987
Education	2,405
Humanitarian	581
Other	14,154

All Figures are based on the sources/numbers in Figure 23 (see the Appendix).

62 Ministry of Internal Affairs of the Russian Federation, *Otdelnye pokazateli migratsionnoi situatsii v Rossiiskoi Federatsii za yanvar-dekabr 2022 goda s raspredeleniem po stranam i regionam*, 2022.

63 Ministry of Internal Affairs of the Russian Federation, *Otdelnyje pokazateli migratsionnoj situatsiji v Rossijskoi Federatsiji za janvar-ijun 2023 goda s raspredelieniem po stranam i regionam*, 2023.

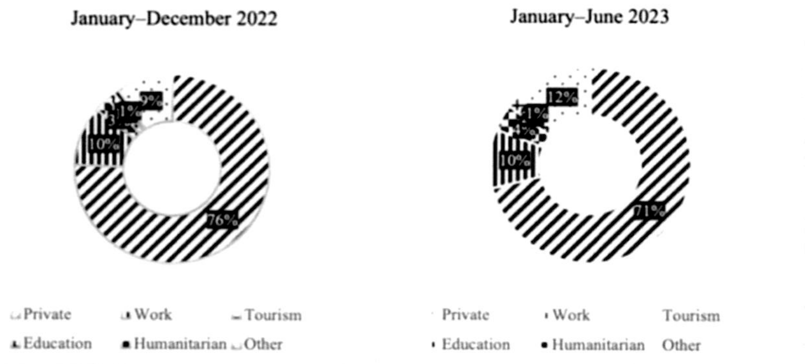

C. Legal Statuses (from the Data of the Russian Ministry of Internal Affairs)

Finally, let us focus on the number of Ukrainian nationals who received any kind of legal status in Russia in 2022 and in the first months of 2023 (see Figure 19 and Figure 22). Ukrainian nationals can enter and remain in Russia without registering for legal status for up to three months. Ukrainians applying for any status in Russia need to undergo mandatory dactyloscopy (the classification of fingerprints) and medical examinations and provide notary-certified translations of relevant documents from the Ukrainian language into Russian. However, Ukrainian nationals will not be able to access any state support or services if they do not regularise their stay through one of the four statuses listed below.

The first is the refugee status (*status bezhentsa*). It is almost non-existent in reality; only five Ukrainian nationals received it in 2022. In total, 26 Ukrainians have received refugee status since 2014. The application for it is lengthy and highly discouraged by Russian officials.

The second is the temporary asylum status (*vremennoe ubezhishche*). Upon receiving this, a person can stay in Russia for one year (with a possibility of extension), apply for the 10,000 RUB onetime cash allowance, work, and study, but cannot leave the Russian territory without losing the status. In 2022, 97,591 Ukrainian nationals received temporary asylum status in Russia, but only 65,374 held it by the end of the year. Some of the previous status holders left the country, and some applied for other statuses or were naturalised.[64] 65,374 is almost the same as the UNHCR number of persons who applied for any kind of status in Russia (see Figure 13), which is 65,400. We can safely conclude that this is where the UNHCR data is coming from.

Third are the temporary or permanent residencies (*razreshenie na vremennoe prozhivanie, vid na zhitelstvo*). These are not very popular due to lengthy procedures

64 Troitskii, *Skolko bezhentsev s Ukrainy*.

with few of the immediate cash and service benefits necessary for war-displaced people and many restrictions on travel and work.

Figure 22: Ukrainian nationals in Russia divided into their legal statuses or a lack thereof (2022).

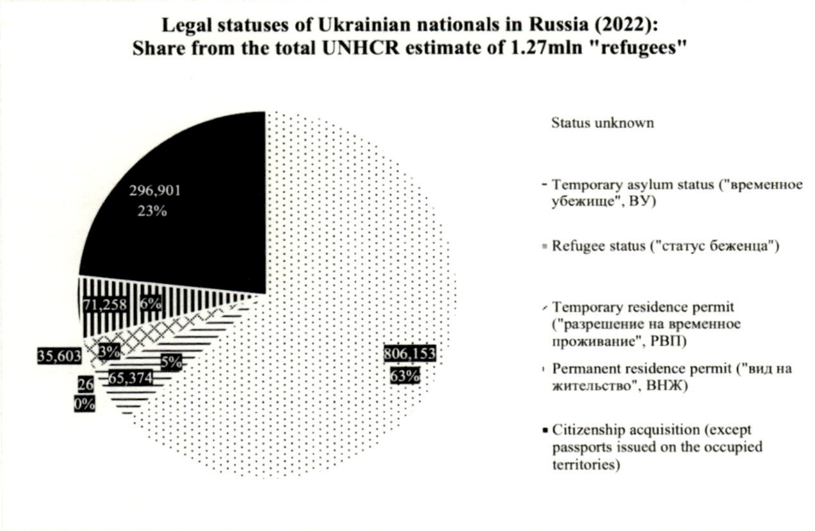

based on data from the Russian Ministry of Internal Affairs as summarised in Figure 19. The percentages are based on the UNHCR total estimate of 1.27 million "refugees from Ukraine in Russia" as of December 2022.

Finally, naturalisation, the fourth option, is the most favoured by Russian officials. Since 2019, Russia has sped up its naturalisation requirements for Ukrainian nationals, especially those from the occupied Donbas region. In May–July 2022, after the occupation of Ukrainian south-eastern territories, the naturalisation procedure for Ukrainian nationals became even more simplified and de facto mandatory in the occupied territories.[65] For war-displaced Ukrainians already on Russian territory, naturalisation is often the only way to access the state services that citizens are entitled to. For instance, full state medical insurance (beyond emergency care), free medication, social benefits, and pensions – all of which are essential for the

---

65 Yale School of Public Health Humanitarian Research Lab, *Forced Passportization in Russia-Occupied Areas of Ukraine: Conflict Observatory Report*, report, 2023, https://hub.conflictobservatory.org/portal/sharing/rest/content/items/e280a7eeb7bf4dc588ed50ee655b9858/data [accessed: 31.07.2024].

elderly, people with disabilities and/or chronic illnesses, and/or those wounded in the war – are only available after receiving Russian citizenship. Similarly, access to legal employment, education, mortgages, and bank loans is facilitated for citizens with permanent residency and difficult to access for foreigners with temporary residency. Overall, 300,000 Ukrainian nationals received Russian citizenship in 2022.[66] Many refuse the push for naturalisation, as they are afraid of the repercussions back in Ukraine, where they left family members and/or property and eventually expect to return. Others are afraid of being drafted into the Russian Army shortly after or not being allowed to leave the Russian territory.

Even though a substantial number of Ukrainians could still be waiting for their legal statuses in Russia, their number is far smaller than both the official Russian and UNHCR numbers of border crossings. According to independent Russian demographer Alexey Raksha and his colleagues, only 0.5–1 million Ukrainian nationals stayed in Russia due to the full-scale invasion.[67] Based on all the data sources discussed above – and particularly the data from the Russian Ministry of Internal Affairs – the number seems to be at most 1 million Ukrainian nationals displaced to the Russian Federation since February 2022. It is more difficult to estimate the number of Ukrainian nationals originating from the territories occupied since 2014, because they might also be Russian passport holders. Their cross-border and intra-Russian travel is harder to track. Still, as the Ukrainian government does not recognise the forced giving out of passports, they remain Ukrainian citizens and retain their right to return to Ukraine at any time.

Conclusions

As suggested by Peter Andreas and Kelly M. Greenhill, "[i]f it is not measured, it doesn't exist. If it is not counted, it doesn't count".[68] The creation, selection, promotion, and proliferation of data are political processes, yet we need data for a problem to be recognised, defined, prioritised, and debated by policymakers and societies.[69] What will happen to Ukrainians displaced to Russia after the war? What kinds of resources will be necessary to support them and ease their return? Distortions in num-

66 Ministry of Internal Affairs of the Russian Federation, *Otdelnye pokazateli migratsionnoi…*, 2022.

67 Nina Polyanskaya, "'Esli my dozhivem do kontsa etogo goda, ya budu udivlen i rad'. Demograf Aleksei Raksha o vliyanii voiny na budushchee rossiyan" ("'If We Survive until the End of This Year, I Will Be Glad and Surprised': Interview with Demographer Aleksei Raksha about the Impact of the War on the Future Of Russians"), *Diskurs* (*Discourse*), 24 March 2023, https://discours.co/articles/social/aleksey-raksha-about-russian-demography [accessed: 31.07.2024].

68 Andreas and Greenhill, *Sex, Drugs and Body Counts*, 1.

69 Ibid., 2.

bers might result from either carelessness or intentionality, so we must be aware of the sources and agendas of data producers and those who circulate it. Russia intentionally inflates the number of those fleeing Ukraine to embarrass its enemy and prove its own 'humanitarianism'. The announcement of a big, shocking, and attention-catching number connected to sensitive issues – and amplified by press coverage – legitimises and perpetuates data that might be difficult to correct later.[70]

The speculations about the number of forcibly displaced Ukrainians (and in particular children) in Russia – ranging from thousands to millions – illustrate that numbers have become yet another war tool. The numbers of border crossings transform into people, and diverse categories of travellers are reported under one label. Numbers provided by the Russian side are repeated by the UNHCR and enter official Ukrainian rhetoric. At the same time, the sources for the data are unreported, unreliable, or based on unknown methodologies. The 'politics of numbers' pose the risk of missing the needs of the individual people behind these numbers because state, international, and civil society actors lack the basis to plan realistic interventions and the necessary resources to identify, reach out to, and support Ukrainians still on Russian territory and to assist them in returning to Ukraine or relocating elsewhere. Even though I conclude that a more realistic estimate of the number of Ukrainian citizens displaced to Russia since the full-scale invasion is neither 5.4 million nor 2.85 million but, rather, one million people at most, each of them still needs this protection and support.

Appendix

Methodological note

The following table is based on daily monitoring of selected official Russian and Ukrainian media sources in search of relevant information about the number of forcibly displaced Ukrainians in Russia. For instance, on the Ukrainian side, this includes the announcements of Iryna Vereshchuk (the Deputy Prime Minister and the Minister for the Reintegration of the Temporarily Occupied Territories); Dmytro Lubinets (the Ukrainian Ombudsman) and his predecessor, Lyudmyla Denisova; the National Information Bureau; and Daria Gerasymchuk (the Children's Ombudswoman). On the Russian side, I monitored TASS announcements and the statements of Maria Lvova-Belova (the Russian Presidential Children's Ombudswoman) and combined these with information on the Russian Ministry of Internal Affairs' website. I obtained the data from UNHCR Russia from their monthly digests. Below, I reference all numbers and sources.

70 Ibid., 26.

References

Figure 23: Combined UNHCR, Russian, and Ukrainian data on the number of Ukrainian citizens displaced to Russia (February 2022–August 2023).

	UNHCR data (based on data from the Russian Ministry for Emergency Situations)[71]	**Official Russian numbers** (based on regular TASS updates)	**Official Ukrainian numbers** (a source is indicated for each number)
18–23 February 2022	105,000	68,500 from the ORDLO (21 February)[72] 93,500 from the ORDLO, including 30,000 Russian citizens (22 February)[73]	No data
24–28 February 2022	148,322	No data	No data
March 2022	285,537	213,152, including 48,788 children (10 March)[74] 400,000 (23 March)[75]	No data
April 2022	688,400	1.13 million, including 200,000 children; most people from the ORDLO[76]	500,000, including 121,000 children[77]
May 2022	1,041,095	1.6 million, including 260,000 children; most people from the ORDLO[78]	No data

71 Data for each month taken from the UNHCR Russia Monthly Digests and the UNHCR Ukraine Data Portal: UNHCR Russia, "Otchety o deiyatelnosti v Rossii".

72 Nesterov, "V Rossii nazvali chislo pribyvshykh iz Donbassa bezhentsev".

73 Izvestiya (News), "Nazvano chislo privyvshykh v RF bezhentsev is Donbassa".

74 Kulikova, "Nazvano chislo pribyvshykh v Rossiyu bezhentsev iz Donbassa".

75 Kiryanov, "V MChS utochnili kolichestvo pribyvshykh v Rossiju bezetszev is Ukrainy i Donbassa".

76 Agafonov, "Pochti 200 000 detiej-bezhenstvev".

77 Statement by Ambassador Sergiy Kyslytsya, the Permanent Representative of Ukraine to the UN, at the UN Security Council meeting on the "Maintenance of peace and security of Ukraine": Sergíy Kyslytsya, "Check against delivery…".

78 Agafonov, "V Rossiyu pribyli uzhe 1,6 mln bezentsev".

June 2022	1,460,650	2.3 million, including 364,000 children; half of all people from the ORDLO[79]	1.2 million, including 240,000 children, among them 2,000 orphans[80]
July 2022	1,952,037	3 million, including 478,000 children[81]	2 million, including a "couple hundred thousand children"[82] 5,600 children according to the Ukrainian Ministry of Internal Affairs[83]
August 2022	2,414,075	3.6 million, including 576,000 children[84]	No data
September 2022	2,820,288	4.2 million, including 654,000 children; almost half of all people from the ORDLO (approximately 2 million)[85]	2.5 million, including 38,000 children[86]
October 2022	2,852,395	4.7 million, including 705,000 children[87]	1.6 million[88]

79 Agafonov, "V Rossii uzhe 2,3 mln bezhentsev".
80 Tyshchenko, "V uriadi povidomyly, skilky ukraintsiv uzhe deportovano do Rosii".
81 Agafonov, "V Rossiyu pribyli uzhe boleje 3 mln bezhentsev s Ukrainy i iz respublik Donbassa".
82 Balachuk, "Okupanty deportuvaly 2 miliony ukraintsiv".
83 Andreeva, "U MVS povidomyly, skilky ukrainskykh ditei deportuvaly v Rosiiu".
84 Izvestiya (News), "Chislo pribyvshykh v RF bezhentsev s territorii Donbassa i Ukrainy prevysilo 3,6 mln".
85 Agafonov, "Chislo bezhentsev v Rossiju prevysilo 4,2 mln chelovek".
86 Baltic News Network (BNN), "Ukrainian official: 2.5 million people forcibly deported to Russia". See also the full notes from the UN Security Council meeting on 07 September 2022.
87 Shevtsova, "Bolee 4,7 mln bezhentsev iz Ukrainy".
88 President of Ukraine, Volodomyr Zelenskyy, Official Website, "Nam potribna vasha pidtrymka, shchob pryskoryty nastannia myru".

November 2022	No updated data published	4.8 million, including 714,000 children [89] In November 2022, based on Decree No. 756,[90] Russian occupying forces forcibly resettled around 115,000 people from Kherson and the Kherson Oblast[91]	6,032 children (Office of the Ombudsman)[92] 11,000 children (President Zelenskyy)[93] 45,995, including 8,140 children (National Information Bureau)[94]
December 2022	No updated data published	5 million, including 721,000 children[95]	More than 1 million Ukrainians (Ministry of Internal Affairs)[96] 2.8 million (Ombudsman Lubinets)[97] 13,000 children (Children's Ombudswoman of Ukraine)[98] 3,400 POWs, 15,000 missing persons[99]
January 2023	No updated data published	5.2 million, including 733,000 children[100]	14,350 children, 20,000 missing persons (Ombudsman Lubinets)[101]
February 2023	No updated data published	5.3 million, including 738,000 children[102]	150,000 children (Ombudsman Lubinets)[103]

89 Agafonov, "Chislo bezhentsev v Rossii prevysilo 4,8 mln chelovek".

90 Ofitsialnoe opublikovanie pravovykh aktov (Official Publication of Legal Acts), Decree of the President of the Russian Federation from 19 October 2022, No. 756.

91 Keffer, "Saldo: iz Khersona s fevralya uekhali bolee 150 tysyatch tchelovek".

92 Ukrainska Pravda (Ukrainian Truth), "Occupiers abduct more than 6,000 Ukrainian children".

93 Pohorilov, "Okupanty deportuvaly 11 tysiach ditei do Rosii".

94 Ombudsman of Ukraine, *Spetsialna dopovid*.

95 Nikolaev, "Chislo bezentsev s Ukrainy i iz Donbassa v Rossii dostiglo 5 mln".

96 MVS Ukrainy (Ukrainian Ministry of Internal Affairs), "DMS oformylo pershe posvidchennia na povernennia v Ukrainu...".

97 Ombudsman Lubinets Dmytro, "Shchonaimenshe 2 800 000 ukraintsiv".

98 Krechetova, "Okupanty deportuvaly".

99 Andalitska, "Nazvano kilkist polonenykh ta znyklykh bezvisty ukrainskykh biitsiv".

100 TASS, "S fevralya 2022 goda v Rossiyu pribyli bolee 5,2 mln bezhentsev s territorii Ukrainy"

101 Lykhogliad, "Zvilnenia polonenykh, povernennia deportovanykh i perehovory z RF".

102 TASS, "Za god s Ukrainy i iz Donbassa na territoriyu RF pribylo 5,3 mln bezhetsev".

103 Ukrinform, "Kilkist nezakonno vyvezenykh u rosiiu ukrainskykh ditei mozhe siahaty 150 tysiach".

March 2023	No updated data published	5.5 million, including 749,000 children[104]	19,514 children (Ministry of Reintegration of Temporarily Occupied Territories)[105], including 4,390 children under state care (Deputy Prime Minister Vereshchuk)[106]
April 2023	No updated data published	No updated data published	100,000 children (National Resistance Centre)[107]
May 2023	No updated data published	No updated data published	No updated data published
June 2023	1,275,315 "refugees from Ukraine recorded in the country" as of 31 December 2022 100,835 refugees from Ukraine who applied for asylum, temporary protection, or similar national protection schemes (as of 31 December 2022)	Up to 5 million people, including up to 1 million without documents and 1.5–2 million "'flowing' wanderers" [108] (*'peretekaemye' skitaltsy*) moving back and forth between "new territories of Russia" and Russia, often without documents. 6 June: explosion of the Kakhovka Dam – 7,000 displaced (Vladimir Saldo, the so-called 'Governor of the Kherson Oblast' appointed by the Russian occupation administration)[109]	20,000 children, including 4,500 children under state care (Deputy Prime Minister Vereshchuk)[110]
July 2023	No updated data	No updated data	No updated data

104 TASS, "V Rossiyu s territorii Donbassa i Ukrainy pribylo 5.5 mln bezhentsev s fevralya 2022 goda".

105 Minreintehratsii (Ukrainian Ministry of Reintegration of Temporarily Occupied Territories), "Natsionalne informatsiine biuro".

106 Ministry of Reintegration of the Temporarily Occupied Territories of Ukraine, "Iryna Vereshchuk".

107 Tsentr natsionalnoho sprotyvu (Centre for National Resistance), "Rosiiany vyvezly ponad 100 tys. ditei zi Skhodu Ukrainy na 'likuvannia'".

108 Emelyanenko, "Rossiya prinyala pyat millionov bezhentsev s Ukrainy".

109 Plamenev, "Saldo soobshchil o 7 tys. evakuirovannykh iz zatoplennykh rayonov Khersonshchiny".

110 Andreeva, "RF deportuvala ponad 4,5 tysiachi ukrainskykh syrit ta ditei bez batkivskoho pikluvannia".

August 2023	No updated data Corrected number: 65,400 refugees from Ukraine who applied for asylum, TP, or similar national protection schemes (as of 31 December 2022)	4.8 million people, including more than 700,000 children (Russian Children's Ombudswoman Lvova-Belova)[111]	700,000 children (Ombudsman Lubinets)[112] 19,546 children have been deported (Children of War official portal)[113]

Bibliography

5:00 AM Coalition, *Deportation of Ukrainian citizens from the territory of active military operations or from the temporarily occupied territory of Ukraine to the territory of the Russian Federation and the Republic of Belarus*, report, 2023, https://zmina.ua/en/publication-en/deportation-of-ukrainian-citizens-from-the-territory-of-active-military-operations-or-from-the-temporarily-occupied-territory-of-ukraine-to-the-territory-of-the-russian-federation-and-the-republic-of/ [accessed: 25.07.2024].

5:00 AM Coalition, *Forced conscription of Ukrainian citizens in the occupied territory of Ukraine by the Russian Federation: facts and legal classification*, report, 2023, https://zmina.ua/wp-content/uploads/sites/2/2023/01/mobilization_eng.pdf [accessed: 25.07.2024].

Agafonov, Ilya, "Chislo bezhentsev v Rossii prevysilo 4,8 mln chelovek" ("The Number of Refugees in Russia Surpassed 4.8 Mil People"), *miloserdie.ru (mercy.ru)*, 22 November 2022, https://www.miloserdie.ru/news/chislo-bezhenczev-v-rossii-prevysilo-48-mln-chelovek/ [accessed: 25.07.2024].

Agafonov, Ilya, "Chislo bezhentsev v Rossiju prevysilo 4,2 mln chelovek" ("The Number of Refugees to Russia Surpassed 4.2 Mil People"), *miloserdie.ru (mercy.ru)*, 19 September 2022, https://www.miloserdie.ru/news/chislo-bezhenczev-v-rossii-prevysilo-42-mln-chelovek/ [accessed: 25.07.2024].

111 Lvova-Belova, *Doklad o deyatelnosti Upolnomochennogo*.

112 Ombudsman Lubinets Dmytro, "Deportatsiia ditei".

113 Dity viiny, https://childrenofwar.gov.ua.

Agafonov, Ilya, "V Rossiyu pribyli uzhe boleje 3 mln bezhentsev s Ukrainy i iz respublik Donbassa" ("More than 3 Mil Refugees from Ukraine and the Donbas Republics Have Already Come to Russia"), *miloserdie.ru (mercy.ru)*, 01 August 2022, https://www.miloserdie.ru/news/v-rossiyu-pribyli-uzhe-bolee-3-mln-bezhenczev-s-ukrainy-i-iz-respublik-donbassa/ [accessed: 25.07.2024].

Agafonov, Ilya, "V Rossii uzhe 2,3 mln bezhentsev" ("There Are Already 2.3 Mil Refugees in Russia"), *miloserdie.ru (mercy.ru)*, 04 July 2022, https://www.miloserdie.ru/news/v-rossii-uzhe-23-mln-bezhenczev/ [accessed: 25.07.2024].

Agafonov, Ilya, "V Rossiyu pribyli uzhe 1,6 mln bezentsev, 260 tysyach iz nikh – deti" ("1.6 Mil Refugees Have Arrived to Russia, 260 Thousand of Them Are Children"), *miloserdie.ru (mercy.ru)*, 01 June 2022, https://www.miloserdie.ru/news/v-rossiyu-pribyli-uzhe-16-mln-bezhenczev-260-tysyach-iz-nih-deti/ [accessed: 25.07.2024].

Agafonov, Ilya, "Pochti 200 000 detiej-bezhenstvev pribyli iz Donbassa v RF, ich chislo prodolzhajet rasti" ("Almost 200 000 Children-Refugees Arrived from Donbas to RF, Their Number Continues To Grow"), *miloserdie.ru (mercy.ru)*, 05 May 2022, https://www.miloserdie.ru/news/pochti-200-tysyach-detej-bezhenczev-pribyli-s-donbassa-v-rf-ih-chislo-prodolzhaet-rasti/ [accessed: 25.07.2024].

Amnesty International, "'Like A Prison Convoy': Russia's Unlawful Transfer And Abuse of Civilians In Ukraine During 'Filtration'", 10 November 2022, https://www.amnesty.org/en/documents/eur50/6136/2022/en/ [accessed: 25.07.2024].

Anastasiadou, Athina, Artem Volgin, and Douglas R. Leasure, "War and Migration: Quantifying the Russian Exodus through Yandex Search Trends", *SocArXiv Papers*, 18 May 2023, 1–25, https://osf.io/preprints/socarxiv/92zam/ [accessed: 25.07.2024].

Andalitska, Inna, "Nazvano kilkist polonenykh ta znyklykh bezvisty ukrainskykh biitsiv" ("The Number of Captured and Missing Ukrainian Soldiers was Announced"), *Unian*, 30 December 2022, https://www.unian.ua/war/rosiyskiy-polon-skilki-ukrajinskih-viyskovih-potrapili-u-polon-12094866.html [accessed: 25.07.2024].

Andreas, Peter, and Kelly M. Greenhill, "Introduction: The Politics of Numbers", in: Peter Andreas and Kelly M. Greenhill (eds.), *Sex, Drugs, and Body Counts: The Politics of Numbers in Global Crime and Conflict*, Ithaca, NY: Cornell University Press, 2010, 1–18.

Andreeva, Viktoriia, "U MVS povidomyly, skilky ukrainskykh ditei deportuvaly v Rosiiu" ("The Ministry of Internal Affairs Reports How Many Ukrainian Children Were Deported to Russia"), *Ukrainska Pravda (Ukrainian Truth)*, 29 July 2022, https://life.pravda.com.ua/society/2022/07/29/249787/ [accessed: 25.07.2024].

Andreeva, Viktoriia, "RF deportuvala ponad 4,5 tysiachi ukrainskykh syrit ta ditei bez batkivskoho pikluvannia – Vereshchuk" ("The RF Deported More than 4.5

Thousand Ukrainian Orphans and Children Without Parental Care – Deputy PM Vereshchuk"), *Ukrainska Pravda (Ukrainian Truth)*, 01 June 2023, https://life.pravda.com.ua/society/2023/06/1/254606/ [accessed: 25.07.2024].

Anti-Discrimination Centre Memorial Brussels, *Violation of the Rights of Children Taken from Ukraine to Russia and Belarus as a Result of Russian Military Aggression*, report, 12 June 2023, https://adcmemorial.org/en/publications/violation-of-the-rights-of-children-taken-from-ukraine-to-russia-and-belarus-as-a-result-of-russian-military-aggression/ [accessed: 25.07.2024].

Balachuk, Iryna, "Okupanty deportuvaly 2 miliony ukraintsiv – prezydent" ("The President: The Occupiers Have Deported 2 Million Ukrainians"), *Ukrainska Pravda (Ukrainian Truth)*, 13 July 2022, https://www.pravda.com.ua/news/2022/07/13/7357898/ [accessed: 25.07.2024].

Baltic News Network (BNN), "Ukrainian official: 2.5 million people forcibly deported to Russia", 08 September 2022, https://bnn-news.com/ukrainian-official-2-5-million-people-forcibly-deported-to-russia-238234 [accessed: 25.07.2024].

Bilkova, Veronika, Cecilie Hellestveit, and Elina Steinerte, *Report on Violations and Abuses of International Humanitarian and Human Rights Law, War Crimes and Crimes against Humanity, Related to the Forcible Transfer and/or Deportation of Ukrainian Children to the Russian Federation*, Organization for Security and Co-operation in Europe, Office for Democratic Institutions and Human Rights, report, 2023, https://www.osce.org/files/f/documents/7/7/542751_1.pdf [accessed: 25.07.2024].

Cardona-Fox, Gabriel, "The Politics of IDP Data", *Refugee Survey Quarterly* 39/4, 2020, 620–633.

Colvin, Victoria, and Phil Orchard, "Forced Deportations and the Ukraine War: Russian Culpability in Atrocity Crimes", *Violence: An International Journal* 3/2, 2023, 1–20.

Crisp, Jeff, "Who Is Counting the Refugees? Displacement Data, Its Limitations, and Potential for Misuse", *Refugee History*, 04 August 2022, https://refugeehistory.org/blog/2022/8/4/who-is-counting-refugees-displacement-data-its-limitations-and-potential-for-misuse [accessed: 25.07.2024].

Crisp, Jeff, "'Who Has Counted the Refugees?' UNHCR and the Politics of Numbers", *New Issues in Refugee Research*, June 1999, https://www.refworld.org/pdfid/4ff58e4b2.pdf [accessed: 25.07.2024].

Derzhavnyi komitet statystyky Ukrainy (State Statistics Committee of Ukraine), "Vseukrainskyi perepys naselennia 2001" ("All-Ukrainian Population Census"), http://2001.ukrcensus.gov.ua/publications/#p1 [accessed: 25.07.2024].

Dity viiny (Children of War), https://childrenofwar.gov.ua [accessed: 25.07.2024].

Dudko, Oksana, "A Conceptual Limbo of Genocide: Russian Rhetoric, Mass Atrocities in Ukraine, and the Current Definition's Limits", *Canadian Slavonic Papers* 64/2–3, 2022, 133–145.

Emelyanenko, Vladimir, "Rossiya prinyala pyat millionov bezhentsev s Ukrainy" ("Russia Accepted Five Million Refugees from Ukraine"), *RG.ru*, 19 June 2023, https://rg.ru/2023/06/19/grazhdane-skitalcy.html [accessed: 25.07.2024].

Fond pomoshchi bezhentsam "Dom s mayakom" (House with a Lighthouse Foundation for Assistance to Refugees), official website, https://mayak.fund [accessed: 12.08.2023].

Getmanova, Daria, and Svitlana Matviyenko, "Producing the Subject of Deportation: Filtration Processes during the Russia–Ukraine War", *Sociologica* (Sociology) 16/2, 2022, 239–252.

Glasman, Joël, and Brendan Lawson, "Ten Things We Know about Humanitarian Numbers", Journal of Humanitarian Affairs 5/1, 2023, 1–10.

Golubev, Sergei, "Rossiyane postavili rekord po vyezdam v Tsentralnuyu Aziyu. Chto govoryat poslednie dannye o peresecheniyakh granitsy" ("Record Entry of Russians into Central Asia: What the Latest Data Says About Border Crossings"), *Mediazona (Mediazone)*, 08 November 2022, https://zona.media/article/2022/11/08/exit [accessed: 25.07.2024].

Hamlin, Rebecca, *Crossing: How We Label and React to People on the Move*, Redwood City: Stanford University Press, 2021.

Hook, Kristina, *The Russian Federation's Escalating Commission of Genocide in Ukraine: A Legal Analysis*, report, July 2023, https://newlinesinstitute.org/wp-content/uploads/20230726-Genocide-Ukraine-Report-NISLAP_.pdf [accessed: 25.07.2024].

Human Rights Centre ZMINA, *Deportation of Custodial Settings from Occupied Territories of Ukraine*, report, 2023, https://zmina.ua/wp-content/uploads/sites/2/2023/07/deportation_f_eng_web.pdf [accessed: 25.07.2024].

Human Rights Centre ZMINA, *Deportation of Residents of Kherson Region: Organized and Independent Departure under Coercion*, report, 2023, https://zmina.ua/wp-content/uploads/sites/2/2023/07/deport_eng_web.pdf [accessed: 25.07.2024].

Human Rights Centre ZMINA, *Deportation of Ukrainian Citizens to the Territory of the Russian Federation: Signs and Context*, report, April 2023, https://zmina.ua/wp-content/uploads/sites/2/2023/05/deport_people_eng_web.pdf [accessed: 25.07.2024].

Human Rights Watch, *"We Must Provide a Family, Not Rebuild Orphanages": The Consequences of Russia's Invasion of Ukraine for Children in Ukrainian Residential Institutions*, report, 13 March 2023, https://www.hrw.org/report/2023/03/13/we-must-provide-family-not-rebuild-orphanages/consequences-russias-invasion [accessed: 25.07.2024].

International Centre for Migration Policy Development (ICMPD), *ICMPD Migration Outlook: Eastern Europe and Central Asia*, 2023, report, 2023, https://www.icmpd.org/file/download/59104/file/230215_ICMPD_Migration_Outlook_EasternEuropeCentralAsia_2023_final.pdf [accessed: 25.07.2024].

International Committee of the Red Cross (ICRC), *ICRC's Central Tracing Agency Bureau for the International Armed Conflict between the Russian Federation and Ukraine*, report, 2023, https://t.me/mkkk_ru/596 [accessed: 25.07.2024].

International Organization for Migration (IOM) UN Migration, *LATVIA. On the Way Back to Ukraine: Surveys with Refugees on Destinations, Length of Stay & Assistance*, report, April–June 2023, https://dtm.iom.int/sites/g/files/tmzbdl1461/files/reports/DTM_2023_LVA_Crossing_back_survey_Ukraine_Q2.pdf [accessed: 25.07.2024].

Ioffe, Yulia, "Forcibly Transferring Ukrainian Children to the Russian Federation: A Genocide?", *Journal of Genocide Research* (Forthcoming), 2022, https://papers.ssrn.com/sol3/papers.cfm?abstract_id=4236369 [accessed: 25.07.2024].

Izvestiya (News), "Chislo pribyvshykh v RF bezhentsev s territorii Donbassa i Ukrainy prevysilo 3,6 mln" ("The Number of Refugees Coming to Russia from the Territory of the Donbas and Ukraine Surpassed 3.6 Mil"), 23 August 2022, https://iz.ru/1383744/2022-08-23/chislo-pribyvshikh-v-rf-bezhentcev-s-territorii-donbassa-i-ukrainy-prevysilo-36-mln [accessed: 25.04.2024].

Izvestiya (News), "Nazvano chislo privyvshykh v RF bezhentsev is Donbassa" ("The Number of Arriving Refugees from the Donbas to the Russian Federation is Announced"), 22 February 2022, https://iz.ru/1295564/2022-02-22/istochnik-nazval-chislo-pribyvshikh-v-rf-bezhentcev-iz-donbassa [accessed: 25.07.2024].

Kamalov, Emil, et al., *Russia's 2022 Anti-War Exodus: The Attitudes and Expectations of Russian Migrants*, PONARS Eurasia, report, September 2022, https://www.ponarseurasia.org/wp-content/uploads/2022/09/Pepm790_Kamalov-Kostenko-Sergeeva-Zavadskaya_Sept2022.pdf [accessed: 25.07.2024].

Keffer, Laura, "Saldo: iz Khersona s fevralya uekhali bolee 150 tysyatch tchelovek" ("Balance: More than 150 Thousand People Left Kherson since February"), *Kommersant (Merchant)*, 21 December 2022, https://www.kommersant.ru/doc/5735376?from=lenta [accessed: 25.07.2024].

Kidmapping map, https://mapping.kids [accessed: 25.07.2024].

Kiryanov, Roman, "V MChS utochnili kolichestvo pribyvshykh v Rossiju bezetszev is Ukrainy i Donbassa" ("The Ministry for Emergency Situations Clarified the Number of Refugees from Ukraine and the Donbas Arriving in Russia], *Lenta.ru*, 23 March 2022, https://lenta.ru/news/2022/03/23/bezhenci/ [accessed: 25.07.2024].

Kokourova, Anastasija, "17 organov vlasti zasekretili statistiku s fevralya proshlogo goda" ("17 Governmental Institutions Made Statistics Secret as of February of Last Year"), *Esli byt tochnym (To Be Precise)*, 18 May 2023, https://tochno.st/materials/zasekretili-statistiku-s-fevralya-proshlogo-goda [accessed: 25.07.2024].

Komitet "Grazhdanskoe sodeistvie" (Civic Assistance Committee), official website, https://refugee.ru [accessed: 12.08.2023].

Komitet "Grazhdanskoe sodeistvie" (Civic Assistance Committee), *Statistika MVD: chislo ofitsialnykh "bezhentsev" upalo na tret za god, prodolzhaetsya padenie interesa k grazhdanstvu RF (Ministry of Internal Affairs Statistics: The Number of Official "Refugees" Fell by a Third over the Year, Interest in Russian Citizenship Continues to Fall)*, report, 28 July 2023, https://refugee.ru/dokladyi/stats-1q-2023/ [accessed: 12.08.2023].

Komitet "Grazhdanskoe sodeistvie" (Civic Assistance Committee), *Pasport RF stal "toksichnym aktivom". Statistika MVD za 2022 god: 277 oftssialnykh "bezhentsev", snizhenie interesa k grazhdanstvu (The Russian Passport Has Become a "Toxic Asset". Ministry of Internal Affairs Statistics for 2022: 277 Official "Refugees", Declining Interest in Citizenship)*, report, 23 February 2022, https://refugee.ru/dokladyi/stats-2022-toxic/ [accessed: 12.08.2023].

Komitet "Grazhdanskoe sodeistvie" (Civic Assistance Committee), *Ubezhyshche dlya 0,04% bezhentsev v mire: rossiiskaya migratsyonnajy statistika za 2021 god i ee analitika (Asylum for 0.04 Percent of World Refugees: Russian Migration Statistics in 2021 and Their Analysis)*, report, 2022, https://refugee.ru/wp-content/uploads/2022/06/migraczionnaya-statistika-za-2021-god-i-ee-kratkaya-analitika.docx.pdf [accessed: 25.07.2024].

Krechetova, Diana, "Okupanty deportuvaly do RF ponad 13 tysiach ukrainskykh ditei – dytiachyi ombudsmen" ("Children's Rights Ombudswoman: The Occupiers Deported More than 13 Thousand Ukrainian Children to the RF"), *Ukrainska Pravda (Ukrainian Truth)*, 09 December 2022, https://life.pravda.com.ua/society/2022/12/9/251776/ [accessed: 25.07.2024].

Kulikova, Evgeniya, "Nazvano chislo pribyvshykh v Rossiyu bezhentsev iz Donbassa" ("The Number of Incoming Refugees from the Donbas to Russia Has Been Announced"), *Lenta.ru*, 10 March 2022, https://lenta.ru/news/2022/03/10/begenci/ [accessed: 25.07.2024].

Kuznetsova, Irina, "To Help 'Brotherly People'? Russian Policy Towards Ukrainian Refugees", *Europe-Asia Studies* 72/3, 2020, 505–527.

Kyslytsya, Sergíy, "Check against delivery...", Facebook post, 19 April 2022, https://www.facebook.com/sergiy.grau/posts/pfbid0af89MyF9htER2DLdiCinmHUWjqTe69A6cJ8TFydh21baneRgCb7n551T71t2Tyeel [accessed: 25.07.2024].

Lawson, Brendan, and Irina Mützelburg, "Humanitarian Numbers in the Russian–Ukrainian War: An Interview with Irina Mützelburg (October 2022)", *Journal of Humanitarian Affairs* 5/1, 2023, 52–61.

Lvova-Belova, Maria, *Doklad o deyatelnosti Upolnomochennogo pri Prezidente Rossiiskoi Federatsii po pravam rebenka v 2022 godu (Report on the Activity of the Russian Federation's Presidential Children's Rights Ombudsman in 2022)*, report, 2023, http://deti.gov.ru/detigray/upload/documents/July2023/7JkHUTqLIsZL45JDp4Xl.pdf [accessed: 12.08.2023].

Lykhogliad, Kateryna, Zvilnenia polonenykh, povernennia deportovanykh i perehovory z RF. Intervju z ombudsmenom Lubintsem" (The Release of Prisoners, the Return of the Deported and Negotiations with the RF. Interview with Ombudsman Lubinets), *Radio Svoboda*, 27 January 2023, https://www.radiosvoboda.org/a/lubinets-poloneni-deportovani-moskalkova/32241301.html [accessed: 25.07.2024].

Malyarenko, Tetyana, and Borys Kormych, "New Wild Fields: How the Russian War Leads to the Demodernization of Ukraine's Occupied Territories", *Nationalities Papers*, 2023, 1–19, https://doi.org/10.1017/nps.2023.33.

Malyarenko, Tetyana, and Borys Kormych, "Russian Policy towards the Economy of Occupied Ukrainian Territories: Crawling de-Modernization", *Eurasian Geography and Economics* 64/2, 2023, 1–18, https://doi.org/10.1080/15387216.2023.2167097.

Matviichuk, Oleksandra, "A Speech to Europe by Oleksandra Matviivhuk", *Documenting Ukraine Blog*, https://www.iwm.at/documenting-ukraine/blog/a-speech-to-europe-2023-by-oleksandra-matviichuk [accessed: 25.07.2024].

Mazurenko, Alona, "Do reestru znyklykh bezvisty vnesly informatsiiu pro ponad 24 tysiatchi osib – upovnovazhenei" ("More than 24,000 Persons Were Registered in the Database of Missing Persons"), *Ukrainska Pravda (Ukrainian Truth)*, 12 July 2023, https://www.pravda.com.ua/news/2023/07/12/7410945/ [accessed: 25.07.2024].

Mediazona (Mediazone), "Kuda vyezzhali grazhdane Rossii" ("Where Russian Citizens Went"), graphic in a Telegram post, 03 February 2023, https://t.me/mediazzona/10585 [accessed: 25.07.2024].

Ministry of Internal Affairs of the Russian Federation, *Otdelnyje pokazateli migratsionnoi situatsiji v Rossijskoj Federatsiji za janvar-ijun 2023 goda s raspredelieniem po stranam i regionam (Selected Indicators of the Migration Situation in the Russian Federation for January-June 2023 with Distribution by Countries and Regions)*, report, n.d., https://мвд.рф/dejatelnost/statistics/migracionnaya/item/40034334/ [accessed: 12.08.2023].

Ministry of Internal Affairs of the Russian Federation, *Otdelnye pokazateli migratsionnoi situatsii v Rossiiskoi Federatsii za yanvar-dekabr 2022 goda s raspredeleniem po stranam i regionam (Selected Indicators of the Migration Situation in the Russian Federation for January–December 2022 with Distribution by Countries and Regions)*, report, 18 January 2023, https://мвд.рф/dejatelnost/statistics/migracionnaya/item/35074711/ [accessed: 14.08.2023].

Ministry of Reintegration of the Temporarily Occupied Territories of Ukraine, "Iryna Vereshchuk: 'Na tymchasovo okupovanykh terytoriiakh ta v rosii perebuvaie 4390 ukrainskykh statusnykh ditei'" ("Iryna Vereshchuk: 'There Are 4,390 Registered Ukrainian Children in the Temporarily Occupied Territories and Russia"), 28 March 2023, https://minre.gov.ua/2023/03/28/iryna-vereshhuk-na

-tymchasovo-okupovanyh-terytoriyah-ta-v-rosii-perebuvaye-4390-ukrayinskyh-statusnyh-ditej/ [accessed: 25.07.2024].

Minreintehratsii (Ukrainian Ministry of Reintegration of Temporarily Occupied Territories), "Natsionalne informatsiine biuro nakopychuie dani pro deportovanykh ukrainskykh ditei…" "National Information Bureau collects data on deported Ukrainian children…"), Telegram post, 28 March 2023, https://t.me/minre_ua/2958 [accessed: 25.07.2024].

Mulheir, Georgette, et al., *Bridging the Gaps: Four Studies on the Situation of Ukrainian Children with Disabilities and Their Families since the War Began, European Disability Forum*, report, 15 February 2023, https://www.edf-feph.org/content/uploads/2023/02/221215-BRIDGING-THE-GAPS-extended-summary-FINAL.pdf [accessed: 25.07.2024].

MVS Ukrainy (Ukrainian Ministry of Internal Affairs), "DMS oformylo pershe posvidchennia na povernennia v Ukrainu…" ("The State Migration Service issued the first certificate of return to Ukraine…"), Telegram post, 01 December 2022, https://t.me/mvs_ukraine/20532 [accessed: 25.07.2024].

National Social Service of Ukraine, "Sotsialnyi zakhyst vnutrishno peremishchenykh osib" ("Social Protection of Internally Displaced Persons"), https://nssu.gov.ua/vpo [accessed: 25.07.2024].

Nesterov, Georgii, "V Rossii nazvali chislo pribyvshykh iz Donbassa bezhentsev" ("Russia Announces the Number of Refugees Arriving from the Donbas"), *Lenta.ru*, 21 February 2022, https://lenta.ru/news/2022/02/21/bortnikov_donbass/ [accessed: 25.07.2024].

Nikolaev, Viktor, "Chislo bezentsev s Ukrainy i iz Donbassa v Rossii dostiglo 5 mln" ("The Number of Refugees from Ukraine and the Donbas in Russia Reached 5 Mil"), *MK.ru*, 19 December 2022, https://www.mk.ru/politics/2022/12/19/chislo-bezhencev-s-ukrainy-i-iz-donbassa-v-rossii-dostiglo-5-mln.html [accessed: 25.07.2024].

Ofitsialnoe opublikovanie pravovykh aktov (Official Publication of Legal Acts), Decree of the President of the Russian Federation from 19 October 2022, No. 756, http://publication.pravo.gov.ru/Document/View/0001202210190002 [accessed: 25.07.2024].

Ofitsialnoe opublikovanie pravovykh aktov (Official Publication of Legal Acts), Federal Laws the Russian Federation from 04 October 2022, No. 372-F3, No. 373-F3, No. 374-F3, and No. 375-F3, http://publication.pravo.gov.ru/search?pageSize=30&index=1&DocumentTypes=82a8bf1c-3bc7-47ed-827f-7affd43a7f27&PublishDateSearchType=1&PublishDate=05.10.2022&NumberSearchType=0&DocumentDateSearchType=0&JdRegSearchType=0&SortedBy=6&SortDestination=1 [accessed: 25.07.2024].

Ofitsialnoe opublikovanie pravovykh aktov (Official Publication of Legal Acts), Resolution of the Government of the Russian Federation from 12 March 2022,

No. 349, http://www.publication.pravo.gov.ru/Document/View/0001202203120005?index=6 [accessed: 25.07.2024].

Ombudsman of Ukraine, *Spetsialna dopovid Upovnovazhenoho Verkhovnoi Rady Ukrainy z prav liudyny shchodo doderzhannia prav osib, iaki postrazhdaly vnaslidok zbroinoi ahresii Rosiiskoi Federatsii proty Ukrainy (Special Report of the Ukrainian Parliament Commissioner for Human Rights on the Observance of the Rights of Persons Affected by the Armed Aggression of the Russian Federation against Ukraine)*, report, 2022, https://ombudsman.gov.ua/storage/app/media/Доповіді/Доповідь.pdf [accessed: 25.07.2024].

Ombudsman Lubinets Dmytro, "Deportatsiia ditei – ne 'dobra sprava', a zlochyn!" ("The Deportation of Children is Not a 'Good Deed', but a Crime"), Telegram post, 31 July 2023, https://t.me/dmytro_lubinetzs/3194 [accessed: 25.07.2024].

Ombudsman Lubinets Dmytro, "Shchonaimenshe 2 800 000 ukraintsiv byly vymusheni vyikhaty chy buly deportovani na terytoriiu RF..." ("At least 2,800,000 Ukrainians were forcibly displaced or deported to the territory of the Russian Federation..."), Telegram post, 04 December 2022, https://t.me/dmytro_lubinetzs/1315 [accessed: 25.07.2024].

Parliamentary Assembly Council of Europe, "Deportations and Forcible Transfers of Ukrainian Children and Other Civilians to Russian Federation or to Ukrainian Territories Temporarily Occupied", Resolution 2495, 2023, https://pace.coe.int/en/files/31776/html [accessed: 25.07.2024].

Plamenev, Ilya, "Saldo soobshchil o 7 tys. evakuirovannykh iz zatoplennykh rayonov Khersonshchiny" ("Saldo Informed about 7 Thou. Evacuated from the Flooded Areas of the Kherson Oblast"), *RBK.ru*, 11 July 2023, https://www.rbc.ru/politics/11/06/2023/6484edde9a79471dc0e4ad79?from=materials_on_subject [accessed: 25.07.2024].

Pohorilov, Stanislav, "Okupanty deportuvaly 11 tysiach ditei do Rosii – Zelenskyy" ("The Occupiers Deported 11 Thousand Children to Russia – Zelenskyy"), *Ukrainska Pravda (Ukrainian Truth)*, 15 November 2022, https://www.pravda.com.ua/news/2022/11/15/7376368/ [accessed: 25.07.2024].

Poia, Anastaiia, "Do Ukrainy povernuly shchonaimenshe 380 ukrainskykh ditei, yaki buly deportovani do RF – Vereshchuk" ("At least 380 Ukrainian Children Deported to the Russian Federation Were Returned to Ukraine"), *Ukrainska Pravda (Ukrainian Truth)*, 10 August 2023, https://life.pravda.com.ua/society/2023/08/10/255831/ [accessed: 25.07.2024].

Polyanskaya, Nina, "'Esli my dozhivem do kontsa etogo goda, ya budu udivlen i rad'. Demograf Aleksei Raksha o vliyanii voiny na budushchee rossiyan" ("'If We Survive until the End of This Year, I Will Be Glad and Surprised': Interview with Demographer Aleksei Raksha about the Impact of the War on the Future Of Russians"), *Diskurs (Discourse)*, 24 March 2023, https://discours.co/articles/social/aleksey-raksha-about-russian-demography [accessed: 25.07.2024].

President of Ukraine, Volodomyr Zelenskyy, Official Website, "Nam potribna vasha pidtrymka, shchob pryskoryty nastannia myru – zvernennia Prezydenta Ukrainy do uchasnykiv sesii Heneralnoi asamblei Orhanizatsii amerykanskykh derzhav (OAD), yaka tryvaie v Limi" ("We Need Your Support to Accelerate the Coming of Peace – The President of Ukraine's Address to the Participants of the General Assembly of the Organisation of American States (OAS), Which Is Taking Place in Lima"), 06 October 2022, https://www.president.gov.ua/news/nam-potribna-vasha-pidtrimka-shob-priskoriti-nastannya-miru-78305 [accessed: 25.07.2024].

Radio Svoboda (Radio Freedom), "Cherez zakryti dilianky kordonu vid pochatku povnomasshtabnoho vtorhnennia povernulos ponad 18 tysiach ukraintsiv – DPSU" ("Over 18 Thousand Ukrainians Have Returned through Closed Border Sections since the Beginning of the Full-Scale Invasion – SBGS"), 08 September 2023, https://www.radiosvoboda.org/a/news-kordon-poverennya-ukrayintsi-rosiya-demchenko-viyna/32538868.html [accessed: 25.07.2024].

Reuters, "Explainer: What is Zelenskiy's 10-point peace plan?", 28 December 2022, https://www.reuters.com/world/europe/what-is-zelenskiys-10-point-peace-plan-2022-12-28/ [accessed: 12.08.2023].

RIA Novosti (RIA News), "Chislo PVR dlya bezhentsev v Rossii dostiglo 807" ("The Number of TAPs in Russia Reached 807"), 24 October 2022, https://ria.ru/20221024/bezhentsy-1826256366.html [accessed: 25.07.2024].

RIA Novosti (RIA News), "Minoborony: bolee 2,7 milliona ukraintsev hotyat evakuirovatsya v Rossiyu" ("The Ministry of Defence: More than 2.7 Million Ukrainians Want to Evacuate to Russia"), 19 March 2022, https://ria.ru/20220319/evakuatsiya-1779069058.html [accessed: 25.07.2024].

Russian Red Cross, "Tsentr Rossiiskogo Krasnogo Kresta po voprosam migratsii" ("The Russian Red Cross Centre for Migration Issues"), https://www.redcross.ru/activity/migratsiya/ [accessed: 25.07.2024].

Schenk, Caress, "Counting Migrants in Russia: The Human Dimension of Administrative Data Production", *International Migration Review*, 2023, 1–28, https://doi.org/10.1177/01979183231154565.

Schenk, Caress, "The Kremlin Has Another Weapon in Its Arsenal: Migration Policy", *The Washington Post*, 11 April 2022, https://www.washingtonpost.com/politics/2022/04/11/russia-ukraine-weaponized-migration/ [accessed: 25.07.2024].

Shevtsova, Veronika, "Bolee 4,7 mln bezhentsev iz Ukrainy i Donbassa pribyli v Rossiyu, sredi nikh 705 tysyach detei" ("More than 4.7 Mil Refugees from Ukraine and the Donbas Came to Russia, Among Them 705 Thousand Children"), *miloserdie.ru (mercy.ru)*, 02 November 2022, https://www.miloserdie.ru/news/bolee-47-mln-bezhenczev-iz-ukrainy-i-donbassa-pribyli-v-rossiyu-sredi-nih-705-tysyach-detej/ [accessed: 25.07.2024].

TASS, "Svyshe 14,1 mlrd rublei vyplatili bezhentsam pribyvshim v Rossiyu s Ukrainy i iz Donbassa" ("Over 14.1 Billion Roubles Paid to Refugees Arriving in Russia from Ukraine and the Donbas"), 05 May 2023, https://tass.ru/obschestvo/1768 3379 [accessed: 25.07.2024].

TASS, "V Rossiyu s territorii Donbassa i Ukrainy pribylo 5.5 mln bezhentsev s fevralya 2022 goda" ("From February 2022 5.5 Mil Refugees from the Territory of the Donbas and Ukraine Came to Russia"), 28 March 2023, https://tass.ru/obschestvo/17 383893 [accessed: 25.07.2024].

TASS, "Chislo pribyvshikh v RF bezhentsev s territorii Ukrainy i Donbassa prevysilo 5,4 mln chelovek" ("The Number of Refugees Coming to Russia from the Territory of Ukraine and the Donbas Surpassed 5.4 Mil People"), 13 March 2023, https://tass.ru/obschestvo/17248303 [accessed: 25.07.2024].

TASS, "Za god s Ukrainy i iz Donbassa na territoriyu RF pribylo 5,3 mln bezhetsev" ("In One Year 5.3 Mil Refugees Came to the Territory of the RF from Ukraine and the Donbas"), 20 February 2023, https://tass.ru/obschestvo/17091725 [accessed: 25.07.2024].

TASS, "Svyshe 2,3 mln bezhentsev pribyli v Rossiyu s Ukrainy, iz DNR i LNR" ("More than 2.3 Mil Refugees Arrived to Russia from Ukraine, from the DNR and the LNR"), 04 July 2022, https://tass.ru/armiya-i-opk/15112613 [accessed: 25.07.2024].

TASS, "S fevralya 2022 goda v Rossiyu pribyli bolee 5,2 mln bezhentsev s territorii Ukrainy" ("More than 5.2 Mil Refugees from the Territory of Ukraine Came to Russia Since February 2022"), 30 January 2022, https://tass.ru/obschestvo/16914 809 [accessed: 25.07.2024].

The Russian Orthodox Church, "Tserkovnaya pomoshch bezhentsam i postradavshim mirnym zhitelyam" ("Church Aid to Refugees and Affected Civilians"), https://помочьвбеде.рф [accessed: 25.07.2024].

Troitskii, Konstantin, *Skolko bezhentsev s Ukrainy nakhoditsya v Rossiiskoi Federatsii? (How Many Refugees from Ukraine Are in the Russian Federation?)*, Komitet "Grazhdanskoe sodeistvie" (Civic Assistance Committee), report, 2023, https://refugee.ru/wp-content/uploads/2023/03/troiczkij-k.e.-skolko-bezhenczev-iz-ukrainy-v-rossijskoj-federaczii_-1-1.pdf [accessed: 25.07.2024].

Tsentr natsionalnoho sprotyvu (Centre for National Resistance), "Rosiiany vyvezly ponad 100 tys. ditei zi Skhodu Ukrainy na 'likuvannia'" ("Russians Transferred More than 100 Thou. Children from the East of Ukraine for 'Medical Treatment'"), 12 April 2023, https://sprotyv.mod.gov.ua/rosiyany-vyvezly-ponad-100-tys-ditej-zi-shodu-ukrayiny-na-likuvannya/ [accessed: 25.07.2024].

Tyshchenko, Kateryna, "V uriadi povidomyly, skilky ukraintsiv uzhe deportovano do Rosii" ("The Government Announced How Many Ukrainians Were Already Deported to Russia), *Ukrainska Pravda (Ukrainian Truth)*, 20 June 2022, https://www.pravda.com.ua/news/2022/06/20/7353670/ [accessed: 25.07.2024].

Ukrainska Pravda (Ukrainian Truth), "Occupiers abduct more than 6,000 Ukrainian children", 07 November 2022, https://www.pravda.com.ua/eng/news/2022/11/7/7375320/ [accessed: 25.07.2024].

Ukrinform, "Kilkist nezakonno vyvezenykh u rosiiu ukrainskykh ditei mozhe siahaty 150 tysiach" ("The Number of Ukrainian Children Illegally Transferred to Russia May Be 150 Thousand"), 17 February 2023, https://www.ukrinform.ua/rubric-ato/3671478-kilkist-nezakonno-vivezenih-u-rosiu-ukrainskih-ditej-moze-sagati-150-tisac.html [accessed: 25.07.2024].

United Nations (UN), "Reports of Russian Federation Forces Putting Ukrainian Civilians in 'Filtration' Camps Must Be Investigated, Senior Officials Tell Security Council", 07 September 2022, https://press.un.org/en/2022/sc15023.doc.htm [accessed: 25.07.2024].

United Nations High Commissioner for Refugees (UNHCR), *Ukraine Regional Refugee Response Plan (January–December 2023)*, report, 2023, https://data.unhcr.org/en/documents/details/97958 [accessed: 25.07.2024].

United Nations High Commissioner for Refugees (UNHCR), "Displacement in the former Soviet region", in: *The State of the World's Refugees 2000: Fifty Years of Humanitarian Action*, report, 2000, 185–209, https://www.unhcr.org/media/state-worlds-refugees-2000-fifty-years-humanitarian-action-chapter-8-displacement-former [accessed: 25.07.2024].

United Nations High Commissioner for Refugees (UNHCR) Operational Data Portal, "Ukraine Refugee Situation", https://data.unhcr.org/en/situations/ukraine/location [accessed: 25.07.2024].

United Nations High Commissioner for Refugees (UNHCR) Russia, "Otchety o deiyatelnosti v Rossii" ("Reports on Operations in Russia"), https://www.unhcr.org/ru/monthlydigest [accessed: 25.07.2024].

United Nations High Commissioner for Refugees (UNHCR) Russia, "Kuda mozhno obratitsya za pomoshchyu litsam, pribyvayushchim na territoriyu RF v svyazi s konfliktom v Ukraine?" ("Where Can People Arriving on the Territory of the Russian Federation in Connection with the Conflict in Ukraine Apply for Assistance?"), 2023, https://www.unhcr.org/ru/28617-helpforukrref.html [accessed: 25.07.2024].

United Nations High Commissioner for Refugees (UNHCR) and World Vision Georgia, *Ukrainian refugees in Georgia: Profile, Intentions and Needs*, report, November 2022, https://data.unhcr.org/en/documents/details/97675 [accessed: 25.07.2024].

Yale School of Public Health Humanitarian Research Lab, *Forced Passportization in Russia-Occupied Areas of Ukraine: Conflict Observatory Report*, report, 2023, https://hub.conflictobservatory.org/portal/sharing/rest/content/items/e280a7eeb7bf4dc588ed50ee655b9858/data [accessed: 25.07.2024].

Yale School of Public Health Humanitarian Research Lab, *System of Filtration: Mapping Russia's Detention Operations in Donetsk Oblast*, report, 25 August 2022, https://hub.conflictobservatory.org/portal/sharing/rest/content/items/7d1c90eb89d3446f9e708b87b69ad0d8/data [accessed: 25.07.2024].

Zhurzhenko, Tatiana, "Terror, Collaboration and Resistance: Russian Rule in the Newly Occupied Territories of Ukraine", *Eurozine*, 17 January 2023, https://www.eurozine.com/terror-collaboration-and-resistance/ [accessed: 25.07.2024].

Gender, War, and Forced Displacement

Social Perceptions and Attitudes

Olena Strelnyk

Russia's war against Ukraine affects all social processes, institutions, and practices. Gender roles and relations are no exception.[1] The impact of the war on the transformation of gender expectations, stereotypes, and roles may be long-lasting, multi-vector, and often contradictory, which poses a challenge for sociological studies. Since the beginning of the full-scale Russian invasion of Ukraine in 2022, a lot of data and reflections have been published, based on both completed research projects and works in progress.

From these data, publications, and reflections, we know that in the context of the war, women play a key role in humanitarian responses but are not as involved in decision-making, especially at the formal level. Meanwhile, women's burden with reproductive work has increased significantly.[2] It was mainly women with children who fled the country, as most men are not allowed to go abroad during martial law.[3] Women are at risk of war-related sexual violence and less reported domestic violence, especially in areas close to warzones.[4] During the war, women, including

1 I express my gratitude to the German Research Foundation (DFG), project number 45202164, which supported my position at the Technical University of Munich, making this essay possible.

2 United Nations Entity for Gender Equality and the Empowerment of Women (UN Women) and CARE International, *Rapid Gender Analysis of Ukraine*, report, 04 May 2022, https://www.unwomen.org/sites/default/files/2022-05/Rapid-Gender-Analysis-of-Ukraine-en.pdf [accessed: 20.03.2024].

3 European Union Agency for Asylum (EUAA), *Forced displacement from and within Ukraine: Profiles, experiences, and aspirations of affected populations*, report, 28 October 2022, 8, https://euaa.europa.eu/sites/default/files/publications/2022-11/2022_11_09_Forced_Displacement_Ukraine_Joint_Report_EUAA_IOM_OECD_0.pdf [accessed: 20.03.2024].

4 For war-related sexual violence, see: Marta Havryshko, "A Weapon of War? Some Reflections on Sexual Violence during the Russian War in Ukraine – Marta Havryshko in Conversation with Regina Mühlhäuser", *The New Fascism Syllabus*, 08 May 2022, http://newfascismsyllabus.com/opinions/ukrainian-dispatches/a-weapon-of-war-some-observations-on-sexual-violence-during-the-russian-war-in-ukraine/ [accessed: 15.03.2023]. For domestic violence, see: Marta Zmysla, "Domashne nasylstvo kriz pryzmu viiny"

those displaced abroad, also face increased risks of sexual harassment and sexual and labour exploitation.[5]

The sociocultural dimensions of gender transformation in the context of war and forced displacement, however, are overall not well researched. Accordingly, in this essay, I focus on how the war challenges gender roles during forced displacement at the level of social perceptions and attitudes. In the first part of the essay, I review the available data on the war's general effects on gender roles at the level of both social attitudes and some practices. The second part considers the gender aspects of the attitudes of the Ukrainian population towards the forcibly displaced abroad. Finally, I discuss the practices of othering internally displaced persons (IDPs) across categories of gender and class. I focus on both IDPs and displaced persons abroad because both groups' experiences demonstrate various manifestations of sociocultural transformations in gender ideals, roles, and expectations in the context of the war and displacement. For this text, I use quantitative and qualitative data from research, including projects I have contributed to, which were conducted between 2022 and 2023, as well as materials from open sources (e.g., officials' statements in the media) and personal archives. I not only review these data but also provide examples of the construction of expectations about women's and men's roles in the context of war and forced displacement.

Gender Roles in the Context of War and Displacement: Is a Retraditionalisation Taking Place?

As many feminist researchers argue, in times of war, traditional representations of gender roles tend to be reinforced, and gender ideas are more likely to be based on the essentialist conceptions of men as 'protectors' and women as 'protected'.[6]

Even though the professional army in Ukraine is open to both men and women, since 24 February 2022, the law and state discourse has assigned the function of

("Domestic Violence through the Lens of War"), *Ukrainska Pravda (Ukrainian Truth)*, 29 November 2022, https://life.pravda.com.ua/columns/2022/11/29/251536/ [accessed: 31.07.2024].

5 Sandra Pertek, Irina Kuznetsova, and Malgorzata Kot, *"Not a single safe place": The Ukrainian refugees at risk of violence, trafficking and exploitation, Findings from Poland and Ukraine*, University of Birmingham, report, 2022, https://www.birmingham.ac.uk/Documents/college-social-sciences/social-policy/iris/2022/sereda-cee.pdf [accessed: 31.07.2024].

6 Cynthia Cockburn, "Gender Relations as Causal in Militarization and War: A Feminist Standpoint", in: Kronsell, Annica, and Svedberg Erika (eds.), *Making Gender, Making War: Violence, Military and Peacekeeping Practices*, New York: Routledge, 2012, 19–34; Cynthia Enloe, *Does Khaki Become You? The Militarization of Women's Lives*, London: Pluto Press, 1983; and Nira Yuval-Davis, *Gender and Nation*, London: Sage, 1997.

protecting the state to men. Most men in Ukraine are prohibited from leaving the country during the war, and only civilian men can be mobilised and/or drafted. This shapes social expectations regarding men's primary role as 'defenders'. However, when considering the impact of war on ideas about masculinity, it is important to take into account the discrepancy between the law and official (state) discourse on the role of men as protectors as opposed to real, often hidden, ideas and practices. These implicit attitudes and practices are evidenced by data on the number of lawsuits for the evasion of mobilisation, the number of men who left or tried to leave the country illegally, and the striking growth of the share of men aged 30 to 45 among university and PhD students in 2022/2023 (under the current legislation, student status is ground for postponing mobilisation).[7]

It is also important to note that the visibility of women in the military[8], in state, public, and media discourses is increasing,[9] which challenges traditional gender order and affects gender perceptions. According to the data of a representative survey from September 2023, only 20 percent of surveyed Ukrainians associate the image of a veteran with men, while 80 percent answered that it could be both a man and a woman.[10]

The available data do not allow us to make unequivocal statements about the retraditionalisation of gender roles; rather, they show the complex and ambiguous nature of these changes in Ukraine. In a representative survey focusing on a group of young people aged 15 to 25, conducted by Info Sapiens (IS), a Ukrainian research agency, at the end of 2022, 58 percent of respondents said that they did not think that there was any change, 28 percent believed that the influence of gender stereotypes during the war strengthened, and only 12 percent reported that it weakened. The study assumes that the respondents associate the increase in this influence with military conscription for men and restrictions on men leaving the country. However, the lessening of these stereotypes may be a consequence of the increased visibility

7 Olena Strelnyk, "Men are defenders, women are defended? How the war affects changes in the attitudes and perceptions of Ukrianian society about gender roles", *Journal of Political and Military Sociology*, special issue, forthcoming 2024.

8 As of June 2023, there were 42,000 women in the military; their number had increased by 2.5 times compared to 2014. 5,000 women were fighting on the frontlines.

9 Olena Strelnyk, "From 'Berehynya' and 'Beauty' to women's agency: Media images of women in the context of Russia's war on Ukraine", in: Maryna Shevtsova (ed.), *Feminist Perspective on Russia's War in Ukraine: Hear Our Voices*, Lanham: Lexington Books, 2024, 19–39.

10 Sotsiolohichna hrupa "Reitynh" (Sociological Group "Rating"), "Dvadtsiat chetverte zahalnonatsionalne opytuvannia: Ukraina v umovakh viiny. Obraz veteraniv v ukrainskomu suspilstvi" ("The Twenty-Fourth National Survey 'Ukraine at War': The Image of Veterans in Ukrainian Society (5–7 September 2023)"), 21 September 2023, https://ratinggroup.ua/research/ukraine/dvadcyat_chetverte_zagalnonac_onalne_opituvanny_ukra_na_v_umovah_v_yni_obraz_veteran_v_v_ukra_nskomu.html [accessed: 31.07.2024].

of women in the army and the fact that women began to perform 'male' roles in displaced and separated families. The respondents of this qualitative study expect that a victory in the war will lead to an increase in gender equality in various spheres; however, they associate this not with the change of roles during the war itself but with further European integration of Ukrainian society.[11]

Before the full-scale war, a high level of economic activity of women,[12] and a rather high level of political representation of women,[13] were combined with mostly traditional distributions of gender roles in families, especially when it came to unpaid care work: mainly women were responsible for childcare and household chores, albeit with a gradual increase in men's participation in this work.[14] At the same time, there was a gradual erosion of gender stereotypes. For example, young people were more likely to support egalitarian views on women's and men's roles.[15]

It seems that the full-scale war did not stop these positive dynamics. For instance, a representative survey conducted in March 2023 showed that, compared to 2021, the share of Ukrainians who believe that "men are better leaders than women" decreased (from 43 to 24 percent), as did the share of those who believe that "a woman's main vocation is to give birth to children" (from 64 to 59 percent).[16]

The war and forced displacement affect the practices of the distribution of roles in families and their discursive justification. Oksana Mikheeva's research, conducted in 2019 in the Donetsk and Luhansk Oblasts, focused on territories both controlled and not controlled by the government of Ukraine. It revealed the prevalence of a patriarchal interpretation of male and female roles in the context of war. She showed that images of aid recipients and victims of war and forced displacement are associated with women, particularly the elderly. The informants

---

11 Inna Volosevych, Olha Prochukhanova, and Olena Strelnyk, *Henderni stereotypy ta roli ochyma molodi: do i pislia pochatku povnomasshtabnoi rosiiskoi ahresii* (*Gender Stereotypes and Roles through the Eyes of Youth: Before and After the Start of the Full-Scale Russian Aggression*), Info Sapiens (IS), report, 2023, https://www.sapiens.com.ua/publications/socpol-research/257/GS_2.pdf [accessed: 31.07.2024].

12 In 2021, the employment rate of women aged 15 to 64 in Ukraine was 55.5 percent (as compared to 63.4 percent in the EU).

13 Women currently make up 21 percent of parliament members.

14 Sotsiolohichna hrupa "Reitynh" (Sociological Group "Rating"), "Henderni roli i stereotypy" ("Gender Roles and Stereotypes"), 2021, https://ratingpro.org/research/gendernye_roli_i_stereotipy_v_ukraine.html [accessed: 31.07.2024].

15 Volosevych, Prochukhanova, and Strelnyk, *Henderni stereotypy ta roli ochyma molodi*, 51

16 Ukrainskyi veteranskyi fond (Ukrainian Veterans Fund) and Sotsiolohichna hrupa "Reitynh" (Sociological Group "Rating"), *Dyskryminatsiia riznykh sotsialnykh hrup u ZSU. Pohliady viiskovykh ta tsyvilnykh hromadian, berezen-kviten 2023* (*The Discrimination of Different Social Groups in the Armed Forces of Ukraine: The Views of the Military and Civilians, March–April 2023*), report, https://nako.org.ua/storage/pdf/2023-06-11--06:58:48-RG_NAKO_ComprehensiveResearch_08062023.pdf [accessed: 31.07.2023].

of her research, both men and women, constructed images of women as responsible for solving problems with documents and obtaining public services, even when the role of the man as the 'breadwinner' was no longer relevant (e.g., in elderly couples). In general, descriptions of and narratives around women focused on passive and sacrificial traits, while informants narrated men's roles in the contexts of duty, military authority, and their responsibilities towards their families and country. At the same time, there was an inversion of traditional gender roles, for example, in situations where men became unemployed and women took on the role of the 'earner'.[17] Similar trends are present in the current situation. A full-scale war and the resulting humanitarian crisis have affected the distribution of gender roles in families and increased the burden on women in unpaid care work.[18] Data obtained after 2022 suggests that receiving humanitarian aid for a family is mostly women's responsibility and, in fact, a new form of reproductive work.[19]

The biggest changes to gender roles take place in displaced and/or separated families (e.g., when a partner serves in the Armed Forces). In these cases, women perform tasks that, before the war, were usually the responsibility of a man. There are also particular challenges for women displaced abroad. Most fled without partners and with children, and they often do not have access to childcare services, are excluded from the usual support networks, suffer psychological issues caused by displacement and family separation, and are now solely responsible for their families.[20]

---

17 Oksana Mikheeva, *Vyity z tini: Vplyv polityky (ne)vyznannia faktiv iz zhyttia liudei z nepidkontrolnykh Ukraini teriroii Lyhanskoi ta Donetskoi oblastei na cholovi ta zhinochi roli u podvsiakdennomu zhytti (Out of the Shadows: The Impact of the Policy of the (Non)recognition of Facts from the Lives of People from the Nongovernment-Controlled Areas of the Luhansk and Donetsk Oblasts on Men's and Women's Roles in Everyday Life)*, PAX, report, spring 2019, https://ac.ucu.edu.ua/wp-content/uploads/2021/01/vyjty-z-tini-doslidzhennya-Oksany-Miheyevoyi-UKU.pdf [accessed: 20.03.2024].

18 Anastasia Bobrova et al., *Pershi dni povnomasshtabnoi viiny v Ukraini: dumky, perezhyvannia, dii (The First Days of a Full-Scale War in Ukraine: Thoughts, Feelings, Actions)*, Centre for Society Research "Cedos", report of initial findings, 2002, https://cedos.org.ua/wp-content/uploads/pershi-dni-povnomasshtabnoyi-vijny-v-ukrayini.pdf, [accessed: 31.07.2024]; and UN Women and CARE International, *Rapid Gender Analysis*.

19 Info Sapiens (IS) and Save the Children (SC), *Gender equality and conflict sensitivity analysis*, report, 2023, 18, unpublished. The study focuses on the impact of the full-scale war and forced displacement on women, men, girls, and boys based on a sample from three Oblasts of Ukraine (Zaporizhzhia, Vinnytsia, and Lviv) and three regions of Romania (Bucharest, Suceava, Iasi). Using individual interviews and focus group discussions, the researchers interviewed 133 participants (95 adults and 38 children). The participants were 92 females and 41 males (22 girls and 16 boys among these) from the local population, IDPs, and forcibly displaced people. The field data were collected in October–November 2022. The report is quoted with the organisation's permission.

20 Ibid.

At the same time, the impact of the war on the division of gender roles and care work in families requires further research. A representative survey from 2023 found that, compared to 2020, the participation of fathers (according to subjective assessments of interviewed men and women) in caring for children of all ages has increased, including in providing daily care and care during illness, buying goods, bringing them to and picking them up from kindergarten and school, and helping with studying, walking, and communicating, among other things. Additionally, the share of men who would like to take paternity leave has increased significantly (from 20 to 50 percent). However, it is difficult to determine whether and how the war influenced these changes.[21]

The Attitude of the Ukrainian Population Towards Forcibly Displaced Persons Abroad: Gender Aspects

Typically, most asylum applicants arriving in the European Union used to be young males. This is not the case for people fleeing Ukraine after the Russian invasion. Rather, these are mostly women and children because most adult men between 18 and 60 are prohibited from leaving Ukraine due to martial law.[22] Some data is available on the gender aspects of the attitudes of the Ukrainian population towards forcibly displaced people. In September 2022, the Kyiv International Institute of Sociology conducted a split-sample survey based on a telephone questionnaire of 2,000 residents of Ukraine (excluding territories not controlled by the Ukrainian government). According to the results of the survey, 90 percent of the respondents have a neutral or positive attitude towards refugees,[23] and only 5 percent condemn them.[24] In addition to the question of the general attitude towards Ukrainian refugees in Europe, detailed scenarios for refugees were provided, as listed below:

---

21 Inna Volosevych and Olha Maksymenko, *Rol cholovikiv u batkivstvi u chas povnomasshtabnoi viiny (The Role of Men in Parenting during the Full-Scale War)*, Info Sapiens (IS) and United Nations Population Fund (UNFPA), report, 2023, https://ukraine.unfpa.org/sites/default/files/pub-pdf/ukr_rol_cholovikiv_u_batkivstvi_u_chas_povnomasshtabnoi_viyny.pdf [accessed: 31.07.2024].

22 EUAA, *Forced displacement from and within Ukraine*.

23 The survey used the term 'refugees'.

24 Anton Grushetsky, *Stavlennia ukraintsiv, iaki zaraz perebuvaiut na terytorii Ukrainy, do ukrainskykh bizhentsiv u Evropi (The Attitudes of Ukrainians Currently Residing in Ukraine Towards Ukrainian Refugees in Europe)*, Kyiv International Institute for Sociology (KIIS), report, 11 November 2022, https://www.kiis.com.ua/?lang=ukr&cat=reports&id=1160&page=1 [accessed: 31.07.2024] [author's trans.].

> A 38-year-old woman has an underage child. She moved to Europe, and her husband stayed in Ukraine. [...] A 25-year-old girl who is unmarried, has no children, and has moved to Europe. [...] A 72-year-old professor who was in Europe for personal reasons at the time of the invasion and has remained there. [...] A 31-year-old man who lives in Ukraine but occasionally works in Poland. He was in Poland at the time of the invasion and decided not to return for now but to continue working in Poland.[25]

Each respondent was asked a general question about their attitudes towards refugees, and only one out of the four questions related to specific groups of refugees. An example question is:

> As you know, many residents of Ukraine fled abroad and became refugees due to the Russian invasion. For example, this is the case of a 25-year-old girl who is unmarried, has no children, and has moved to Europe. Some residents of Ukraine who stayed behind are sympathetic to her and do not condemn her for leaving and not yet returning. Other people, on the contrary, are upset by this choice and condemn her for leaving and not returning. And what is your general attitude towards her?[26]

According to the results of the survey, there is a differentiation in attitudes depending on the category of refugee. The most understanding attitude is towards women with young children whose husbands stayed in Ukraine. In this case, 90 percent of people chose "do not condemn" and only six percent chose "condemn", which corresponds to the attitude towards refugees in general. This perception is somewhat worse if underage children are removed from the description. In cases of women without children, the results were 87 percent "do not condemn" and nine percent "condemn". With men, the attitude also becomes more negative. Even if we are talking about an elderly man who was in Europe before the invasion, the results were 83 percent "do not condemn" and 10 percent "condemn". The most negative attitude (among the considered categories) was towards a young man who was in Europe at the time of the invasion and stayed there. In this case, 75 percent do not condemn him, while 19 percent condemn him.[27] Although such variations are not striking, they nevertheless indicate differences in the perceptions of the roles of women and men in the context of war and displacement.

These attitudes apply especially to men displaced abroad. Since most men are prohibited from leaving the country during martial law, they may face the prejudice that they have crossed the border illegally. In Facebook groups centred on Ukrainians

25 Ibid.

26 Ibid.

27 Ibid.

living, for example, in Germany, a male refugee's request for advice or help is often received aggressively with reproaches and questions of how and why he ended up abroad.[28]

In cases of displacement abroad, public opinion, as we can see, is most favourable to women, especially those with children. At the same time, women may face prejudices and stigma if their behaviour does not correspond to public ideas about 'real' victims of the war. For example, 'inappropriate behaviour' among refugee women is often connected to beauty practices. Manicures have turned into one such marker of behaviour that contradicts the image of a female victim of the war. "It hurt me to watch how for several weeks the discourse of 'terrible Ukrainian [women] refugees' who ask for asylum and then dare to get a manicure was spread", writes Kateryna Babkina for *Deutsche Welle*, suggesting that the authors of such messages may be Russian information 'technologists' specialising in influencing public sentiment.[29] Mariya Shcherbyna rightly points out that on the one hand, beauty practices are part of the image of a 'real woman', but on the other, they contradict the image of a 'real victim'. The search for beauty professionals by refugee women on social networks results in hate speech and new forms of control over a woman's body.[30]

'Us' and 'Them': Gender and Class in the Othering of IDPs

Quantitative studies conducted from 2016 to 2022 reveal that the Ukrainian population had a generally positive attitude towards IDPs. However, negative attitudes and their regional bias were also noticeable. In particular, in 2016, 39 percent of Kyiv residents suggested that the arrival of IDPs caused increases in crime, while in other regions this indicator did not exceed 16 percent. Similarly, 21 percent of Kyiv residents considered that the arrival of IDPs led to increased social tensions in the community, which is twice as much as the percentage of that view in any other region. Lastly, residents of Kyiv often saw IDPs as competition for jobs, affordable housing, and free places in kindergartens. Meanwhile, the residents of Western Ukraine, especially outside the regional centres, also supported negative stereotypes about

28 This is based on the author's observation of at least three of the most popular Facebook groups for Ukrainians in Munich from June 2022 to September 2023.

29 Kateryna Babkina, "Manikiur iak zbroia masovoho urazhennia" ("A Manicure as a Weapon of Mass Destruction"), *Deutsche Welle*, 16 May 2022, https:/www.dw.com/uk/kateryna-babkina-manikiur-yak-zbroia-masovoho-urazhennia/a-61816902 [accessed: 31.07.2024] [author's trans.].

30 Mariya Shcherbyna, "Beauty practices and Ukrainian women refugees: another double bind", presentation at the conference *Women and their body*, 15 March 2023–17 March 2023, Center for the History of Women Philosophers and Scientists, Paderborn.

IDPs. They emphasised their pro-Russian political views, reluctance to work, aggressive attitude towards the locals, a posture of superiority, and desire to hold a special status due to their life circumstances.[31]

The start of the full-scale war caused an unprecedented wave of forced internal displacement. As of 23 May 2023, the International Organisation of Migration estimated that 5.1 million people were internally displaced in Ukraine. This represents a decrease compared to 5.9 million as of 5 December 2022.[32] The share of males in the population of IDPs has steadily decreased during the first year of the full-scale war. For example, in March 2022, 46 percent of IDPs were male, as compared to 30 percent in August 2022[33]. In May 2023, the share of males among IDPs was 42 percent..[34] Some studiesclaim that men avoid official registration as IDPs due to the intention to avoid mobilisation.[35]

In a representative survey conducted by Info Sapiens (IS) in May 2022, 61 percent of respondents reported that they have a positive and sympathetic attitude towards IDPs, and only 5 percent reported a negative one. Almost one in three respondents (32 percent) reported that they help IDPs with food, and one in five (20 percent) said they assist financially or by volunteering.[36] However, a quantitative methodology cannot always provide a complete picture of attitudes towards IDPs, often due to the latent features of these attitudes. A 2022 study by IS and Right to Protect, which combined quantitative and qualitative methodologies, identified several conflict situations between local populations and IDPs caused by different reasons.[37]

---

31 Texty.org.Ua, "Opytuvannia dlia OON: ukraintsi pozytyvno stavliatsia do vymushenykh pereselentsiv" ("Survey for the UN: Ukrainians Have a Positive Attitude towards Displaced People"), 10 June 2016, https://texty.org.ua/fragments/68267/Opytuvanna_dla_OON_ukrajinci_pozytyvno_stavlatsa_do-68267/ [accessed: 31.07.2024].

32 International Organization of Migration (IOM), *Ukraine Internal Displacement Report: General Population Survey*, report, round 13, June 2023, https://dtm.iom.int/reports/ukraine-internal-displacement-report-general-population-survey-round-13-11-may-14-june-2023? [accessed: 31.07.2024]; and International Organization of Migration (IOM), *Ukraine Internal Displacement Report: General Population Survey*, report, round 12, 23 January 2023, 1, https://dtm.iom.int/reports/ukraine-internal-displacement-report-general-population-survey-round-12-16-23-january-2023 [accessed: 31.07.2024].

33 EUAA, *Forced displacement from and within Ukraine*, 34.

34 IOM, *Ukraine Internal Displacement Report: General Population Survey*, report, round 13, June 2023, 9.

35 CARE International, *Rapid Gender Analysis: Ukraine*, report, October 2023, 36, https://careevaluations.org/wp-content/uploads/RGA_Ukraine_2023_ENG.pdf [accessed: 31.07.2024].

36 Info Sapiens (IS), "61% ukraintsiv stavliatsia do vymushenykh pereselentsiv pozytyvno ta spivchutlyvo, ale 5% – nehatyvno" ("61% of Ukrainians Have a Positive and Sympathetic Attitude towards Forcibly Displaced People, but 5% Have a Negative Attitude"), 06 June 2022, https://sapiens.com.ua/ua/publication-single-page?id=232 [accessed: 31.07.2024].

37 Info Sapiens (IS) and Right to Protect, *Relationship Practices, Conflicts, and Trigger Themes among Ukrainian IDPs and Host Communities, as Well as Returnees and Home Communities,*

Othering newly arrived people is something that may occur in any migration or displacement situation; however, this process has specific qualities in the context of the war and, in particular, when considering gender expectations towards men. One can assume that although not all men, or even most of them, are on the frontlines, gendered expectations that men should or have to fight are quite strong.[38] According to a study by the nongovernmental organisation (NGO) Centre for Society Research "Cedos", which was conducted during the first months of the full-scale war, some IDPs said they experienced negative attitudes from locals. This was especially true for men because of the idea that men are 'defenders' and should fight, rather than stay in safe areas. According to some respondents, these prejudices even made it harder to access housing.[39]

Data on the characteristics of such tensions and conflicts are available in other studies. According to the IS and Right to Protect study, 53 percent of IDPs and 59 percent of locals stated that they, with differing degrees of frequency, "have come across cases when men are accused of not fighting (hiding from the Military Commissariat)".[40] In a study conducted by IS and Save the Children (SC) in October–November 2022, women, especially those whose loved ones were at the front, spoke emotionally about their expectations regarding men's gender roles during the war. They constructed distinctions between 'us' (locals) and 'them' (IDPs) around the issue of men's military service, viewing this as "our ('real') men fight" while "their ('unreal') men refuse to go to the front".[41]

Negative images of displaced men are also present in official rhetoric. By default, it is assumed that local men are ready for military service, and the negative image of male IDPs is constructed around their reluctance to serve in the Armed Forces of Ukraine. For example, during a press conference, Pavlo Svadovskyi, the head of the centre responsible for the registration of men of draft age in the Volyn Oblast, said,

---

report, 2022, https://www.sapiens.com.ua/publications/socpol-research/255/R2P_Key%20research%20findings_peacebuilding_ENG-1.pdf [accessed: 31.07.2024].

38 No direct data are available on what proportion of men and women share these expectations. It is also worth considering the dynamic nature of the population's attitude towards state mobilisation policies, which can influence attitudes towards male IDPs as well. I assume that public opinion is not consolidated on this issue, and with the passage of time, as issues became clear (the protracted nature of the war, systemic problems with the treatment and rehabilitation of the military, the sometimes forced nature of mobilisation, as well as the actual inability of military personnel to demobilise during the war), the share of men who are willing to serve in the Armed Forces has decreased significantly.

39 Bobrova et al., *Pershi dni povnomasshtabnoi viiny v Ukraini*.

40 IS and Right to Protect, *Relationship Practices, Conflicts, and Trigger Themes*, 72.

41 IS and SC, *Gender equality and conflict sensitivity analysis*, 42–43.

"[t]hey [male IDPs] don't want to fight. Of course, not all internally displaced persons [...] but most of them have no desire to register and defend the country".[42]

Othering IDPs, and in particular men, sometimes takes the form of hate speech. In March 2022, the mayor of Chernivtsi, Roman Klichuk, wrote this post on his Facebook page:

> WARNING
> If you have witnessed inappropriate attacks on you or your acquaintances, have encountered rude behaviour from IDPs or other people, from today onwards, you should CALL AND REPORT THIS.
> The police and a group of "educators" are ready to expedite the dispatch of those who like to "fight" to the front![43]

1,700 users shared this post. However, many critical comments said that the message provokes enmity between residents of different regions of Ukraine.

Othering male IDPs is not only based on gender but also class. The negative image of a male IDP is often one of a 'silver-spooner' (*mazhory*)[44]: he drives an expensive car and 'sits in bars'. Some of the messages showing hate speech towards IDPs have markers of intentional misinformation, probably to create social discord. However, some of them seem genuine and appear in public spaces and in public statements of officials. For example, in the spring of 2022, a billboard was installed in the city of Truskavets reading: "'Refugee'-silver-spooners [*Bizhentsi-mazhory*]. We hosted you hospitably. If you get drunk, we will beat you up and send you to the front".[45]

In March and April 2022, I also heard a few testimonies about so-called 'guidelines for the decent behaviour of IDPs' (this is mostly a typed text) placed in the public

---

42 Volynski novyny (Volyn News), "Na Volyni – skladna sytuatsiia z viiskovym oblikom pereselentsiv-cholovikiv" ("In Volyn, There is a Difficult Situation with the Military Registration of Displaced Men"), 25 October 2022, https://www.volynnews.com/ua/news/all/bazhannia-zakhyshchaty-krayinu-nemaye-na-volyni-skladna-sytuatsiia-z-viyskovym-oblikom-pereselentsiv-cholovikiv/ [accessed: 31.07.2024].

43 Roman Klichuk, official Facebook page, "UVAHA ...", Facebook post, 04 March 2022, https://www.facebook.com/klichuk.roman/posts/363680165764257 [accessed: 31.07.2024] [author's trans.]

44 The expression derives from 'born with a silver spoon in their mouth', referring to the person's wealthy and privileged background.

45 Daria Kurennaia, "Vid movy vorozhnechi do 'zustrichaemo svoikh': iak zminiuvalosia stavlennia ukraintsiv do vymushenykh pereselentsiv" ("From the Language of Hostility to 'Meeting Our People': How the Attitude of Ukrainians towards Forced Displaced Changed"), 23 November 2022, https://v-variant.com.ua/article/stavlennia-ukraintsiv-do-pereselentsiv/ [accessed: 31.07.2024] [author's trans.]. In the section featuring "we will beat you up", profanity is used.

spaces (e.g., hotels) of communities with high numbers of IDPs and addressed primarily to men.[46] They contained the following items, formulated in an aggressive tone with a threat of violence:

> 1. Did you sign up for territorial defence, did you register with the military? 2. You have two days for this. 3. Women, children, elderly people: we will certainly help them, and you fight; our men are on the frontlines. 4. The money you spend in our restaurants should go to the needs of the army and real refugees. 5. Women who do not have small children should volunteer. 6. These rules should become golden for you. If you don't follow the rules, the boys of the Territorial Defence, the police, and the Military Commissariat will explain them to you more intelligibly.[47]

The image of a displaced woman, while gender-specific, can be constructed as class-based as well. For example, Borys Filatov, the mayor of Dnipro, wrote a Facebook post about IDPs in May 2022, after he visited Chernivtsi in Western Ukraine:

> Girls with highlighted hair, with dogs under their arms, and in Juicy Couture plush costumes ... Boys [...] with laptops, who occupied all public catering establishments. Children screaming and running on the tables, with the complete indulgence of their parents. Total traffic violations by cars.[48]

More than 8,000 users and several media sources shared the post.[49]

---

46 I received two photographs as testimonies of such posters placed in a region with a high concentration of IDPs (in the city of Morshyn). According to one of the informants, who provided the photo in June 2022, she saw such posters frequently ("all over the city"). According to other evidence, these posters were no longer there in April 2022.

47 The original list contains eight items. Authors unknown, posters with so-called 'guidelines for the decent behaviour of IDPs', based on photographs of the posters received from anonymous sources, Morshyn, Ukraine, June 2022. [author's trans.].

48 Borys Filatov, personal Facebook page, Facebook post, 23 April 2022, https://www.facebook.com/100002157183088/posts/5050845398330650 [accessed: 21.03.2023] [author's trans.]. As of 22 November 2023, the post is not available.

49 Dariia Demianyk, "'Ia vse ponymaiu, no...'. Fylatov v shoke ot povedenyia pereselentsev v Chernovtsakh ("'I Understand Everything, but...': Filatov Shocked by the Behaviour of IDPs in Chernivtsi"), *Glavkom*, 25 April 2022, https://glavcom.ua/ru/news/ya-vse-ponimayu-no-filatov-v-shoke-ot-povedeniya-pereselencev-v-chernovcah-840742.html [accessed: 31.07.2024].

Conclusions

The war has affected gender expectations, stereotypes, and roles. In this essay, I focused primarily on the negative results of such processes. Using the example of the Ukrainian population's attitude towards forcibly displaced persons and the practices of othering IDPs, I showed how the war reinforces patriarchal ideas of gender roles. However, this is only a fragment of social reality. The impact of the war on social attitudes towards women's and men's roles is more complex and controversial. On the one hand, there is evidence of the reinforcement of traditional gender conceptions. This applies particularly to men, who, at least at the level of official state discourse, are expected to primarily perform the role of the 'defender' of the state. These expectations are expressed in the othering practices of male IDPs and those displaced abroad. On the other hand, data from sociological studies also indicate a positive trend in the decline of Ukrainian society's support for gender stereotypes and traditional gender-role expectations, which continues even during the war. One can also assume there is a trend of erasing patriarchal gender expectations of Ukrainian society about gender roles, not least due to forced displacement and family separation, as a result of which women acquire new roles and responsibilities. The nature and sustainability of these changes, however, require further research.

Bibliography

Authors unknown, posters with so-called 'guidelines for the decent behaviour of IDPs', based on photographs of the posters by anonymous sources, Morshyn, Ukraine, June 2022.

Babkina, Kateryna, "Manikiur iak zbroia masovoho urazhennia" ("A Manicure as a Weapon of Mass Destruction"), *Deutsche Welle*, 16 May 2022, https:/www.dw.com/uk/kateryna-babkina-manikiur-yak-zbroia-masovoho-urazhennia/a-61816902 [accessed: 29.07.2024].

Bobrova, Anastasia, et al., *Pershi dni povnomasshtabnoi viiny v Ukraini: dumky, perezhyvannia, dii (The First Days of a Full-Scale War in Ukraine: Thoughts, Feelings, Actions)*, Centre for Society Research "Cedos", report of initial findings, 2002, https://cedos.org.ua/wp-content/uploads/pershi-dni-povnomasshtabnoyi-vijny-v-ukrayini.pdf, [accessed: 29.07.2024].

CARE International, *Rapid Gender Analysis: Ukraine*, report, October 2023, 36, https://careevaluations.org/wp-content/uploads/RGA_Ukraine_2023_ENG.pdf [accessed: 29.07.2024].

Cockburn, Cynthia, "Gender Relations as Causal in Militarization and War: A Feminist Standpoint", in: Kronsell, Annica and Svedberg Erika (eds.), *Making Gen-*

der, Making War: Violence, Military and Peacekeeping Practices, New York: Routledge, 2012, 19–34.

Demianyk, Dariia, "'Ia vse ponymaiu, no...'. Fylatov v shoke ot povedenyia pereselentsev v Chernovtsakh ("'I Understand Everything, but...': Filatov Shocked by the Behaviour of IDPs in Chernivtsi"), *Glavkom*, 25 April 2022, https://glavcom.ua/ru/news/ya-vse-ponimayu-no-filatov-v-shoke-ot-povedeniya-pereselencev-v-chernovcah-840742.html [accessed: 29.07.2024].

Enloe, Cynthia, *Does Khaki Become You? The Militarization of Women's Lives*, London: Pluto Press, 1983.

European Union Agency for Asylum (EUAA), *Forced displacement from and within Ukraine: Profiles, experiences, and aspirations of affected populations*, report, 28 October 2022, 8, https://euaa.europa.eu/sites/default/files/publications/2022-11/2022_11_09_Forced_Displacement_Ukraine_Joint_Report_EUAA_IOM_OECD_0.pdf [accessed: 29.07.2024].

Filatov, Borys, personal Facebook page, Facebook post, 23 April 2022, https://www.facebook.com/100002157183088/posts/5050845398330650 [accessed: 21.03.2023].

Grushetsky, Anton, *Stavlennia ukraintsiv, iaki zaraz perebuvaiut na terytorii Ukrainy, do ukrainskykh bizhentsiv u Evropi* (*The Attitudes of Ukrainians Currently Residing in Ukraine Towards Ukrainian Refugees in Europe*), Kyiv International Institute for Sociology (KIIS), report, 11 November 2022, https://www.kiis.com.ua/?lang=ukr&cat=reports&id=1160&page=1 [accessed: 29.07.2024] [author's trans.].

Havryshko, Marta, "A Weapon of War? Some Reflections on Sexual Violence during the Russian War in Ukraine – Marta Havryshko in Conversation with Regina Mühlhäuser", *The New Fascism Syllabus*, 08 May 2022, http://newfascismsyllabus.com/opinions/ukrainian-dispatches/a-weapon-of-war-some-observations-on-sexual-violence-during-the-russian-war-in-ukraine/ [accessed: 29.07.2024].

International Organization of Migration (IOM), *Ukraine Internal Displacement Report: General Population Survey*, report, round 13, June 2023, https://dtm.iom.int/reports/ukraine-internal-displacement-report-general-population-survey-round-13-11-may-14-june-2023? [accessed: 29.07.2024].

International Organization of Migration (IOM), *Ukraine Internal Displacement Report: General Population Survey*, report, round 12, 23 January 2023, https://dtm.iom.int/reports/ukraine-internal-displacement-report-general-population-survey-round-12-16-23-january-2023 [accessed: 29.07.2024].

Info Sapiens (IS) and Save the Children (SC), *Gender equality and conflict sensitivity analysis*, report, 2023, unpublished.

Info Sapiens (IS), "61% ukraintsiv stavliatsia do vymushenykh pereselentsiv pozytyvno ta spivchutlyvo, ale 5% – nehatyvno" ("61% of Ukrainians Have a Positive and Sympathetic Attitude towards Forcibly Displaced People, but 5% Have a Negative Attitude"), 06 June 2022, https://sapiens.com.ua/ua/publication-single-page?id=232 [accessed: 29.07.2024].

Info Sapiens (IS) and Right to Protect, *Relationship Practices, Conflicts, and Trigger Themes among Ukrainian IDPs and Host Communities, as Well as Returnees and Home Communities*, report, 2022, https://www.sapiens.com.ua/publications/socpol-research/255/R2P_Reserch_full_report_ENG.pdf [accessed: 29.07.2024].

Klichuk, Roman, official Facebook page, "UVAHA ...", Facebook post, 04 March 2022, https://www.facebook.com/klichuk.roman/posts/363680165764257 [accessed: 29.07.2024].

Kurennaia, Daria, "Vid movy vorozhnechi do 'zustrichaemo svoikh': iak zminiuvalosia stavlennia ukraintsiv do vymushenykh pereselentsiv" ("From the Language of Hostility to 'Meeting Our People': How the Attitude of Ukrainians towards Forced Displaced Changed"), 23 November 2022, https://v-variant.com.ua/article/stavlennia-ukraintsiv-do-pereselentsiv/ [accessed: 29.07.2024].

Mikheeva, Oksana, *Vyity z tini: Vplyv polityky (ne)vyznannia faktiv iz zhyttia liudei z nepidkontrolnykh Ukraini teriroii Lyhanskoi ta Donetskoi oblastei na cholovi ta zhinochi roli u podvsiakdennomu zhytti* (*Out of the Shadows: The Impact of the Policy of the (Non)recognition of Facts from the Lives of People from the Nongovernment-Controlled Areas of the Luhansk and Donetsk Oblasts on Men's and Women's Roles in Everyday Life*), PAX, report, spring 2019, https://ac.ucu.edu.ua/wp-content/uploads/2021/01/vyjty-z-tini-doslidzhennya-Oksany-Miheyevoyi-UKU.pdf [accessed: 20.03.2024].

Pertek, Sandra, Irina Kuznetsova, and Malgorzata Kot, *"Not a single safe place": The Ukrainian refugees at risk of violence, trafficking and exploitation, Findings from Poland and Ukraine*, University of Birmingham, report, 2022, https://www.birmingham.ac.uk/Documents/college-social-sciences/social-policy/iris/2022/sereda-cee.pdf [accessed: 29.07.2024].

Shcherbyna, Mariya, "Beauty practices and Ukrainian women refugees: another double bind", presentation at the conference *Women and their body*, 15 March 2023–17 March 2023, Center for the History of Women Philosophers and Scientists, Paderborn.

Sotsiolohichna hrupa "Reitynh" (Sociological Group "Rating"), "Dvadtsiat chetverte zahalnonatsionalne opytuvannia: Ukraina v umovakh viiny. Obraz veteraniv v ukrainskomu suspilstvi" ("The Twenty-Fourth National Survey 'Ukraine at War': The Image of Veterans in Ukrainian Society (5–7 September 2023)"), 21 September 2023, https://ratinggroup.ua/research/ukraine/dvadcyat_chetverte_zagalnonac_onalne_opituvanny_ukra_na_v_umovah_v_yni_obraz_veteran_v_v_ukra_nskomu.html [accessed: 29.07.2024].

Sotsiolohichna hrupa "Reitynh" (Sociological Group "Rating"), "Henderni roli i stereotypy" ("Gender Roles and Stereotypes"), 2021, https://ratingpro.org/research/gendernye_roli_i_stereotipy_v_ukraine.html [accessed: 29.07.2024].

Strelnyk, Olena, "Men are defenders, women are defended? How the war affects changes in the attitudes and perceptions of Ukrainian society about gender roles", *Journal of Political and Military Sociology*, special issue, 2024 (forthcoming).

Strelnyk, Olena, "From 'Berehynya' and 'Beauty' to women's agency: Media images of women in the context of Russia's war on Ukraine", in: Maryna Shevtsova (ed.), *Feminist Perspective on Russia's War in Ukraine: Hear Our Voices*, Lanham: Lexington Books, 2024, 19–39.

Texty.org.Ua, "Opytuvannia dlia OON: ukraintsi pozytyvno stavliatsia do vymushenykh pereselentsiv" ("Survey for the UN: Ukrainians Have a Positive Attitude towards Displaced People"), 10 June 2016, https://texty.org.ua/fragments/68267/Opytuvanna_dla_OON_ukrajinci_pozytyvno_stavlatsa_do-68267/ [accessed: 29.07.2024].

Ukrainskyi veteranskyi fond (Ukrainian Veterans Fund) and Sotsiolohichna hrupa "Reitynh" (Sociological Group "Rating"), *Dyskryminatsiia riznykh sotsialnykh hrup u ZSU. Pohliady viiskovykh ta tsyvilnykh hromadian, berezen-kviten 2023* (*The Discrimination of Different Social Groups in the Armed Forces of Ukraine: The Views of the Military and Civilians, March–April 2023*), report, https://veteranfund.com.ua/analitics/social-group-discr/ [accessed: 29.07.2024].

United Nations Entity for Gender Equality and the Empowerment of Women (UN Women) and CARE International, *Rapid Gender Analysis of Ukraine*, report, 04 May 2022, https://www.unwomen.org/sites/default/files/2022-05/Rapid-Gender-Analysis-of-Ukraine-en.pdf [accessed: 29.07.2024].

Volosevych, Inna, and Olha Maksymenko, *Rol cholovikiv u batkivstvi u chas povnomasshtabnoi viiny* (*The Role of Men in Parenting during the Full-Scale War*), Info Sapiens (IS) and United Nations Population Fund (UNFPA), report, 2023, https://ukraine.unfpa.org/sites/default/files/pub-pdf/ukr_rol_cholovikiv_u_batkivstvi_u_chas_povnomasshtabnoi_viyny.pdf [accessed: 29.07.2024].

Volosevych, Inna, Olha Prochukhanova, and Olena Strelnyk, *Henderni stereotypy ta roli ochyma molodi: do i pislia pochatku povnomasshtabnoi rosiiskoi ahresii* (*Gender Stereotypes and Roles through the Eyes of Youth: Before and After the Start of the Full-Scale Russian Aggression*), Info Sapiens (IS), report, 2023, https://www.sapiens.com.ua/publications/socpol-research/257/GS_2.pdf [accessed: 29.07.2024].

Volynski novyny (Volyn News), "Na Volyni – skladna sytuatsiia z viiskovym oblikom pereselentsiv-cholovikiv" ("In Volyn, There is a Difficult Situation with the Military Registration of Displaced Men"), 25 October 2022, https://www.volynnews.com/ua/news/all/bazhannia-zakhyshchaty-krayinu-nemaye-na-volyni-skladna-sytuatsiia-z-viyskovym-oblikom-pereselentsiv-cholovikiv/ [accessed: 29.07.2024].

Yuval-Davis, Nira, *Gender and Nation*, London: Sage, 1997.

Zmysla, Marta, "Domashne nasylstvo kriz pryzmu viiny" ("Domestic Violence through the Lens of War"), *Ukrainska Pravda* (*Ukrainian Truth*), 29 November 2022, https://life.pravda.com.ua/columns/2022/11/29/251536/ [accessed: 29.07.2024].

Reassessing the Past?

National Identity and Memory Among Ukrainian Refugees in Poland

Ivan Kozachenko

"But we are Kyivan Rus, not *them*! They are just a horde!" I heard a middle-aged Ukrainian woman exclaiming at the overcrowded Krakow Main railway station in early March 2022. Following the illegal and unprovoked Russian invasion, this station had become the key locus for Ukrainian refugees[1] on their way to the European Union. Given the circumstances, this phrase may seem absurd – why would anyone discuss distant history during a hard and chaotic journey? Surprisingly, however, this phrase makes perfect sense. The conflict between Russia and Ukraine has been driven not only by the geopolitical ambitions of the Putin regime but is also deeply embedded in the nation-building processes and memory politics of the warring countries. Never-ending debates[2] on historical events and figures, the origins and role of languages, and the demarcations of sameness and otherness have been a crucial part of life for Ukrainians and Russians since the Euromaidan Revolution of 2014. Therefore, for many people fleeing the war – one so absurd and so sudden – a conversation about history may provide an explanation of the ongoing events, a self-healing narrative, and a sense of belonging.

Through participant observation and interviews, this paper explores the following two research questions: How are refugees' narratives of the war and displacement related to Ukrainian discourses on identity and memory? And, in the

1 Although called 'refugees' throughout this text, the EU has applied the Council Directive 2001/55/EC on Temporary Protection to Ukrainians fleeing the war. Thus, in contrast to the guarantees of asylum seekers, Ukrainians are normally granted a right to healthcare and work. Poland also provided new arrivals with a one-time payment and a monthly subsistence for children. See: European Commission, Migration and Home Affairs, "Temporary Protection", https://home-affairs.ec.europa.eu/policies/migration-and-asylum/common-european-asylum-system/temporary-protection_en [accessed: 31.07.2024].

2 Oxana Shevel, "The Battle for Historical Memory in Postrevolutionary Ukraine", *Current History* 115/783, 2016, 258–263; and David R. Marples, "Decommunization, Memory Laws, and 'Builders of Ukraine in the 20th Century'", *Acta Slavica Iaponica (Japanese Slavic Journal)* 39, 2018, 1–22.

given situation, what are the refugees' perceptions of Russia and Poland? In this exploration, the study draws on two sets of literature. The first concerns Ukrainian national 'imagination' and the second concerns refugee identities and belonging. While Ukrainian nation-building will be discussed separately, it is necessary to point out that in refugee and migration studies, language and emotional attachment are seen as crucial for fostering a sense of belonging.[3] These can be explored at different levels, but in this study, linguistic identities and emotional attachments are investigated in relation to national identity and memory. Moreover, this study considers the cultural and communicative dimensions of memory. Jan Assmann points out that cultural memory is created by elites and passed through institutions, while communicative memory exists and is transmitted at the level of small social groups.[4]

To lay out its argument, this paper first discusses the key features of Ukrainian nation-building after 1991. Next, it outlines the research methodologies this study is based on. Third, it explores how the invasion and displacement affect refugees' sense of belonging to Ukraine. Finally, the paper investigates refugees' perceptions towards the aggressor country, Russia, and the receiving country, Poland.

National 'Imagination' and Memory in Ukraine Before the Invasion

Since its independence in 1991, Ukraine has been continuously portrayed as a 'cleft country'.[5] The divide was seen as both regional – pro-Russian Southern and Eastern Ukraine versus pro-European Western Ukraine – and symbolic, where oscillating identities are polarised between 'supranational' and 'national' projects. The former refers to the achievements of the Russian Empire and Soviet Union and can be called 'Russophile' and 'Sovietophile'. Although these can be seen as contradicting each other, earlier research has indicated that in contemporary discourses, they are combined in a postmodern fashion.[6] These narratives centre on the crucial role

3 Montserrat Guibernau, *Belonging: Solidarity and Division in Modern Societies*, Cambridge: Polity, 2013; and Cathrine Brun and Anita Fábos, "Making Homes in Limbo? A Conceptual Framework", *Refuge* 31/1, 2015, 5–17, here 5.

4 Jan Assmann, "Communicative and Cultural Memory", in: Peter Meusburger, Michael Heffernan, and Edgar Wunder (eds.), *Cultural Memories: The Geographical Point of View*, Dordrecht: Springer, 2011, 15–27.

5 Samuel P. Huntington, *The Clash of Civilizations and the Remaking of World Order*, New York: Simon and Schuster, 1996; and Ivan Katchanovski, *Cleft Countries: Regional Political Divisions and Cultures in Post-Soviet Ukraine and Moldova*, New York: Columbia University Press, 2006.

6 Ivan Kozachenko, "Fighting for the Soviet Union 2.0: Digital nostalgia and national belonging in the context of the Ukrainian crisis", *Communist and Post-Communist Studies* 52/1, 2019, 1–10.

of the USSR in the victory in World War II, Russian Orthodox religiosity, and the Russian language. The language holds a key function, as 'Russian speakers' are often discursively equated with 'Russians'. At its extreme, this discourse denies Ukrainian agency and describes Eastern Slavs as a 'triune nation' of Ukraine, Belarus, and Russia. Vladimir Putin's oft-repeated assertion that Ukrainians and Russians are "one people" is an example of such an extreme ideology.[7] In contrast to the 'supranational' project, the 'national' one presents a different perspective.

Taras Kuzio asserts that Ukrainian 'national' identity is based on the portrayal of Ukraine as a peaceful European country that has its origins in Kyivan Rus and is an integral part of Europe.[8] Thus, this identity is also related to the supranational European project. Within this perspective, the Soviet period is portrayed as a time of repression and suffering. Here, the Holodomor – a genocidal famine of 1932/1933 – is a key symbol of Ukrainian martyrdom. In their more conservative forms, 'national' narratives pay specific attention to Ukrainian freedom fighters during WWII – the Ukrainian Insurgent Army (UPA) and the Organisation of Ukrainian Nationalists (OUN). Volodymyr Kulyk argues that the Russian annexation of Crimea and the aggression in the Donbas made nationalist figures of this time more attractive in Ukraine.[9] At the same time, based on an extensive empirical study, he asserts that since the Euromaidan Revolution, Ukrainian national identity has become more civic and inclusive. Overall, the events that followed the revolution and the February invasion have demonstrated that Ukraine is not as divided as previously argued. Moreover, Russian soldiers were met with fierce resistance and not with flowers, as the Kremlin seemingly anticipated. So how do displaced Ukrainians relate to these identities and memories? In exploring this question, I employed a qualitative research methodology.

Methodology and Case Selection

This analysis draws on participant observation and in-depth interviews with 12 refugees residing in the Lesser Poland, Silesian, Greater Poland, and Masovian Voivodeships provinces of Poland. The participants are from the eastern oblasts of Ukraine (Kharkiv, Dnipro, and Luhansk) and the southern ones (Kherson and Odesa), as well as from the capital city of Kyiv. I recruited them by contacting

---

7 Vladimir Putin, "On the Historical Unity of Russians and Ukrainians", *Presidential Library*, https://www.prlib.ru/en/article-vladimir-putin-historical-unity-russians-and-ukrainians [accessed: 31.07.2024].

8 Taras Kuzio, "National Identity and History Writing in Ukraine", *Nationalities Papers* 34/4, 2006, 407–427, here 409.

9 Volodymyr Kulyk, "National Identity in Ukraine: Impact of Euromaidan and the War", *Europe-Asia Studies* 68/4, 2016, 588–608, here 604.

refugee assistance points, administrators of free Polish language courses, and cultural event organisers (who plan fundraisers, meetings with writers and poets, charity concerts, etc.). I did so to interview people who rely on volunteer and state assistance, as well as those who apparently plan a longer stay and, thus, learn the language of the receiving country. Lastly, those people who attend cultural events can be assumed to have a more secure life situation with free time for attendance and the ability to pay for tickets or donate money to charitable causes.

I conducted five interviews in person and the rest via communication applications (Viber, WhatsApp, or Messenger). Ten of the participants were women. While this somewhat reflects the fact that men between 18 and 60 years of age are not allowed to leave Ukraine as they can be drafted into the army, I must stress that I approached many men, but almost all refused to be interviewed. This could be due to uneasiness around the circumstances through which they left Ukraine or how or why they have avoided conscription. These two factors have contributed to the gender imbalance in the sample. Moreover, many older people who rely on help from assistance points were also not eager to participate in the study. They explained that they were afraid to give a 'wrong answer' or do something that would compromise their already vulnerable position.

The interview guide included topics on the participants' biographies, the circumstances of their departure from Ukraine, their attitudes towards the countries under study, national histories, and the reasons for the Russo–Ukrainian War, as well as questions about the refugees' current life situation. For each interview, I obtained informed consent. This included a clear explanation of the research aims and objectives, the researcher's affiliation and contact details, guidelines on anonymity and confidentiality, as well as an outline of how data will be dealt with. I analysed the collected data using a framework technique[10] that allows for the identification of thematic clusters and variations within them. The results of the analysis will be presented in the following paragraphs.

Ukraine

This study reveals that the events of the war have caused a renegotiation of belonging to Ukraine among the participants. Additionally, it demonstrates that essentialist narratives play an important role in their interpretations of events. Moreover, those who previously spoke Russian have switched or are switching to Ukrainian. The data suggests that for most participants, the war and the experience of displacement have

10 Jane Ritchie and Liz Spencer, "Qualitative Data Analysis for Applied Policy Research", in: Michael A. Huberman and Matthew B. Miles (eds.), *The Qualitative Researcher's Companion*, Thousand Oaks: Sage, 2002, 305–329.

strengthened their sense of national belonging. Many described how proud they felt about their country, which fights a brutal and cynical aggressor so well. When asked why Ukraine performs so well, many answered that the war started in 2014, and since then, many people have realised what may be coming next. Along with mentioning effective Ukrainian policies and the importance of Western help, participants normally added that it is also due to a lasting Ukrainian military tradition. As one of the participants explained: "[in Ukrainian] You know, this line 'we are of the Cossack origin' in the Ukrainian anthem is really true. I feel proud how we are resisting the aggressor. [...] Russia will lose" (F, 32, 7 February 2023). This essentialism is manifested by a strong belief that Ukraine exists as an entity with lasting features and traits. For instance, most participants saw Ukrainians as 'naturally' free people who cannot live under oppression, and that this is something that really differentiates them from Russians. References to Cossackdom[11] often occurred in the interviews. In such cases, the direct democracy of the Cossacks is presented as further evidence of the built-in dedication of Ukrainians to this form of governance. Cossacks, indeed, elected their leader – the Hetman – at a general assembly that was a very different practice from those of the Russian Empire, where absolute monarchy took hold for a significant historical period.

The participants described how painful it was to leave Ukraine and that they never fully realised how important the country is to them. Perhaps unsurprisingly, given their experiences, their vivid descriptions of their journeys westward dominated the interviews. The pain of leaving family members behind, overcrowded train stations, crying children, stressed adults, and episodic violence are typical parts of these stories. One participant recalls her departure from one of the eastern cities in March last year:

> [in Russian] When we reached this first platform, there was just an insane amount of people. One soldier even had to shoot in the air in order to make people stop pushing [...] and people were just squeezing their children through the windows of the train, so they could leave to safety. My grandmother was in Auschwitz, and she was telling me stories [about] how they were transported by overcrowded trains. I never could imagine that something similar would happen to me [starts crying] (F, 39, 19 February 2023).

This part of the interview shows not only how stressful and traumatic the journey was but also illustrates how participants connect this experience with the communicative memory of their family. In two other interviews, the participants

11 TRAFO – Blog for Transregional Research, "The Cossack Myth in Eastern Europe – Interview with Denys Shatalov", 09 December 2019, https://trafo.hypotheses.org/21007 [accessed: 31.07.2024].

mentioned that their relatives were repressed by the Soviet regime and that they never had any illusions about it. They point out, however, that it was hard for them to imagine that Russia would go in the same direction and that it would be them fleeing from danger and possible persecution.

The Ukrainian language serves as a powerful symbol of national belonging. While five participants indicated that they were Ukrainian speakers, four stated that they either switched to Ukrainian or were trying to speak Ukrainian as much as possible. They also said that writing online posts or asking questions in relevant social media groups is nearly exclusively conducted in Ukrainian now, and that Russian is not tolerated by fellow Ukrainians. These narratives are deeply interconnected with perceptions of the aggressor country, Russia.

Russia

The perception of Russia among the respondents comes down to several key themes. First, there is a clear pattern that not only the Putin regime but also the Russian people are to blame for the invasion. Second, there is a distancing from the Russian language, which is related to the switch to Ukrainian. Moreover, an overwhelming majority of participants considered Russian culture and literature as something toxic for Ukraine. And third, a small group of participants who had previously held pro-Russian views has turned away from this country. This, however, has not made those participants more pro-Ukrainian. It is necessary to provide several illustrations of these findings.

The annexation of Crimea and the war in the Donbas already made these participants perceive Russia as an aggressor country, but this view was mainly about the Russian state. However, a lack of resistance among Russian society to the February invasion – and even a noticeable support for it – made them see Russian people in a negative way. One participant from Southern Ukraine notes:

> [in Ukrainian] I know that Russia is a police state, and it is hard to protest over there as you can be arrested immediately. But, if they are against the war, they could just stop going to work *en masse*. Just stay at home and it would be enough; if not to stop the war, then change the situation dramatically. But they never did it. [...] After our victory, there should be a 5-metre fence between our countries, and we should forget about them (F, 35, 17 February 2023).

The distancing from the Russian language is often related to an unwillingness to be identified as Russian. These behaviours are also directly connected to the concept of social identity as a perceived membership in a certain social group: "[in Ukrainian]

I do not use Russian in public as I do not want to be identified as Russian. [...] I was at the airport recently, and there were Russian people nearby, and I felt anger and disgust" (Male, 63, 15 February 2023). Similarly, they question the value of Russian culture and literary classics for Ukraine. Many participants wonder how such a presumably great culture can have bred the people who are committing crimes in Bucha or Izium.

However, not all participants share such sentiments. Two people expressed more downbeat views. In their vision, Ukraine is a pawn in a global geopolitical game and does not have any agency. They view the Orange and Euromaidan Revolutions as American conspiracies against Russia. While they admitted that before the invasion they had quite strong pro-Russian views, the brutality of the invasion has significantly undermined these. In these cases, however, it does not mean that the participants have a stronger sense of belonging to Ukraine now. As one of the respondents explains:

> [in Russian] I used to be pro-Russian, but that is not the case anymore after everything I went through. I think that they made a huge mistake by invading Ukraine. [...] They do not have a monopoly on either the Russian language or on Soviet history. We should remember Soviet times and continue to celebrate Soviet holidays like the Day of the Motherland Defenders, which is today. [...] I think that Ukraine will lose this war. I just cannot see it winning it [...] I am not going back [to Ukraine] (M, 41, 23 February 2023).

These lapsed pro-Russian sentiments show that some people are somewhat 'lost in-between' national loyalties. This interview also shows a degree of Soviet nostalgia and the view that Soviet memory should be preserved in Ukraine. Most of the participants in this study, however, have opposite views. For them, the Russian invasion has shattered a positive cultural memory of the Soviet past. Notably, the admission of previous susceptibility to Soviet mythology is common within this group: "[in Russian] I somewhat believed in the myth of the noble Russian soldier, but what I saw were thieves and rapists" (F, 47, 11 February 2023). Notably, the perceptions of the homeland are also related to the intentions of staying abroad or returning, as those who expressed positive views towards Ukraine were more likely to stress that they would return as soon as the war ended.

Poland

The most pronounced themes in the discussion of Poland are the appreciation of help and the cultural and geographic proximity of the country, new knowledge about the country, and an admission of the hardships of living in Poland. The participants of this study almost universally express gratitude to Poland and Polish people for their support and help.

After their hard journeys, the participants received a very warm welcome upon crossing the border. They stress that much of the help came from ordinary people who were not members of nongovernmental organisations (NGOs) or representatives of national or international organisations. A young woman from Southern Ukraine described her experience as follows:

> [in Ukrainian] We have arrived in Przemyśl. There was an ocean of people, but everything was very well organised. You could meet a volunteer every five metres, asking you what you need. There were hundreds of baby buggies waiting to be taken by those in need. We came with two cats, and the door on one carrier was broken. There was a vet inspecting animals, and she not only inspected our cats but also gave them shots, and gave us a new carrier. I am so touched by this help and will always be grateful for it (F, 35, 17 February 2023).

As mentioned earlier, the participants appreciate the cultural and geographical proximity of Poland. The ease of learning Polish along with the positive attitude contribute towards emotional dimensions of belonging, like those described by Catherine Brun and Anita Fábos.[12] Another common theme is the desire and ability to live somewhere close to Ukraine. One of the participants explains that most of her friends who have left lived in the parts of Poland that are close to Ukraine to come back quickly "when we win".

Seven out of the 12 participants had never previously visited Poland or any other country in the European Union. The participants who had never visited Poland before provided extended stories about how limited they were in their knowledge of the country. A reoccurring narrative is that they imagined Poland as not being markedly different from Ukraine, and while not having had previous contact with Polish people, they were perceived as arrogant and disdainful towards Ukrainians:

> [in Russian] I always thought of Polish people as arrogant and hostile towards Ukrainians. You know, this *Polskiy pan* [Polish master][13] sort of thing. I think that you get this sort of information from school, from literature... And it was completely wrong. Polish people are very nice and very similar to us.

12 Brun and Fábos, "Making Homes in Limbo?", 5.

13 This is a reference to the discrimination of Ukrainians in the Polish Commonwealth as well as the exploitation of the Ukrainian peasantry by Polish nobility after the partitions of Poland. The negative portrayal of the Polish nobility in *Taras Bulba* by Nikolai Gogol or that of the 'Polish seducer' Pan Mussyalovich in Fyodor Dostoevsky's *Bratya Karamazovy* (*The Brothers Karamazov*) may serve as good examples here.

> [...] Poland has an amazing history. I recently learnt that it has 402 castles. Imagine that (F, 71, 1 February 2023).

This and many other quotes point out that there were strong prejudices towards Poland and the Polish people. Thus, their help and warmth were surprising for many displaced Ukrainians. Some even go as far as saying that they previously considered Russians as 'fraternal people', but Poles better fit this description now.

There are also some negative aspects of residing in Poland for the participants. These mainly come down to the lack of state support. This is especially evident in the case of people relying on various assistance schemes. The participants explained that initially, it was easier when the Polish state was providing monetary compensation for those who hosted Ukrainians. These payments stopped in the summer of 2022, and it became significantly more difficult to find accommodation. The arrival of Ukrainians also increased rental prices across Poland, making them unaffordable for many refugees. Furthermore, there are pronounced class divisions. Ukrainians with high skills quickly found employment and took advantage of the open labour market. This is not the case for people representing the working class. Many research participants are young mothers who need flexible working schedules, which is not possible due to their lack of language skills or the professions in demand. Thus, even with the appreciation of support, for many participants, hardship is a big part of their daily routine.

Conclusions

The Russian invasion and forced displacement have significantly altered the sense of belonging among the people who participated in this study. For most of them, it strengthened their sense of belonging to Ukraine. It is evident that the invasion has dramatically weakened what can be called a pro-Russian 'supranational' identity. Participants also reported that they became more critical of the Soviet past and its mythology, which is so actively used by Russia. There is also a pronounced role of linguistic identities, where speaking or switching to Ukrainian is a crucial manifestation of national identity. The heroic resistance of Ukraine reinforces the participants' sense of pride in being Ukrainian. In describing their homeland, participants primarily rely on essentialist visions of the nation. They have also fundamentally 'reimagined' Russia and Poland, with a clear distancing from the former. Notably, their negative views are now towards both the Russian state and the Russian people. This is quite different from the case of Poland. The absolute majority of participants are deeply touched by the support of the Polish people. However, many experienced hardship while staying in Poland. As the war continues, it is hard to predict how the

Ukrainian community in Poland will look in the future. Their attitudes towards the homeland and the aggressor country, however, seem to have a lasting nature.

Bibliography

Assmann, Jan, "Communicative and Cultural Memory", in: Peter Meusburger, Michael Heffernan, and Edgar Wunder (eds.), *Cultural Memories: The Geographical Point of View*, Dordrecht: Springer, 2011, 15–27.

Brun, Cathrine, and Anita Fábos, "Making Homes in Limbo? A Conceptual Framework", *Refuge* 31/1, 2015, 5–17.

European Commission, Migration and Home Affairs, "Temporary Protection", https://home-affairs.ec.europa.eu/policies/migration-and-asylum/common-european-asylum-system/temporary-protection_en [accessed: 29.07.2024].

Guibernau, Montserrat, *Belonging: Solidarity and Division in Modern Societies*, Cambridge: Polity, 2013.

Huntington, Samuel P., *The Clash of Civilizations and the Remaking of World Order*, New York: Simon and Schuster, 1996.

Katchanovski, Ivan, *Cleft Countries: Regional Political Divisions and Cultures in Post-Soviet Ukraine and Moldova*, New York: Columbia University Press, 2006.

Kozachenko, Ivan, "Fighting for the Soviet Union 2.0: Digital nostalgia and national belonging in the context of the Ukrainian crisis", *Communist and Post-Communist Studies* 52/1, 2019, 1–10.

Kulyk, Volodymyr, "National Identity in Ukraine: Impact of Euromaidan and the War", *Europe-Asia Studies* 68/4, 2016, 588–608.

Kuzio, Taras, "National Identity and History Writing in Ukraine", *Nationalities Papers* 34/4, 2006, 407–427.

Marples, David R., "Decommunization, Memory Laws, and 'Builders of Ukraine in the 20th Century'", *Acta Slavica Iaponica (Japanese Slavic Journal)* 39, 2018, 1–22.

Putin, Vladimir, "On the Historical Unity of Russians and Ukrainians", *Presidential Library*, https://www.prlib.ru/en/article-vladimir-putin-historical-unity-russians-and-ukrainians [accessed: 29.07.2024].

Ritchie, Jane, and Liz Spencer, "Qualitative Data Analysis for Applied Policy Research", in: Michael A. Huberman and Matthew B. Miles (eds.), *The Qualitative Researcher's Companion*, Thousand Oaks: Sage, 2002, 305–329.

Shevel, Oxana, "The Battle for Historical Memory in Postrevolutionary Ukraine", *Current History* 115/783, 2016, 258–263.

TRAFO – Blog for Transregional Research, "The Cossack Myth in Eastern Europe – Interview with Denys Shatalov", 09 December 2019, https://trafo.hypotheses.org/21007 [accessed: 29.07.2024].

Ukrainian Forcibly Displaced Persons in Germany
Post-Migration Strategies

Natalia Zaitseva-Chipak

Return migration has received limited attention in migration studies, and the literature remains fragmented. This is partially due to the difficulty of recording return migration in many countries and the lack of adequate data. However, to grasp the phenomenon, it is necessary to define several trends in the research. The first concentrates on labour migrants who intend to return or have returned to their home countries and their self-reported motives.[1] The second looks at forced returnees (due to a legal decision of the receiving country) and the motives for compliance or resistance by migrants subjected to assisted or forced return.[2] A third focuses on migrants returning from Europe to post-conflict countries.[3] This literature proposes different classifications of respondents' self-reported motives. Michael Sinnige, Marieke van Houte, and Arjen Leerkes argue for a regulative,

1 Thomas Niedomysl and Jan Amcoff, "Why return migrants return: Survey evidence on motives for internal return migration in Sweden", *Population, Space and Place* 17/5, 2011, 656–673; Eva A. Duda-Mikulin, "*Should I stay or should I go now?* Exploring Polish women's returns 'home'", *International Migration* 56/4, 2018, 140–153; and Lemlem F. Weldemariam, Ayansina Ayanlade, Marion Borderon, and Karoline Möslinger, "Dynamics and factors influencing return migration to Sub-Saharan Africa: A systematic review", *Heliyon* 9/8, 2023, e18791.

2 Michael Sinnige, Marieke van Houte, and Arjen Leerkes, "Talking about return: Governmental caseworkers' regulative, normative and cultural-cognitive strategies during 'return conversations' with irregularised migrants", *International Migration* 61/1, 2023, 288–303.

3 Marieke van Houte and Tine Davids, "Moving Back or Moving Forward? Return Migration, Development and Peace-Building", *New Diversities* 16/2, 2014, 71–87, https://newdiversities.mmg.mpg.de/wp-content/uploads/2015/01/2014_16-02_06_vanHoute.pdf [accessed: 12.04.2024]; Dany Bahar, Cem Özgüzel, Andreas Hauptmann, and Hillel Rapoport, "Migration and Post-Conflict Reconstruction: The Effect of Returning Refugees on Export Performance in the Former Yugoslavia", IZA Institute of Labor Economics, Discussion Paper no. 12412, 2019, https://docs.iza.org/dp12412.pdf [accessed: 12.04.2024]; and Richard Black and Saskia Gent, "Sustainable Return in Post-conflict Contexts", *International Migration* 44/3, 2006, 5–38, https://doi.org/10.1111/j.1468-2435.2006.00370.x [accessed: 31.07.2024].

normative, and cultural-cognitive understanding.[4] Meanwhile, Thomas Niedomysl and Jan Amcoff stress the importance of economic issues (e.g., job opportunities and income options for returning individuals) and social reasons as key motivators in understanding why migrants return.[5] This perspective considers the potential impact on a life course.

The case of the current displacement of Ukrainian citizens to European Union countries differs from many others in size, and legislation applied to Ukrainian refugees. It is also an ongoing conflict. Therefore, the motivations for staying or moving back may include many elements (including physical and psychological trauma, as well as the risk of loss of life and property and the potential for rapidly deteriorating living conditions in the country of origin) and can radically change with time. Simultaneously, in their attempts to predict refugee movements to adjust their refugee policies, the Ukrainian government as well as the governments of the receiving countries started to ask questions about the refugees' intentions to return as early as March 2022.[6] Most of these enquiries are quantitative and often limited to one or a few questions. They do not consider emotional reactions or present the complexity of factors and how the interlocutors prioritise them. Accordingly, this study conducts qualitative exploratory research on Ukrainian refugees' self-reported motives to prolong their stay in Germany or to return to Ukraine.

According to the United Nations High Commissioner for Refugees (UNHCR), since the beginning of the Russo–Ukrainian War, as of April 2024, Germany has accepted about 1.4 million forcibly displaced persons (FDPs) from Ukraine, and more than 1,053,000 people have registered for temporary protection or similar national protection programmes.[7] This is a staggering figure. Incoming migrants to Germany have also received numerous benefits: financial aid, health insurance, housing, compensation for utilities and travel, and free German language courses. This strains the country's social system. It is enough to multiply the cost of these benefits by the number of FDPs to understand that this support is worth billions of euros.

However, these costs are temporary. Soon, Ukrainian FDPs could adapt and be able to join the German economy, which could become a potentially powerful factor in its growth. For example, 2023 EU survey data indicates that about 40 percent of

4 Sinnige, Houte, and Leerkes, "Talking about return".

5 Niedomysl and Amcoff, "Why return migrants return".

6 Holger Liljeberg, Sindy Krambeer, and Yvonne Blunck, *Geflüchtete aus der Ukraine, Bundesministerium des Innern und für Heimat – März 2022* (*Refugees from Ukraine, Federal Ministry of the Interior and for Home Affairs – March 2022– March 2022*), INFO GmbH Markt und Meinungsforschung (INFO GmbH Market and Opinion Research), report, 4 April 2022, https://rathaus.jena.de/sites/default/files/2022-04/BMI_Umfrage_Gefl%C3%BCchtete_aus_der_Ukraine.pdf [accessed: 12.04.2022].

7 Numbers given as of 12 April 2024, https://data.unhcr.org/en/situations/ukraine [accessed: 31.07.2024].

Ukrainian FDPs have already integrated into the labour markets of EU countries. In general, at the end of 2022, Ukrainian FDPs increased the available labour force in the EU by 0.5 percent.[8] Given that most of the migrants are women (of working age) with children,[9] these contributions are significant, not only for the near but also for the more distant future.

At the same time, the loss of these people will be detrimental to postwar Ukraine. Even today, Ukrainian demographers fear the country's depopulation.[10] This, in turn, could be a critical factor slowing down the country's reconstruction, as it requires labour, skilled workers, and young people. Currently, it is difficult to predict what most Ukrainians who moved to Germany due to the war will want in the future. Quantitative sociological studies show that the majority of surveyed FDPs plan to return home after the war ends but under different conditions.[11] According to the Razumkov Centre's opinion poll conducted in August 2022, 36 percent of respondents intend to return when they are convinced that it is safe to stay in the area where they lived, 35 percent immediately after the end of the war, 13 percent a year or several years after the end of the war, seven percent once the company they worked for resumes work or they are sure that they will find another job at home, 11 percent generally in the near future, and 7 percent do not plan to return to Ukraine at all (among these last respondents, 18 percent of them have a permanent job in the host country).[12] Of course, this is an equation with many unknown variables. People's motivations also depend on the duration of the war, the extent of the destruction in Ukraine and their region, the amount of support for the country's

---

8 See the UNHCR document titled "Lives on Hold: Intentions and Perspectives of Refugees fr om Ukraine #3", 22 February 2023, for further details. https://data.unhcr.org/en/documents/details/99072 [accessed: 31.07.2024].

9 According to the data from Deutsches Institut für Wirtschaftsforschung (German Institute for Economic Research): Nykyta Zholkver, "Ukrainskie bezhentsy v Germanii. Kakie oni?" ("Ukrainian refugees in Germany: What are they like?"), *Deutsche Welle* (*German Wave*), 15 December 2022, https://www.dw.com/ru/ukrainskie-bezency-v-germanii-kakie-oni/a-64107524?maca=rus-rss-ru-all-1126-rdf [accessed: 31.07.2024].

10 Ukrainske radio (Ukrainian Radio), "'90% bizhentsiv z Ukrainy ne povernetsia dodomu' — dyrektorka Instytutu demohrafii ta sotsdoslidzhen im. Ptukhy Ella Libanova" ("'90% of refugees from Ukraine will not return home" – Ella Libanova, Director of the Ptukha Institute for Demography and Social Studies"), 09 February 2023, http://www.nrcu.gov.ua/news.html?newsID=100692 [accessed: 13.04.2024]; and World Population Review, "Ukraine Population 2024 (Live)", https://worldpopulationreview.com/countries/ukraine-population [accessed: 31.07.2024].

11 Razumkov Centre, "Nastroi ta otsinky ukrainskykh bizhentsiv (lypen–serpen 2022r.)" ("Attitudes and assessments of Ukrainian refugees (July–August 2022)"), 30 August 2022, https://razumkov.org.ua/napriamky/sotsiologichni-doslidzhennia/nastroi-ta-otsinky-ukrainskykh-bizhentsiv-lypen-serpen-2022p [accessed: 31.07.2024].

12 Ibid.

reconstruction after the war, the pace of economic development, the reliability of the social system, and sufficient guarantees of future security.

Ukrainian demographer Ella Libanova claims that, based on the experience of other war-induced displacement experiences, usually only a third of those who left return.[13] High indicators of readiness to return in opinion polls can be attributed to the feeling of patriotism or the discomfort of admitting the desire to stay to strangers. Moreover, questions about the return plans of Ukrainian FDPs are often asked by people who are in a stable and secure situation and who debate whether Ukrainians will return to a country that was devastated by the largest war in recent European history.

To be able to predict future return migration, it is necessary to consider multiple factors. It is possible to start with Abraham Maslow's pyramid of needs: security (of health, property, future, etc.) is at the core of human needs. However, the weight of these issues may turn out to be less significant than that of the longing for home and familiar circles of communication and culture or difficulties with adapting.

Research has shown that even those FDPs who declare their readiness to return home consider different scenarios for the future, which may delay their return or force them to stay in Germany for a long time. Therefore, methodologically, the prediction of the behaviour of Ukrainian FDPs cannot be based on a single question measuring the strength of their intentions to return. It should include complex indicators that consider various aspects of their motivations, including those related to security as well as psychological, economic, cultural, and social reasons, among others. What other conditions do Ukrainians, forcefully displaced by the war, consider when building their post-migration strategy? Their final choice is still an open question.

My research aims to determine a list of decision-making motives that is as complete as possible. Additionally, it intends to establish the significance of such motives and to understand the mechanisms of choice formation. Finally, it sets out to model (or predict) which choices different social groups of FDPs from Ukraine could be inclined to make. I argue that understanding the intentions of FDPs from Ukraine will allow both Germany and Ukraine to build their social and economic policies in an effective and balanced manner.

This is especially important given that quantitative forecasts can be accurate only up to a certain point and do not allow us to fully predict FDPs' future choices. Addi-

13 Iryna Krykunenko, "Zazvychai povertaietsia tretyna. Skilky ukraintsiv zalyshatsia za kordonom ta yak blekauty zminiuiut demohrafiiu – Libanova" ("Usually a Third Returns: How Many Ukrainians Will Stay Abroad and How Blackouts Change Demographics – Libanova"), *New Voice* (*NV*), 11 December 2022, https://nv.ua/ukr/ukraine/events/skilki-ukrajinciv-zalishitsya-pislya-peremogi-naslidki-dlya-ukrajini-ekspert-ostanni-novini-50289318.html [accessed: 31.07.2024].

tionally, pure numbers do not provide a clear understanding of how such choices are made – that is, what factors are taken into account and what the impact of each of them is. By contrast, in the paradigm of 'interpretive sociology' (which, incidentally, originated in Germany as *verstehende Soziologie*)[14], we can focus on the inner worldviews of people and better understand how their choices form.

Given that both countries will be interested in this development potential and will (likely) compete for human resources in the future, it is important to examine which influences could shape such decisions. Additionally, this study helps identify areas of Germany's aid policies towards Ukrainian FDPs that, in my opinion, require improvement.

Methodology

To answer my research questions, I interviewed 15 female Ukrainians who experienced displacement to Germany. The respondents were of different ages (four aged 20 to 34, ten aged 35 to 55, and one over 55), from different regions (three from Ukrainian rear regions (places far from the frontline), nine from frontline territories, and three from occupied territories), and from areas of different sizes (two from the capital, eight from large cities or regional centres, four from small towns, and one from a rural area). The participants currently live in different places in Germany (including large and small cities and rural areas). The sample included people who experienced living in refugee camps, with German families, and in housing provided by local authorities. I conducted semi-structured online interviews. The main blocks of questions covered the experience of living through war and displacement, the specifics of living conditions in Germany, their future strategies, post-migration intentions (adapting or returning), motives for migration or a refusal to migrate, and forecasts of Ukraine's development (specifically their degree of optimism). I conducted the interviews between 5 December 2022 and 30 January 2023.

The Intentions of Ukrainian FDPs in Germany (at the Time of This Research)

My study, of course, does not claim to be representative, but it confirms the results of previous quantitative studies: my respondents mostly declared their desire to re-

14 Interpretive sociology studies the meaning of behaviour (its causes and motives), as opposed to positivist sociology, which focuses on action. Interpretive sociology also relies on qualitative data, while positivist sociology tends to use quantitative data.

turn to Ukraine.[15] Only one respondent made a final decision to stay in Germany. Her main motive is that her city is in the occupied territories and was destroyed by the war. One of the families I interviewed has already returned to Ukraine, but because of the recent attacks on energy infrastructure, they do not rule out coming back to Germany. Interestingly, the forcefully displaced women I interviewed who plan to return to Ukraine show two key behavioural strategies. Some of them seem to be 'putting their lives on hold' – that is, they are waiting out the war in a safe environment and plan to return to Ukraine once the war is over to start rebuilding their lives there. Others, however, are trying to use their new opportunities to become more resourceful in the future. For example, they plan to learn or are learning a language that will be an added competitive advantage at home, or they are acquiring experiences in Germany that they can transfer to their communities in Ukraine. The first group is less likely to adapt in Germany and more likely to leave, while the second group is likely to adapt better and will therefore have more reasons to remain.

Meanwhile, a minority of the respondents admitted that they are at a crossroads and are hesitant about their future life strategies:

> Some people want to return to Ukraine. Some don't. Everyone is very uncertain. Everyone is stressed (F, 42, from a rear region).
>
> I can't say 100 percent that I'm ready to live here and 100 percent that I'm ready to return to Ukraine. At the moment, I can't say. But my mother wants to go home, so she's sitting and waiting for spring to come, when they are promising that everything will be over, and she can return home, and everything will be fine (F, 35, from a frontline region).

There are two key strategies for making decisions that align with the aforementioned behavioural strategies. Some try to think according to algorithms by which they will make their decisions (i.e., they define the conditions under which they will leave or stay), while others believe that it is inappropriate to try to make decisions until the war is over and the situation in Ukraine is stable. The first group tends to work more actively on influencing their conditions in Germany because the conditions in Ukraine are beyond their control. For this reason, they have a higher chance of adapting to their new place of residence and will most likely refuse to return:

> If the war ends in two months, that's one situation. If it ends in two years, that's a different situation. It depends on what my position here will be at that moment. If I can find a job and know German to some degree, I might try to stay here. But this is not a fact, it's not 100 percent certain (F, 38, from an occupied region).

15 Razumkov Centre, "Nastroi ta otsinky".

The second group is more likely to passively observe how circumstances will develop.

Intentions to stay in Germany or return to Ukraine also significantly correlate with the sociodemographic backgrounds of the FDPs as well as how much their regions of origin are affected by the war and their proximity to the frontline. Residents from regions less affected by the war are more likely to declare their intention to return, as their regions have not suffered large-scale destruction or occupation.

A significant number of women left Ukraine in the first weeks of the war, when its consequences were unclear: the occupation was spreading rapidly, rocket attacks destroyed residential buildings across the country, and the state's ability to provide the population with the most basic necessities was unpredictable. With the stabilisation of the frontline in late summer of 2022, and reports that life in the rear regions farthest from the front was relatively safe (or at least not as risky as previously thought), the opportunity to live in their own home, with their family, and in a familiar social circle and cultural environment became a strong arguments for returning. Many Ukrainian FDPs were inclined to return at this point, but the recent attacks on energy infrastructure changed their plans.

Another distinct point is that FDPs who have higher chances of adaptation tend to stay in Germany. This includes, for example, those who are fluent in German or work in a field that is in demand in Germany. Such people have higher chances of building a career or obtaining a higher-quality education in the country. Young people (17–25 years old), for instance, are much more likely to express an intention to stay. They often speak the German language, have an easier time adapting, have not yet started a family, and have opportunities to receive higher education in the country. I frequently heard from middle-aged people (26–54 years old) that they planned to return to Ukraine but insisted that their children should remain abroad (at least until they graduate). Some parents with school-age children who expressed a willingness to return to Ukraine explained that they are ready to sacrifice their desire for the sake of their children having a better future in a stable Europe:

> I plan to take the language exam in March, leave my son and mom here, and return to Ukraine to find a job, to live in Ukraine for some time and to come visit my son [here] (F, 42, from a rear region).

> My older daughter went back to Germany because she's studying and working there [she knows the language], and I stayed in Ukraine with my younger children (F, 41, from a rear region).

In contrast, middle-aged Ukrainian women who have built a career, started a family, and had a home in Ukraine are more likely to return:

> I would like to return home. I'm afraid now about when this will be. I've never had such aspirations [to go abroad]. I have a house there. I had a perfectly good job that I loved, I had a life there that suited me perfectly. I see no reason to lose it. If everything is restored, I want to restore it [my previous life] as well (F, 34, from an occupied region).

Reasons for Choosing a Country to Live in and Motivations to Remain Abroad

First, I should note that each of the respondents emphasised that their main motivation for going abroad was security concerns. Respondents from the frontline regions of Ukraine fled from the occupation forces and active bombardment; those from the rear regions left the country because of difficulties in caring for elderly parents or young children amid constant air raids and fears of the unpredictable risks of war:

> There was only one argument for leaving: to feel safe and not to hear those sounds and not to see what was happening. Not to feel that fear (F, 35, from a frontline region).

Ukrainians could count on taking refuge in many Western countries. The choice of Germany as a destination for these FDPs often stemmed from three factors:

- Social contacts in Germany: Family or friends removed the factor of uncertainty and facilitated adaptation in the first weeks of the war. They offered housing and advised on how to apply for refugee status and social aid. However, eventually, the majority of respondents left the homes of their loved ones and sought support from the state.
- Access to medical care: The ability to receive health insurance was important for half of the FDPs I interviewed. This issue was especially relevant for elderly people with chronic diseases, parents with young children, and people who needed surgical interventions.
- The availability of social benefits: This was particularly relevant for the period of adaptation (i.e., when they were learning a language and searching for a job).

My interviewees also provided a wide range of reasons for staying in Germany after the end of the war. Their level of optimism or pessimism about the future of Ukraine plays a key role in this decision. FDPs are scared by the prospect of returning to a country with a ruined economy, a lack of jobs, and only vague prospects for recovery:

> You see, after the war, the situation will be unstable, it won't end on the last day of the war. Especially in my city. It's a small, economically depressed city. And I don't understand at all what will happen there when the war ends (F, 38, from an occupied region).

> There will be an unstable economic situation, part of the country has already been destroyed, and the people who used to live there are already losing their jobs. New ones will appear after these cities are rebuilt, but that's another issue. It's not yet clear what will be left of our city, what will happen there (F, 20, from a rear region).

Some FDPs see going back to Ukraine not as a return to a familiar environment but as a step into the unknown. Due to their long absence from the country, they often lost not only their jobs but also their emotional closeness with their social environments. By contrast, they perceive Germany as a zone of stability and a country of economic prosperity. Here, finding a job with decent pay is more probable.

This leads to another important motive for staying in Germany: social security. The war in Ukraine has led to inflation and a devaluation of the hryvnia (the Ukrainian currency). Consequently, as of July 2022, almost half of Ukrainians received pensions no higher than what equals to about 80 euros per month;[16] internally displaced person (IDP) payments amount to about 53 euros per adult and 80 euros per child per month.[17] After the war, Ukraine will face depopulation (especially the outflow of young people), economic devastation, the need to pay off debts, and a likely reduction of international support. Therefore, the situation of social security may worsen. FDPs are not sure that they will be able to maintain a decent standard of living in postwar Ukraine. Germany, however, has already demonstrated the ability to provide decent social security, including a sufficient degree of social benefits and health insurance (e.g., FDPs can have chronic diseases treated or undergo surgery free of charge):

> Socially, we are more protected here. We have health insurance. In Ukraine, I receive the minimum pension. I worked for thirty years in agriculture, but I have the minimum pension, and my husband has a little more. And we will not be able to live off our pensions – or rather, even now we're not able to live [off them]. People who moved from Donetsk, Luhansk, and Odesa... They told

16 This is according to the Pension Fund of Ukraine: Pensiinyi fond Ukrainy (Pension Fund of Ukraine) (Facebook page), "Rozpodil pensioneriv po vydakh..." ("Distribution of pensioners by type..."), Facebook post, 15 July 2022, https://www.facebook.com/pfu.gov.ua/posts/412375920933627 [accessed: 31.07.2024].

17 This is according to the Ukrainian Ministry of Reintegration of Temporarily Occupied Territories: https://minre.gov.ua/2023/11/01/vyplaty-vpo-teper-pryznachatymutsya-na-sim%ca%bcyu/ [accessed: 31.07.2024].

> me what kinds of benefits our social security system gave them. A person gets two thousand hryvnia [about 50 euros] for moving, three thousand hryvnia [about 75 euros] for a child. I understand that there is a war… and the budget is low, but is it possible to survive on such amounts, to find an apartment, and to find a job? Now you can't even find a job (F, 69, from a rear region).

In the context of social protection, my interviewees specifically mentioned better-protected labour rights and housing. Germany has provided private housing for a considerable number of Ukrainian FDPs. This factor is especially important for those who lost their homes in Ukraine. They often do not believe that their housing will be rebuilt or that the state will be able to find them decent housing if they return; it will not be easy to accumulate the necessary funds under conditions of postwar devastation. Rents in Ukraine are also quite high. For example, according to the statistics of the trading platform OLX, in 2022, the average price per square metre on the secondary market in Ukraine was 24,277 hryvnia (606 euros if one is buying).[18] According to the Stated Service of Ukraine, the average monthly rent for a one-room apartment in Ukraine in January 2023 was 5,994 hryvnias (150 euros), and the average salary in 2022 was 14,577 hryvnias (364 euros).[19] Therefore, for FDPs who have lost their homes, access to a place to live encourages them to stay in Germany:

> I had several of these impulses during the period that I've been here. I wanted to return to Ukraine. But I was restrained by the fact that I had nowhere to return to. I told myself that if I had a place to live, if I had a house in Lviv or Kyiv, I probably would have returned by now (F, 38, from an occupied region).

On the other hand, losing their housing in Germany may encourage FDPs to return to Ukraine.

For some FDPs, working or studying in Germany can be a significant deterrent to a possible return. Part of my interviewees say that they may delay returning home if they find employment and self-realisation in Germany. This factor becomes even more important given the uncertainty of employment prospects and the low level of salaries in Ukraine:

---

18 Mariia Babenko, "Kvartyra za 30 tysiach dolariv: yak zminiuiutsia tsiny na zhytlo u Kyievi ta v Ukraini" ("Apartment for 30 Thousand Dollars: How Housing Prices in Kyiv and Ukraine Are Changing"), *Fokus* (*Focus*), 15 February 2023, https://focus.ua/uk/economics/550204-kvartira-za-30-tysyach-dollarov-kak-menyayutsya-ceny-na-zhile-v-kieve-i-po-ukraine [accessed: 31.07.2024].

19 See by category reports of the State Statistics Service of Ukraine at: https://www.ukrstat.gov.ua/ [accessed: 31.07.2024].

> If I get a job and am able to provide for myself, why would I go back to Ukraine? (F, 35, from a frontline region).

In this context, educational opportunities in Germany deserve special attention. The possibility of receiving a high-quality European education and an internationally recognised diploma attracts young people. They see this, in turn, as allowing them to build a career in the West:

> A European university is the best education. And not even that is important, but the fact that you can stay here afterwards (F, 20, from a rear region).

However, some of the research participants expressed wanting to leave just their children in Germany temporarily so that they can study (e.g., obtain a diploma or improve their language skills):

> I kept thinking that we were about to return home. Then my son started school, and it turned out to be such a good opportunity for him. Because now in Ukraine, the situation in education, in my opinion, is haphazard. This is logical, because there is a war in the country. But in Germany, he studies in an integration class. He already speaks German. He has improved his English a lot. I plan to return to Ukraine if there's no major crisis. And I plan to leave my son here for another year to learn German (F, 41, from a rear region).

Based on these responses, we can conclude that another key factor in my respondents' decision-making is German-language proficiency. People who are educated in Germany have a language level that is close to native and better access to job opportunities, career development, and education. Overall, they are better adapted and, therefore, more likely to stay in Germany.

The people I interviewed occasionally, yet infrequently, mentioned a few other motives for remaining in Germany:

- A higher level of personal safety (e.g., lower crime rates, the absence of land mines, and low risks of war in Germany):

  > These are life-threatening risks because the whole of Ukraine is mined. If after the Second World War a lot of places were not cleared of mines, after this war it will take years (F, 35, from a frontline region).

  > [My] main fear is that the war in Ukraine, even if it temporarily stops, will eventually start again (F, 35, from a frontline region).

- Newly established social contacts (e.g., the emergence of a circle of friends and loved ones)
- More opportunities to travel within Europe (e.g., the proximity to France, Switzerland, and other countries)

Some respondents noted that some FDPs choose to stay in Germany because they can return to Ukraine at any time. Conversely, they fear that if they return and the events in Ukraine unfold negatively, access to Germany will be denied to them:

> You can always return to Ukraine, but to here [Germany], unfortunately, you can't (F, 35, from a frontline region).

The condition of the infrastructure in Ukrainian cities on the frontlines is another extremely important factor. With the absence of electricity, water, or heating, FPDs tend to delay their return home. Finally, the willingness to stay in Germany gradually increases as they become familiar with and adapt to the new location. Therefore, the longer the war lasts, the less likely it is that some FDPs will return to Ukraine:

> One gets used to a place. I don't know whether I'll stay here or not [because my city is occupied now], but I'm already starting to get used to the life I have here (F, 38, from an occupied region).

Motivations for Returning to Ukraine

The range of motivations for returning to Ukraine is broad, intertwining social, pragmatic, psychological, and ideological considerations. Socially, the main motivation for returning is the desire to reunite with family and re-enter a former circle of friends:

> [My] main goal is to return to my relatives, to my husband, to my family, to my parents (F, 41, from a rear region).

Often, moving to Germany is impossible or undesirable for all family members (especially men and older people who did not leave the country during the war and do not want to start life anew in another country or adapt to foreign customs):

> My husband will definitely not be able to live in Germany because he feels very secure in Ukraine. And he won't work as an ordinary worker, he'll definitely fail in this. It'll be a complete loss of social status for him (F, 38, from an occupied region).

This desire is reinforced by the fact that Ukrainians in Germany are in a kind of linguistic bubble. Because they do not know the language, their communication is limited. My respondents also claim that it is difficult for them to protect their rights without sufficient language proficiency. According to a survey conducted in Germany in November 2022, close to a quarter of the surveyed Ukrainian refugees admitted experiencing discrimination.[20] In my interviews, among many other situations, refugee women with school-age children complained that their children were bullied by children from Russian families. Without knowledge of the German language, it is difficult for them to explain the situation to teachers to defend their children:

> [There's a] very limited social circle. [My] parents do not speak any [foreign] language. When they go outside, they can't even ask where to go or how to get there. Their life is centred solely around their grandchildren in the apartment. My father doesn't like it very much, and every day he says that he wants to return to Ukraine (F, 42, from a rear region).

Respondents also report that without the help of an interpreter, it is difficult for them to get medical advice, find necessary information, and properly study. All this creates an extremely stressful and uncomfortable situation for them:

> The main problem is that it's very difficult to explain something, to achieve something, to find something if you don't know the language. In the beginning, volunteers helped. Now, there is no such help. So now, it's my problem, my personal problem (F, 38, from an occupied region).

Additionally, the vast majority of my respondents' in-person communication happens with other FDPs, or, at best, with representatives of the Ukrainian diaspora or with volunteers. Meanwhile, communication with locals is extremely limited. Consequently, FDPs do not establish friendships, do not learn about the local culture, and often misinterpret the behaviour of others:

> In general, it seems to me that Germans are very closed [off] people. If you didn't go to school or kindergarten with them, I don't know how to make friends with them. They're very emotionally closed [off]. And to arrange a

20 Viktoriya Sereda, Olena Havrysh, Jörg Fischer, and Kariem Soliman, *Aus der Ukraine nach Thüringen geflohen: Ergebnisse einer landesweiten Befragung* (*Having Fled from Ukraine to Thuringia: Results of a Nationwide Survey*), Institut für kommunale Planung und Entwicklung e.V. (IKPE) (Institute for Communal Planning and Development e.V.), report, November 2022, DOI:10.13140/RG.2.2.14478.02884 [accessed: 31.07.2024].

> meeting with them, well, it's just a joke among Ukrainians that you have to make an appointment [with them] (F, 42, from a rear region).

The poor cultural adaptation of many FPDs, in turn, reflects this. Even after nine months of living in Germany, the local culture seems incomprehensible and alien to them:

> I can't say for sure that I want to stay here, that I have everything here. No. Everything here is someone else's. At the moment, it's all foreign. When you're as old as I am, 40, and you have lived all your life in another country, with other rules, with other views, then, of course, when you come here, you will not be yourself (F, 38, from an occupied region).

It is also difficult for them to protect their rights in everyday life. However, as they learn the language, this problem gradually improves. Social ties expand, and they find shared meanings and values with the local population:

> My son says [...] that it was hard for him at first. Not because he was in a different environment, but because he missed his friends. He lost his social circle. And until he had such a solid circle of friends [again], he said that he wanted to return. And now... now he doesn't have these conversations. And he thinks that he'll study here at some point in the near future (F, 42, from a rear region).

Among the psychological factors that motivate my respondents to want to leave, the most significant is the feeling of homesickness. Often, they openly declare that Germany has done the impossible in terms of material support. Rationally, they understand that most of their needs have been met. However, it is difficult for them to cope with some of their emotions:

> My husband tells me, you're now in a beautiful city, the children drink iodised water. The air there is beautiful, enriched with iodine. What else is missing, why are you so upset? I didn't want this. Nothing makes me happy anymore. I don't want anything anymore. I'm no longer happy with the sea or the free ice cream the Germans offer us. I don't want anything. I want to go home (F, 41, from a rear region).

Some FPDs, however, want to return home for patriotic reasons. They understand that Ukraine's success is linked to whether it will be able to retain its human capacities for reconstruction:

> Ukraine needs to be rebuilt. That is, we're needed there (F, 41, from a rear region).

War and migration forced these people to take a fresh look at their lives and their country:

> I used to consider myself a patriot, but I didn't think I was that patriotic [...] You see, when it's like, "Well, yes, I love my country, but here this isn't right, and this isn't good, and in general I want to go live in Germany, marry a German, and forget [this place]". And now I live in Germany, and I want to go home, to Ukraine (F, 20, from a rear region).

Ukrainian FDPs also discovered that they had overestimated the quality of life in Germany and underestimated it in Ukraine. According to the respondents, it turned out that Ukraine has much more progressive state bureaucratic procedures (many more are digitised and conducted without special appeals to officials) and banking systems (which allow you to get a bank card instantly and online and to conduct financial transactions within one or two minutes). Similarly, they often also consider Ukraine to have better services and more affordable entertainment and facilities:

> Germany is far behind Ukraine in many ways. They don't know what an ID card is, they don't know what it means to transfer money and receive it within a minute, they don't understand many things (F, 41, from a rear region).

> It's a very bureaucratic country, everything takes a long time. There is less digitalisation than in Ukraine. I mean, everything is faster there [in Ukraine]. Here, everything is so outdated (F, 38, from an occupied region).

> It's hard for me to communicate with their government agencies. With their letters. With the waiting time. With the constant confusion (F, 42, from a rear region).

Also, according to the informants, despite its lower social standards, in Ukraine there are fewer bureaucratic restrictions and more opportunities to develop your business and generate capital:

> We have less social protection, less of all these perks from the state, but in Ukraine, it's freer to live, in the sense that in business you can do whatever you want (F, 42, from a rear region).

> Germany is very good at providing social assistance, but the taxes here are so crazy. I mean, they won't let you die, but they won't let you get rich either (F, 35, from a frontline region).

As a result, people with a high level of entrepreneurial activity and ideas for their own businesses, those who strive to achieve a higher than average social and financial status, consider Ukraine a more promising country to live in and are more likely to plan to return home.

The most important pragmatic factor that encourages Ukrainians to return home is the low prospect of maintaining a high social status in Germany (i.e., getting a white-collar job). FDPs often believe that it will take them several years to reach the required language level, so a career in their field is not available to them. Additionally, they believe that the local market currently offers only blue-collar jobs. Most Ukrainians completed higher education, and many of them had successful white-collar careers before the war and are not ready to lose their status:

> It's hard without knowledge of the language, it seems like you're unlikely to find the kind of job you'd like to find. It's more like service work, or working in a factory somewhere (F, 35, from a frontline region).

> You can't work in your field here (F, 69, from a rear region).

In only a few cases did FDPs from Ukraine explain their desire to return home as motivated by being dissatisfied with their living conditions in Germany or by limited access to social services. These instances included:

- A lack of kindergarten places for their children (and thus, an inability for mothers to learn the language and work)
- A lack of permanent housing (and instead living in camps or having difficulties finding an apartment)
- Long waiting times for medical appointments

National Identity and Intentions to Return to Ukraine

The potential return to Ukraine also correlates with the informants' sense of identity. Although this factor is rarely reflected by the research participants as an argument for migration, it is noticeable that those who actively identify themselves as Ukrainian are more likely to return home than those who do not spontaneously mention this identity. Those who plan to return to Ukraine interpret their 'Ukrainianess' as an active position: one of being actively involved in the country's life and interested in its history and politics. A willingness to help compatriots is an important civic identity that reinforces a national one. Those who have doubts about returning to Ukraine have a less pronounced civic identity. They are less interested in the history of Ukraine and politics in general and less active in volunteering.

At the same time, the interviews show that the war had a significant impact on the identity shifts of Ukrainian women in Germany. Many respondents claim that their level of patriotism and pride for their country and people has increased, as has their interest in national and international politics and history. They also admit that their readiness for civic participation and volunteering also grew. Some of the Russian-speaking respondents confess to switching (at least in public communication) to the Ukrainian language. Such a rethinking of one's identity is an important factor that motivates displaced persons to keep strong ties with Ukraine and to return after the end of the war. However, another important point that strongly correlates with the refugees' return strategy is the experience of internal displacement. Those for whom it was negative question the prospect of return because they connect it to their quality of life after the war.

Conclusions

As of the beginning of 2023, the Ukrainian FDPs who I interviewed for this research mostly plan to return to Ukraine. However, these intentions are unstable and might change depending on the duration of the war. The respondents' answers show that the longer Ukrainians stay in Germany, the more they tend to adapt to their new location and feel less inclined to return home.

The desire to stay in Germany is often based on pragmatic considerations of which country will provide a more effective life strategy and better prospects. The main motivations here are the opportunity to live in a stable and predictable environment, a higher level of safety (no mined areas, a lower risk of future hostilities), social security, housing, quality and affordable education for children and young people, access to free healthcare, and high wages. The motives for returning to Ukraine are primarily social: the desire to reunite with family and return to the usual circle of friends. Due to the lack of language skills, many of the respondents experienced an acute sense of isolation and limited opportunities: a lack of integration into local society, poor cultural adaptation, and the inability to protect their rights on their own. The ability to maintain a high social status (i.e., the former prestige they had in their community in Ukraine, a white-collar profession, or a career generally) is also essential.

At the same time, emotional motives to return to Ukraine are strong as well. These include a sense of homesickness, patriotism, and a desire to contribute to the reconstruction of their country. Other pragmatic motives, such as convenient government and banking services, inexpensive entertainment and amenities, and greater prospects for small businesses, are the least important in these considerations.

The motivation for choosing a country to live in is quite complex. The dominance of certain motives depends on the extent to which the war has affected the territories of the former residences of the Ukrainian FDPs. Those whose regions are occupied or destroyed are less likely to return. In this case, their property and usual social environment have been lost, rebuilding life from scratch appears exhausting, and the risks that come with returning to a postwar country are high. The prewar social status of Ukrainian women also matters strongly. There seems to be a belief among refugee women that Germany is more promising for young people (who can get an education there), workers in blue-collar occupations, the elderly, and people in need of social support. Conversely, Ukraine may be more promising for an economically active population, white-collar workers, and entrepreneurs (especially from areas not affected by the war). However, these factors are only relevant if there are available jobs and decent wages.

The motivation to return is not a stable construct; rather, it is in flux. If the war continues and Ukrainians manage to learn the language of their host country, find a job or study position, and adapt to their new environment, their decision to return may change. In the context of formulating state social policy to attract human resources, Ukraine and Germany should keep in mind that the availability of medical services (e.g., free healthcare or free health insurance), housing programmes,[21] and educational and employment opportunities are all important conditions that could influence the migration intentions of Ukrainian women. Germany has provided these opportunities in its migration policy. However, aspects such as employment, education (the education of children and retraining of adults), and housing require more attention. At the same time, the extent of a refugee's adaptation and their cultural and social integration also largely determine their desire to live in Germany. Therefore, compulsory German language courses are a useful instrument for helping Ukrainians settle in Germany. This, however, is not enough.

In addition to getting from zero to gradually improving language skills, Ukrainians also need cultural adaptation, inclusion in social relations, and more active interaction with and integration into their new environments. An example of this could be the involvement of Ukrainians in activities with the German population (e.g., through volunteer work, internships at enterprises, or joint events):

21 Even now, forcibly displaced Ukrainians are having trouble finding accommodation in big German cities (e.g., Munich). However, in Ukraine, the issue of compensation for lost housing has not yet been resolved.

> I would even go to some kind of job training. Once a week... I don't know, some nearby factory to do something, do some public works. At least it would help me get acquainted with the culture, to meet the locals (F, 34, from an occupied region).

An equally important aspect that my interviewees report as overlooked in Germany is the lack of sufficient counteraction to the aggressive behaviour of some immigrants from Russia towards Ukrainians:

> The son of one of our classmates from the language course is 11 or 13 years old and goes to a city school, where, in addition to Germans and other refugee children, he is also studying with Russian children. The Russian children used to disgrace the children, strip them naked in winter, throw away their clothes, trample [children] on the ground, beat them, insult them. An ordinary child would have just burst into tears, but the boy to whom this all happened, he wiped his tears away and went straight for the person who insulted him with his fists. German teachers reacted with, "Oh, God, what have you done?" They don't understand that there is a conflict between two states! They do not understand this! They don't see it! (F, 20, from a rear region).

Forced migrants also request information and counselling services from mentors for successful adaptation and integration. To a certain extent, this role could be fulfilled by a unified digital platform (with information for FDPs on where and how to prepare documents, receive social services, or find housing or work in Germany) or chatbots that could answer the most common questions and provide guidance on the proper actions in difficult situations. However, a human mentor would also be effective in the cultural adaptation of FDPs.

It is important to make refugees from Ukraine understand what Germany's strategy is for them in the future. They need to understand whether the country is interested in them staying or whether it prefers them to return to Ukraine. Germany's migration policy after the war is also an open but crucial factor in the decision-making processes of forcibly displaced Ukrainians. For example, will the country accept Ukrainian men who could not leave Ukraine earlier due to martial law restrictions but, after the war, would like to join their families? It is crucial to provide a clear understanding of the conditions under which it will be possible for Ukrainians to stay in the country as permanent residents.

At the same time, my respondents' accounts suggest that it will be important for Ukraine to prove its capability and prospects during its postwar development. The country will need active reforms, like fighting corruption, introducing health insurance, and enacting tax and judicial reform:

> I will return if we really change as a country. If the system becomes similar to the one in European countries, particularly in Germany. [Only] if there are some programmes to restore the country's economic situation, to change the insurance system, to change the taxation system. [Not] if everything remains as it was, with a lot of corrupt officials, with these crony-brother-in-law relationships. Well, there's no such thing here [in Germany]. Here, almost everyone is equal. Nobody brings you a box of chocolates and says, "Here, do this for me (F, 38, from an occupied region).

Based on my findings, I argue that Ukraine's ability to guarantee its security in the future is critical, so joining the EU and NATO (or building closer alliances with them) is a priority. Among other things, this will hopefully attract domestic and foreign investment, create new jobs and decent wages, and improve social protection. I believe that a sense of social justice will also provide an incentive for increased citizen engagement. For the Ukrainian government, launching programmes to encourage the return of FDPs, such as compensation for lost or damaged property and preferential mortgage programmes, will be important. My findings suggest that these programmes are especially relevant for young people.

Moreover, it is important to restore the infrastructure of frontline cities, as refugees tend to return to their earlier places of residence rather than to new ones. Particular attention should be paid to the reconstruction and economic recovery of small towns, as they have a high chance of becoming economically depressed. Finally, it is, in my view, important to clearly articulate the need for the return of every citizen, and the Ukrainian government should appeal to the patriotism of the forcibly displaced and emphasise their value and potential contribution to the country's recovery. Any shaming of citizens who left the country during the war should stop in Ukraine.

Bibliography

Babenko, Mariia, "Kvartyra za 30 tysiach dolariv: yak zminiuiutsia tsiny na zhytlo u Kyievi ta v Ukraini" ("Apartment for 30 Thousand Dollars: How Housing Prices in Kyiv and Ukraine Are Changing"), *Fokus (Focus)*, 15 February 2023, https://focus.ua/uk/economics/550204-kvartira-za-30-tysyach-dollarov-kak-menyayutsya-ceny-na-zhile-v-kieve-i-po-ukraine [accessed: 29.07.2024].

Bahar, Dany, Cem Özgüzel, Andreas Hauptmann, and Hillel Rapoport, "Migration and Post-Conflict Reconstruction: The Effect of Returning Refugees on Export Performance in the Former Yugoslavia", IZA Institute of Labor Economics, Discussion Paper no. 12412, 2019, https://docs.iza.org/dp12412.pdf [accessed: 29.07.2024].

Black, Richard, and Saskia Gent, "Sustainable Return in Post-conflict Contexts", *International Migration* 44/3, 2006, 5–38, https://doi.org/10.1111/j.1468-2435.2006.00370.x [accessed: 29.07.2024].

Duda-Mikulin, Eva A., "*Should I stay or should I go now?* Exploring Polish women's returns 'home'", *International Migration* 56/4, 2018, 140–153.

Krykunenko, Iryna, "Zazvychai povertaietsia tretyna. Skilky ukraintsiv zalyshatsia za kordonom ta yak blekauty zminiuiut demohrafiiu – Libanova" ("Usually a Third Returns: How Many Ukrainians Will Stay Abroad and How Blackouts Change Demographics – Libanova"), New Voice (NV), 11 December 2022, https://nv.ua/ukr/ukraine/events/skilki-ukrajinciv-zalishitsya-pislya-peremogi-naslidki-dlya-ukrajini-ekspert-ostanni-novini-50289318.html [accessed: 29.07.2024].

Liljeberg, Holger, Sindy Krambeer, and Yvonne Blunck, *Geflüchtete aus der Ukraine, Bundesministerium des Innern und für Heimat – März 2022 (Refugees from Ukraine, Federal Ministry of the Interior and for Home Affairs – March 2022 – March 2022)*, INFO GmbH Markt und Meinungsforschung (INFO GmbH Market and Opinion Research), report, 4 April 2022, https://rathaus.jena.de/sites/default/files/2022-04/BMI_Umfrage_Gefl%C3%BCchtete_aus_der_Ukraine.pdf [accessed: 29.07.2024].

Niedomysl, Thomas, and Jan Amcoff, "Why return migrants return: Survey evidence on motives for internal return migration in Sweden", *Population, Space and Place* 17/5, 2011, 656–673.

Pensiinyi fond Ukrainy (Pension Fund of Ukraine) (Facebook page), "Rozpodil pensioneriv po vydakh..." ("Distribution of pensioners by type..."), Facebook post, 15 July 2022, https://www.facebook.com/pfu.gov.ua/posts/412375920933627 [accessed: 29.07.2024].

Razumkov Centre, "Nastroi ta otsinky ukrainskykh bizhentsiv (lypen–serpen 2022r.)" ("Attitudes and assessments of Ukrainian refugees (July–August 2022)"), 30 August 2022, https://razumkov.org.ua/napriamky/sotsiologichni-doslidzhennia/nastroi-ta-otsinky-ukrainskykh-bizhentsiv-lypen-serpen-2022p [accessed: 29.07.2024].

Sereda, Viktoriya, Olena Havrysh, Jörg Fischer, and Kariem Soliman, Aus der Ukraine nach Thüringen geflohen: Ergebnisse einer landesweiten Befragung (Having Fled from Ukraine to Thuringia: Results of a Nationwide Survey), Institut für kommunale Planung und Entwicklung e.V. (IKPE) (Institute for Communal Planning and Development e.V.), report, November 2022, DOI:10.13140/RG.2.2.14478.02884 [accessed: 29.07.2024].

Sinnige, Michael, Marieke van Houte, and Arjen Leerkes, "Talking about return: Governmental caseworkers' regulative, normative and cultural-cognitive strategies during 'return conversations' with irregularised migrants", International Migration 61/1, 2023, 288–303.

Ukrainske radio (Ukrainian Radio), "'90 % bizhentsiv z Ukrainy ne povernetsia dodomu' — dyrektorka Instytutu demohrafii ta sotsdoslidzhen im. Ptukhy Ella Libanova" ("'90% of refugees from Ukraine will not return home" – Ella Libanova, Director of the Ptukha Institute for Demography and Social Studies"), 09 February 2023, http://www.nrcu.gov.ua/news.html?newsID=100692 [accessed: 29.07.2024].

UNHCR, "Lives on Hold: Intentions and Perspectives of Refugees from Ukraine # 3", 22 February 2023, https://data.unhcr.org/en/documents/details/99072 [accessed: 29.07.2024].

van Houte, Marieke, and Tine Davids, "Moving Back or Moving Forward? Return Migration, Development and Peace-Building", New Diversities 16/2, 2014, 71–87, https://newdiversities.mmg.mpg.de/wp-content/uploads/2015/01/2014_16-02_06_vanHoute.pdf [accessed: 27.07.2024].

Weldemariam, Lemlem F., Ayansina Ayanlade, Marion Borderon, and Karoline Möslinger, "Dynamics and factors influencing return migration to Sub-Saharan Africa: A systematic review", *Heliyon* 9/8, 2023, e18791.

World Population Review, "Ukraine Population 2024 (Live)", https://worldpopulationreview.com/countries/ukraine-population [accessed: 29.07.2024].

Zholkver, Nykyta, "Ukrainskie bezhentsy v Germanii. Kakie oni?" ("Ukrainian refugees in Germany: What are they like?"), *Deutsche Welle (German Wave)*, 15 December 2022, https://www.dw.com/ru/ukrainskie-bezency-v-germanii-kakie-oni/a-64107524?maca=rus-rss-ru-all-1126-rdf [accessed: 29.07.2024].

What the Telegram Channels of Ukrainian Migrants in Germany 'Talk' and 'Keep Silent' About

Taisiia Ratushna

In today's globalised and digitalised world, forced migration takes on new features as new means of communication and interaction have emerged that can significantly influence it. Online social media and social networks currently play a role in migration processes. Migrants use various digital applications to access information, resources, and news, as well as for purposes such as communication, emotional management, intercultural relations, identification, and participation, among others.[1]

Of course, such media cannot eliminate all the negative consequences of forced migration and solve migrants' problems, such as being far from their homes and habitual way of life, the separation of families, or the difficulties along the migration route. However, because social networks are primarily aimed at finding and maintaining contacts and providing interconnection between users, this makes them an important resource for migrants. They help to obtain necessary information, communicate with people in similar situations, share emotions and experiences, and, finally, just feel support or find distractions. Migrants and representatives of the host country can also use them to establish social ties. To some extent, this eases adaptation to the new environment and helps with integration.

Migrants are often imagined as rootless or uprooted people, as they have been forced to break away from their homeland, communities, and family and can quickly or gradually lose contact with them. However, modern communication technologies have fundamentally changed this situation. The internet blurs geographical distance and gives a sense of presence in the 'here and now' – a sense of community and unity. Therefore, digital social media and social networks are appearing more frequently

1 Koen Leurs and Madhuri Prabhakar, "Doing Digital Migration Studies: Methodological Considerations for an Emerging Research Focus", in: Ricard Zapata-Barrero and Evren Yalaz (eds.), *Qualitative Research in European Migration Studies*, Cham, Switzerland: Springer Open, 2018, 247–66, https://doi.org/10.1007/978-3-319-76861-8_14.

in migration studies.[2] These studies help to understand how forced migrants build their social networks and see their 'inner world'. However, there is not yet a single explanatory theoretical model to describe the interaction of forced migrants on social networks. In this context, it seems necessary to study different cases and expand the empirical base for further theoretical development. One such case is the use of social media by forced migrants from Ukraine in host countries, particularly in Germany, which, according to official data, has received more than a million Ukrainians.

Since the beginning of Russia's full-scale war against Ukraine on 24 February 2022, the flow of forced migrants and asylum seekers from Ukraine to EU countries has increased rapidly. According to the United Nations High Commissioner for Refugees (UNHCR), in December 2022, the recorded number of forced migrants from Ukraine across Europe amounted to 7,896,825 people, and 4,885,650 refugees registered for temporary protection or in similar national protection schemes in Europe.[3] In early March, almost 50,000 people crossed the border with the EU every day; these figures gradually decreased, but the migration flow has not stopped. Poland received the largest number of forced migrants at the beginning of the invasion. A large number of Ukrainians also moved to Germany, the Czech Republic, Romania, Hungary, Slovakia, and other countries.[4]

Since 24 February 2022, mobile communication and the internet have provided forced migrants from Ukraine with the opportunity to keep abreast of events and receive up-to-date information about what is happening in their country of origin and abroad through a smartphone. Mobile operators in Ukraine and the EU have created special initiatives to support Ukrainians (e.g., free SIM cards, free calls and SMS to Ukraine, roaming benefits, and other offers for subscribers). This allowed many forced migrants to stay in touch with their families, quickly find information in their countries of arrival, and share it through groups on social networks.

---

2 Elaine McGregor and Melissa Siegel, "Social Media and Migration Research", *UNU-MERIT Working Papers*, December 2013, https://www.merit.unu.edu/publications/wppdf/2013/wp2013-068.pdf [accessed: 31.07.2024]; Lee Komito, "Social Media and Migration: Virtual Community 2.0", *Journal of the American Society for Information Science and Technology* 62/6, 2011, 1075–1086, https://doi.org/10.1002/asi.21517; and Cornelius J. P. (Nelus) Niemandt, "A network society, social media, migration and mission", *Missionalia* 41/1, 2013, https://doi.org/10.7832/41-1-19.

3 United Nations High Commissioner for Refugees (UNHCR) Operational Data Portal, "Ukraine Refugee Situation", https://data.unhcr.org/en/situations/ukraine [accessed: 31.07.2024].

4 Liliana Filipchuk, Natalia Lomonosova, Olena Syrbu, and Yulia Kabanets, "Vymushena mihratsiia i viina v Ukraini (24 liutoho — 24 bereznia 2022)" ("Forced Migration and War in Ukraine (24 February–24 March 2022)"), *Cedos*, 29 March 2022, https://cedos.org.ua/researches/vymushena-migracziya-i-vijna-v-ukrayini-24-lyutogo-24-bereznya-2022/ [accessed: 31.07.2024].

Social networks became a tool for self-organisation, as they created information 'bridges' between those who needed help and those who were willing and able to provide it. The most popular of them (e.g., Facebook, Telegram, X (formerly Twitter), etc.) have groups, chats, chatbots, and channels for Ukrainians, where they can find the necessary information, useful links, current announcements for support, and volunteer and charitable initiatives. They can also ask for help or advice, post requests, and find like-minded people, among other things.

This research paper studies the role played by the internet and, in particular, social media groups for forced migrants from Ukraine in Germany and explores the 'inner world' of such communities and the peculiarities of their communication. The study considers Telegram channels created in Germany to help forced migrants from Ukraine after 24 February 2022. According to a Kyiv International Institute of Sociology study conducted in the summer of 2022, this social network has become one of the leaders in the information space of Ukraine.[5] This is due to two main reasons. First, Telegram is easy to navigate, use, and administer. Second, this messenger platform has been present in Ukraine for a long time as a channel of personal communication with family members and friends. Its popularity increased during the COVID-19 pandemic when it was used to establish remote work in many institutions and organisations in both the private and public sectors. Additionally, trust in this platform also increased because Ukrainian government institutions and state organisations, after the beginning of the full-scale war, started using Telegram channels and creating chatbots to notify the population.

This study considers specifically two Telegram channels created in Germany to help forced migrants from Ukraine: "Berlin helps Ukrainians"[6] (with 23,000 followers and 450–900 messages per day) and "Ukraine in Tübingen Reutlingen"[7] (with 1,960 followers and 35–100 messages per day). The channels are both information-rich cases. The first channel represents a large urban setting, and the second represents a smaller provincial town. Additionally, the former is in the north of Germany, and the latter is in the south. In the first stage of this study, I thematically analysed

---

5 Civil Network OPORA, *Democracy, Citizen Rights and Freedoms and Mediaconsumption in Times of War: July 2022*, report, 17 August 2022, https://www.oporaua.org/en/viyna/24256-pid-chas-povnomasshtabnoyi-viini-v-ukrayini-zris-popit-na-silnu-ruku-shvidki-ta-strukturovani-novini-i-reguliuvannia-mediaprostoru-opituvannia-24256 [accessed: 31.07.2024].

6 The users' direct speech, used for subsequent analysis, was extracted from an openly accessible channel within the Telegram messenger platform: https://t.me/berlinhelpsukrainians. The number of channel participants and the daily frequency of messages were recorded as of August 2022.

7 The users' direct speech, used for subsequent analysis, was extracted from an openly accessible channel within the Telegram messenger platform: https://t.me/ReutlingenTubingen. The number of channel participants and the daily frequency of messages were recorded as of August 2022.

the channels: I selected messages two days a month for six months (March–August 2022) and categorised them into thematic blocks. In the second stage, I added further categories to the thematic blocks based on keywords.

Russian is the main language of these Telegram channels, with a much lower frequency of Ukrainian and rare posts in German or English. The predominance of the Russian language is due to many of the forced migrants coming from the Russian-speaking regions of Ukraine (east and south), which suffered the most from the Russian invasion. German and English were used mostly in March and April, usually in offers of assistance and accommodation. Linguistic borrowing from German is also present in messages through transliterations into Russian or Ukrainian, mainly in reference to institutions, authorities, or documents.[8] Such borrowing suggests that users cannot find immediate equivalents in Ukrainian or Russian for these words.

Through an analysis of the two channels, I identified the ten key topics used.[9] Below, I sketch out my initial impressions of these topics and their change over time to provide insight into the 'inner worlds' of communication on migration and integration processes as conducted over these Telegram channels.

Communication Topics

1. Arrival and Transportation

In March, most messages in this category were about transport and opportunities to get to Germany from Ukraine and Poland, with many questions about how to get to different German cities and about volunteer aid with transportation. For example, a user wrote: "Is anyone maybe driving tomorrow from Shehynia [the border crossing point between Ukraine and Poland] to Berlin? Morning–afternoon. 3 people need to be taken…". There were also messages about the volunteers in the arrival centres and the addresses of the centres themselves. In general, the messages are emotional, including many exclamation marks, emojis, and requests for help: "what to do", "where

8 For example, words such as *Jobcenter* (джобцентр, *dzhobtsentr*), *Sozialamt* (соціаламт, *sotsialamt*), *Termin* (термін, *termin*), *Fiktion* (фікшион, *fikshyon*), *Anmeldung* (анмельдунг, *anmeldunh*), *Kindergeld* (кіндергельд, *kinderheld*), and others were often used.

9 Specifically, the topics are the following: arrival and transportation; housing, humanitarian aid, and household items; registration, documents, and legal issues; social assistance, work, and integration courses; childcare, education, and children's leisure; medical and psychological assistance; banking services and online shopping; leisure, sports, and beauty; communication, activities, and local events; and appointments, postal services, correspondences, parcels, and digital services.

to look", and "who can help me". These messages show confusion and some loss of orientation in the new situation.

During April and May, most of the messages were concerned with travel within Germany and public transport. In July and August, meanwhile, users discussed public transport issues (especially at the end of August, before the expiration of the 9-Euro-Ticket).

2. Housing, Humanitarian Aid, and Household Items

In March and April, many users sought housing in Germany. They exchanged information about accommodation with German families and contacts of volunteers who could help find temporary housing. In early March, users reported accommodation for one night or a brief period in shelters. In May and June, users wrote about the need to leave the temporary housing provided by volunteers and find permanent accommodation. Some of the reports also contained complaints about prolonged stays in refugee camps and the inability to find their own residences. In the Berlin channel, there were many messages about the *Wohnberechtigungsschein* (WBS)[10] and how to obtain it. For example, one user wrote: "Hello, has anyone applied for a WBS already? Could you let me know how it generally went?"

In May, the number of requests for assistance in finding accommodation increased, likely because some German families who sheltered Ukrainians at the beginning of the war, as well as the forced migrants themselves, expected that such accommodation would be temporary and were not prepared for long-term cohabitation. Users shared links to housing search sites and reminders that housing in Germany is difficult to find, even for locals.

Meanwhile, in March and April, users also requested humanitarian aid, food, clothing, and information about volunteer groups and aid centres. From May to August, as Ukrainians found housing, they inquired about buying furniture and household appliances. Some phrases during this time indicate that users were happy to have found their own private space: "we found our apartment", "we managed to find our housing", and "we already moved into our apartment".

3. Registration, Documents, and Legal Issues

Obtaining a temporary protection status and registration, as well as filling out documents, were the most prevalent concerns in this category on both Telegram channels from March to May. There were a large number of related questions and answers. The Berlin channel even developed certain standard answers and links to sources on

10 A permit for subsidised housing in Germany.

these topics and posted them in pinned messages. Some of the inquiries were directed to such pinned messages. Users, however, still wrote the requests. The rapid growth of followers of the channels explains this situation: there was an addition of 'newcomers' who did not want to reread many earlier messages.

In late May and June, a new wave of messages about filling in documents flooded both Telegram channels due to the registration of a considerable number of Ukrainian forced migrants at the *Jobcenter*.[11] In the summer, both Telegram channels also received many requests from users to clarify how to apply for 21 days of vacation, to provide information on whether they were eligible, and to explain other specifics.

4. Social Assistance, Work, and Integration Courses

A large number of discussions in both Telegram channels were related to the issues of receiving social assistance, unemployment allowances, and child benefits. In the messages, users mainly shared their own experience with the necessary documents, the schedules and features of the relevant institutions, and their correspondences with them. They asked about the amounts of financial aid and the timing of the payments. The channels also posted links to official announcements on the websites of the relevant institutions and translations of essential information.

Many questions appeared around work permits, especially in the Berlin Telegram channel, as in early March it was not clear what status forced migrants from Ukraine would receive. By mid-April, users often asked whether Ukrainians had free access to the labour market. In both channels, but especially in the Berlin one, Ukrainians showed readiness to look for work immediately after arriving in Germany. Users even discussed whether this was the right approach. For example, some participants (who had emigrated to Germany earlier) pointed out that without language skills and the recognition of diplomas, they could find only unskilled, low-wage jobs, so they "should not rush", but first focus on language learning and a confirmation of their qualifications.

Part-time employment (i.e., *minijobs*) was also an important topic. The participants asked whether they would lose their social allowances if they had a *minijob*. On this topic, users suggested that if social allowances are reduced to less than 100 euros, it may not be worth taking such work. On the other hand, users who already

11 Ukrainians who registered in Germany after 24 February could receive financial assistance on the basis of the law on support for asylum seekers. The situation changed on 1 June 2022. Since then, Ukrainians of working age are only allowed to receive general support from the *Jobcenter* (employment office), which gives an unemployment allowance (*Arbeitslosengeld II* or ALG II for short, also known as *Hartz IV*).

had experience in *minijobs* indicated that their main motivation was not financial, but the opportunity to integrate faster.

Language courses also came up in both channels,[12] especially in May and June. Participants searched for and shared the locations of language courses and recommended those with smaller queues. Course schedules and the problem of childcare for young children were important topics. Many mothers of children aged three to six worried that they could not attend the courses because they did not have a kindergarten spot and would, for this reason, lose their social allowance.

5. Childcare, Education, and Children's Leisure

In March and April, users inquired about accommodation with children, acquiring children's clothes and food, and locating medical treatment. According to the users' posts, the difficult journey and the seasonal increase in respiratory infections caused many children to become sick. From April on, users increasingly asked about childcare and/or spots in kindergartens and schools. Mostly, they shared their own experiences and discussed difficulties. For many, the biggest problem was a lack of kindergarten spots.

The situation with schools appeared better, as users mostly asked how to find schools with integration classes and what vaccinations children need for registration. Some parents shared that their children were in their final grades and wanted to complete the school year online to receive Ukrainian educational documents.

Lastly, many users inquired about leisure activities for children. Most forced migrants from Ukraine are women with children, and this question was highly prevalent. This topic, however, was also somewhat controversial. Some users in the Berlin group were outraged by questions about where to take children for free entertainment (e.g., zoos, swimming pools, museums, other attractions, etc.). Specifically, they found entertainment irresponsible, while people in Ukraine suffered. One user wrote, "Are you looking for protection or entertainment here, how can one even think about this when children back home are sitting in basements being bombed…". Other users pointed out that those children who have already reached a safe place should have leisure activities as part of their normal lives.

6. Medical and Psychological Assistance

In March and April, users inquired about medical care, asking where to go and how to find a doctor, make an appointment, and arrange insurance, among other things.

12 Attending language integration courses is an important prerequisite for receiving financial aid from the *Jobcenter*.

Often, they requested a Russian-speaking doctor, as many users did not know German and, simultaneously, many German doctors did not know Ukrainian. (It is easier to find a doctor who speaks Russian, as most people from the former Eastern Bloc studied it.)

In May and June, the users who had experience with the German medical system posted about the differences between the Ukrainian and German systems. Supporters of the German system stressed the quality of service, the modern equipment, and the positive attitudes of medical workers towards the patient. Opponents listed the long waiting times for an appointment, the high cost of the services, particularly dental work, that are not covered by health insurance, and the inability to choose the types of diagnostics, among other things. For example, one user wrote: "...back home [in Ukraine], you come to a hospital, [to] a clinic with a problem... It doesn't matter what kind of problem... Immediately, they take a general blood test, then the diagnosis... Here [in Germany], you have to be dying to get even a blood test...". Most of the critical posts seemed to stem from a lack of experience with the German healthcare system, and other users provided answers.

In spring, there were also offers for free psychological support and aid. Moreover, these included both online assistance from psychologists in Ukraine and in-person help from specialists in Germany, as well as forced migrants from Ukraine who were psychologists.

7. Banking Services and Online Shopping

Many posts in the channels, both in spring and summer, were related to banking services, as most forced migrants from Ukraine needed to open German bank accounts to receive social allowances. The users mainly discussed the conditions of different banks and the advantages of some over others. Users also asked about online banking and money transfers to and from Ukraine. Many messages in spring had requests and offers to privately exchange Ukrainian currency and US dollars for euros. An agreement between the National Bank of Ukraine and the Deutsche Bundesbank only happened in late May. Following this, in June, users asked how the exchange process worked.

When discussing banking services, users often compared them with Ukrainian ones. In their opinion, banking services in Ukraine are more modern, digitalised, and faster.

8. Leisure, Sports, and Beauty

The groups received the topics of leisure, beauty, and sports with mixed feelings. For example, when one participant in the Berlin group asked about free classes in a fitness club for Ukrainians, a dispute began about whether it is appropriate for asylum seekers to ask for such things. Some users responded that these services are not necessary and therefore should not be free. Others, meanwhile, argued that this is a health concern and an opportunity to distract oneself from the war and adapt to the new environment.

Participants in the Berlin group responded negatively to requests for hairdressers and other beauty industry workers. They argued that such issues are not relevant "when there is a war in your country". However, such responses were only typical for the first months of the war (from March to May), while from June onwards, finding hairdressers no longer caused negative reactions. In the group "Ukraine in Tübingen Reutlingen", meanwhile, this confrontation did not occur; on the contrary, users shared the contacts of hairdressers from Ukraine or recommended the hairdresser they visited.

In these situations, forced migrants, as opposed to representatives of the host society, imposed stringent expectations on themselves. They denied themselves and others in the same situation so-called 'unnecessary' things, services, expenses, and forms of leisure, especially at the initial stage of adapting to new conditions.

9. Communication, Activities, and Local Events

In April and May, the Berlin channel shared events organised specifically for forced migrants from Ukraine, as well as explanations about the peculiarities of local life. For example, users posted about the traditions around celebrating Easter and other holidays or the particularities of various institutions on holidays and weekends. However, such posts decreased over time.

The group "Ukraine in Tübingen Reutlingen" also shared updates about local life and meeting opportunities for Ukrainians. There were frequent invitations to a local club for forced migrants from Ukraine in Reutlingen called Dialog. Beyond communication and various events, the club helped with documents and translation, among other things. This channel, more often than the Berlin channel, published about local events, fairs, and holidays, indicated specific locations, and featured invitations in German.

10. Appointments, Postal Services, Correspondences, Parcels, and Digital Services

Both groups discussed the concept of the *Termin* in March and April. Seemingly, Ukrainians found making appointments and meetings with institutions and organisations several days or weeks in advance somewhat strange. In Ukraine, this practice is not widespread, and most institutions and organisations provide services to visitors without an appointment.

German post offices and correspondence practices were an important topic for forced migrants from Ukraine. The channels found the large amount of paper letters from most institutions and organisations unusual. This also applied to sending documents (e.g., bank cards, pin codes, health insurance cards, etc.) by mail. Largely, this can be explained by the fact that Ukraine underwent noticeable digitalisation in the last three years, reducing paperwork and transitioning to the provision of most public services through digital apps (e.g., Diia).

Lastly, there were also frequent requests for carriers shipping or delivering goods from Ukraine and back. This was not only for transporting personal belongings but also to send humanitarian aid to Ukraine.

What Do the Telegram Channels of Ukrainian Migrants in Germany 'Keep Silent' About?

Certain topics were 'not welcome' in the channels. If these topics came up, the moderators[13] warned that they could ban these users or exclude them from the groups. Specifically, these topics include language, religion, ethnicity, and politics.

Users brought up language more than once because most of the messages were in Russian. However, any disputes about whether to use Russian or switch to Ukrainian ended with a moderator's warning about the inadmissibility of language conflicts and the possible blocking of participants involved in the dispute. "Ukraine in Tübingen Reutlingen" asked users to join a specially created channel, "Fludilka", for such conversations. Meanwhile, moderators also prohibited discussing religion and ethnicity. Any intolerant statements, as seen by the moderators or other participants, received warnings and explanations that Germany is a tolerant country, everyone has the same rights, and everyone should be equally respected. These rules did not always apply to Russians, and derogatory neologisms such as 'rusnya', 'ruscists', and 'orcs' were often used for them.

The moderators discouraged discussing political issues, but there were some reports about rallies and other events supporting Ukraine, references to current world events, and updates on victories by the Armed Forces of Ukraine. Users, meanwhile, almost never mention gender. Although most Ukrainian forced migrants are women with children, there are men in both Telegram channels, and they are active participants. Occasionally during conflicts, users asked these men what they were doing abroad, why they were not defending the country, or for which reasons they left

13 The initiators and moderators of the channels were mostly immigrants from the former Soviet Union and Ukrainian immigrants who had moved to Germany from 2014 onwards. They had experience with migration and could give valuable advice to newcomers, so creating the channels was a form of solidarity and support.

Ukraine. This was generally used to insult them. Such posts, however, were an exception.

Moderators, and sometimes participants themselves, did not react well to posts that compared and complained. Complaints were not taboo, but users told their authors that they were ungrateful and disrespectful to the host country and that they needed to adapt to new living conditions. Sometimes they said so directly: "adapt or go back", "no one is keeping you here", or "we have to live here like others". However, such complaints did not decrease in number.

For example, Ukrainians often complained about the German bureaucracy and the long waits for solutions to what they considered "very simple issues". Answers such as "you just have to be patient", "wait", and "take your time" were not very reassuring. Having only temporary protection, Ukrainian forced migrants cannot plan their lives in the long term, and many of them have not chosen a further strategy: to stay or return to Ukraine. Nonetheless, 'temporariness versus permanence' was a topic that the channel participants avoided. Most users did not say that they wanted to stay in Germany forever, although sometimes in messages about finding housing, there were mentions of having nowhere to return to (e.g., their house was destroyed or located in a warzone or occupied territory). However, according to research, a considerable number of Ukrainian forced migrants are not considering a long-term stay in Germany. According to studies, 7[14] to 26 percent[15] do not plan to return to Ukraine,[16] but the rest see their situation as migrants as temporary and would like to go home. For this reason, time is a valuable resource for them. They want to solve their problems in the 'here and now' without postponing them into the future.

As with dissatisfaction with bureaucratic and other waiting times, a comparable situation was true in the service sector. Ukrainians are accustomed to 24/7 shops and the possibility to get numerous services even on weekends and holidays, so it was difficult for them to get used to the conditions in Germany. Therefore, they were

---

14 Razumkov Tsentr (Razumkov Centre), *Nastroi ta otsinky ukrainskykh bizhentsiv (Lypen–Serpen 2022p.) (Attitudes and Assessments of Ukrainian Refugees (July–August 2022))*, report, 30 August 2022, https://razumkov.org.ua/napriamky/sotsiologichni-doslidzhennia/nastroi-ta-otsinky-ukrainskykh-bizhentsiv-lypen-serpen-2022p [accessed: 31.07.2024].

15 Institut für Arbeitsmarkt- und Berufsforschung, Bundesinstitut für Bevölkerungsforschung, Bundesamt für Migration und Flüchtlinge, and Das Sozio-oekonomische Panel, "Refugees from Ukraine in Germany: Fleeing the War and Starting Life in a New Country Summary: Background and Results", 2023, https://www.bib.bund.de/EN/Research/Migration/Projects/pdf/2023-01-02-Ukraine-Summary-ENG.pdf?__blob=publicationFile&v=5 [accessed: 31.07.2024].

16 However, this data is relative, as the situation may change according to individual life circumstances. Moreover, the decision to return to their homeland is a sensitive topic for migrants, which increases the possibility of obtaining socially acceptable answers. Lastly, due to different sampling methods and wording of questions in the questionnaires, we cannot compare the results of these studies.

very nostalgic and said that they could now see how much they used to have. This led to them over appreciating the Ukrainian level of development in many areas (but especially in the service sector).

The posts show that some Ukrainian forced migrants do not identify themselves as refugees. They sometimes wrote about this directly: "I'm not a refugee, I just have temporary protection" or "...Paragraph 24 is not refugee status; it's different". They also still considered Ukraine their home: "at my home in Ukraine", "I need to go back home [meaning to Ukraine]", and "if I go home to Ukraine for a while, will I be accepted back in Germany?" In addition, when describing their life in Germany, Ukrainian forced migrants often used phrases that denoted their identity not as migrants but as Ukrainians (e.g., "here for us Ukrainians", "here we are accepted as Ukrainians...", etc.). Even the names of the Telegram channels emphasise belonging to Ukraine and the users being Ukrainians, especially the name of the channel "Ukraine in Tübingen, Reutlingen", where the first word, "Ukraine", is written in Cyrillic (Україна), while the rest of the words are in German and the Latin alphabet. Accordingly, this suggests that a part of the 'motherland' has moved to Germany. Thus, their experiences in and memories of their homeland continued to influence how forced migrants perceived their place in the new environment.

Conclusions

The Telegram channels of Ukrainian forced migrants in Germany demonstrate an interesting example of self-organisation and mutual assistance. Nevertheless, the initiative to create such groups, rules, and processes of virtual interaction and communication between participants largely depends on the moderators. These channels accumulate useful information for forced migrants that can help solve some of their problems and record and share their experience of interacting with an unfamiliar environment. However, the large number of messages per day and the uniformity of questions and answers make these channels a kind of 'time sink'. To find relevant information, it is often necessary to read many 'surplus' messages that create 'information noise'.

How much these groups help to integrate their users into the new society is also debatable. In the groups, users communicate 'among themselves' and not with representatives of the host society. Additionally, such groups have a 'core' of participants, but they are overall unstable and in flux, suggesting little cohesion. Thus, the Telegram channels of Ukrainian forced migrants are an auxiliary tool for adaptation and orientation in new conditions, allowing users to feel 'less lonely', to see what problems others have and how they solve them, and to ask for advice or get help.

Social media platforms offer forced migrants a digital arena for social interaction and the exchange of experiences, thereby fostering a sense of belonging and community, which can play a significant role in maintaining their identity.

Bibliography

Civil Network OPORA, *Democracy, Citizen Rights and Freedoms and Mediaconsumption in Times of War: July 2022*, report, 17 August 2022, https://www.oporaua.org/en/viyna/24256-pid-chas-povnomasshtabnoyi-viini-v-ukrayini-zris-popit-na-silnu-ruku-shvidki-ta-strukturovani-novini-i-reguliuvannia-mediaprostoru-opituvannia-24256 [accessed: 29.07.2024].

Filipchuk, Liliana, Natalia Lomonosova, Olena Syrbu, and Yulia Kabanets, "Vymushena mihratsiia i viina v Ukraini (24 liutoho — 24 bereznia 2022)" ("Forced Migration and War in Ukraine (24 February–24 March 2022)"), *Cedos*, 29 March 2022, https://cedos.org.ua/researches/vymushena-migracziya-i-vijna-v-ukrayini-24-lyutogo-24-bereznya-2022/ [accessed: 27.07.2024].

Institut für Arbeitsmarkt- und Berufsforschung, Bundesinstitut für Bevölkerungsforschung, Bundesamt für Migration und Flüchtlinge, and Das Sozio-oekonomische Panel, "Refugees from Ukraine in Germany: Fleeing the War and Starting Life in a New Country Summary: Background and Results", 2023, https://www.bib.bund.de/EN/Research/Migration/Projects/pdf/2023-01-02-Ukraine-Summary-ENG.pdf?__blob=publicationFile&v=5 [accessed: 29.07.2024].

Komito, Lee, "Social Media and Migration: Virtual Community 2.0", *Journal of the American Society for Information Science and Technology* 62/6, 2011, 1075–1086, https://doi.org/10.1002/asi.21517.

Leurs, Koen, and Madhuri Prabhakar, "Doing Digital Migration Studies: Methodological Considerations for an Emerging Research Focus", in: Ricard Zapata-Barrero and Evren Yalaz (eds.), *Qualitative Research in European Migration Studies*, Cham, Switzerland: Springer Open, 2018, 247–266, https://doi.org/10.1007/978-3-319-76861-8_14.

McGregor, Elaine, and Melissa Siegel, "Social Media and Migration Research", *UNU-MERIT Working Papers*, December 2013, https://www.merit.unu.edu/publications/wppdf/2013/wp2013-068.pdf [accessed: 29.07.2024].

Niemandt, Cornelius J. P. (Nelus), "A network society, social media, migration and mission", *Missionalia* 41/1, 2013, https://doi.org/10.7832/41-1-19.

Razumkov Tsentr (Razumkov Centre), *Nastroi ta otsinky ukrainskykh bizhentsiv (Lypen–Serpen 2022p.)* (*Attitudes and Assessments of Ukrainian Refugees (July–August 2022)*), report, 30 August 2022, https://razumkov.org.ua/napriamky/sotsiologichni-doslidzhennia/nastroi-ta-otsinky-ukrainskykh-bizhentsiv-lypen-serpen-2022p [accessed: 29.07.2024].

United Nations High Commissioner for Refugees (UNHCR) Operational Data Portal, "Ukraine Refugee Situation", https://data.unhcr.org/en/situations/ukraine [accessed: 29.07.2024].

Minority Experiences

The Identity Migration of Religious Actors during the War in Ukraine (since 2014)

Denys Brylov and Tetiana Kalenychenko

From the beginning of the independent history of Ukraine, following the dissolution of the Soviet Union in 1991, Ukrainian society experienced a religious renaissance, which also began to define identity. Identities did not always remain purely religious but could also have a cultural and traditional character, such as the self-definition of a Ukrainian as a Christian, mainly Orthodox, despite the country's multireligious and multicultural map. The formation and clash of religious identities in Ukrainian society closely relate to the political context of a dramatic period of history, which started in the late 1980s and early 1990s. The revival of the Ukrainian Greek Catholic Church (UGCC) and the split in Ukrainian Orthodoxy into the Ukrainian Orthodox Church (in canonical unity with the Moscow Patriarchate, UOC-MP), the Ukrainian Orthodox Church Kyiv Patriarchate (UOC-KP) in 1992, and the Ukrainian Autocephalous Orthodox Church (UAOC, before 2018) determined the dynamics of the formation of religious identity in Ukraine for many years as the dominant religious groups.

Having reached a certain level of stability by the end of the 1990s, this process sharply escalated in connection with the Russian occupation of Crimea and the armed conflict and Russian aggression in Eastern and Southern Ukraine since 2014. The key event in this period was the unification of two Orthodox churches – the UOC-KP and the Ukrainian Autocephalous Orthodox Church (UAOC) – at the Unification Council of 2018 into the Orthodox Church of Ukraine (OCU) and its receipt of autocephaly from the Ecumenical Patriarchate in January 2019.[1] The 'church issue' became rapidly politicised against the background of the rise of patriotic sentiment in Ukrainian society.

The full-scale Russian invasion on 24 February 2022 further exacerbated the problem of the transformation of religious identities. Currently, dramatic changes

1 For a brief history of the creation of the OCU, see their official website: Pravoslavna Tserkva Ukrainy (Orthodox Church of Ukraine), "Pravoslavna Tserkva Ukrainy: shliakh kriz viky" ("Orthodox Church of Ukraine: The Path through the Centuries"), https://www.pomisna.info/uk/tserkva/istoriya/ [accessed: 14.04.2024].

are taking place among the believers and the clergy of the UOC-MP, which, seemingly, is experiencing the most serious crisis of its entire existence.[2] Questions about the connection between religious identity and political positions also arose before representatives of Protestant denominations, closely associated with their Russian coreligionists. In our study, we focus precisely on these transformations of religious identity occurring under the conditions of the Russo–Ukrainian War. We chose the crisis of the UOC-MP and the questions of the Protestant denominations as the two case studies of this article since both the believers of the UOC-MP and the Protestants are religious groups that have close ties with Russian believers and are also spread over all regions of Ukraine, both those under the control of the Ukrainian government and those that are occupied.

As a theoretical approach, we use the model proposed by Rawi Abdelal, Yoshiko M. Herrera, Alastair Iain Johnston, and Rose McDermott, who define 'collective identity' as a social category that varies along two dimensions: 'content' and 'contestation'. Content describes the meaning of a collective identity. The content of social identities may take the form of four, non-mutually exclusive types:

- Constitutive norms refer to the formal and informal rules that define group membership
- Social purposes refer to the goals that the members of a group share
- Relational comparisons refer to defining an identity group by what it is not, that is, the way it views other identity groups, especially when such views about others are a defining part of the first group's identity
- Cognitive models refer to the worldviews or understandings of political and material conditions and interests that a particular identity shapes

Contestation, meanwhile, refers to the degree of agreement within a group over the content of the shared identity.[3]

This article is based on an analysis of audio and video materials available on the internet and social media (as open-access content), press articles, media messages, and anonymous in-depth interviews with senior UOC-MP and OCU clergy. Data gathered during field research on the religious situation in Ukraine conducted from 2021 to 2023 complement these sources.

---

2 Denys Brylov and Tetiana Kalenychenko, "Ukrainian Religious Actors and Organizations after Russia's Invasion: The Struggle for Peace", *Berkley Center*, 27 September 2022, https://berkleycenter.georgetown.edu/events/ukrainian-religious-actors-and-organizations-after-russia-s-invasion [accessed: 31.07.2024].

3 Rawi Abdelal, Yoshiko M. Herrera, Alastair Iain Johnston, and Rose McDermott, "Identity as a Variable", *Perspectives on Politics* 4/4, 2006, 695–711, here 696.

The Religious Situation in Ukraine on the Eve of the Russo-Ukrainian War

Historically, Ukraine has been a polyconfessional country, in which, already in the era of Kyivan Rus (10th–13th centuries), powerful religious traditions such as pagan beliefs, Christianity, Judaism, and Islam coexisted. Today, more than 100 faith communities are represented in Ukraine, which includes 37,049 religious organisations, 93 religious centres, and 301 religious administrations.[4]

According to official statistics, Ukraine is home to the third largest Orthodox population in the world, following Russia and Greece. Orthodoxy in Ukraine, however, is not a monolith. Perhaps the most important religious dynamic at play across the country is the fragmentation of the Orthodox Church into two (or more) competing factions: the UOC-MP and the OCU. A 2023 study reported that 61 percent of Ukrainian respondents identified as Orthodox, with six percent aligning with the UOC-MP and 42 percent with the OCU. At the same time, it is important to note that a sharp decline in the number of those who profess to be faithful to the UOC-MP occurred after the start of Russia's full-scale war (from 13 percent in 2021 to six percent in 2023).[5]

The level of religiosity among Ukrainians has an expressively regional character. According to the sociological data of the Razumkov Centre, a Kyiv-based think tank, in 2018, these regional specificities still played an important role: up to 91 percent of residents of western regions and up to 59 percent of residents of southern regions considered themselves believers.

The connection between religious and national identities differs regarding the region and denomination of a person. Survey data from the Razumkov Centre show that since 2000, 54 percent of Western Ukraine inhabitants were sure that religion should be nationally oriented (21 percent of respondents opposed it), while merely 12 percent of respondents from Eastern Ukraine supported this idea (61 percent opposed it). A majority of UGCC believers also support this idea (66 percent), while OCU members are less unified (48 percent agree), and UOC members mainly oppose it (with only 26 percent supporting). Between 2000 and 2020, the group of supporters of national-religious identity did not grow significantly, while the number

4 See the report by the State Service of Ukraine for Ethnic Policy and Freedom of Conscience on the network of religious organisations as of 1 January 2021 on their website: Derzhavna sluzhba Ukrainy z etnopolityky ta svobody sovisti (DESS) (State Service of Ukraine for Ethnic Policy and Freedom of Conscience), *Zvit pro merezhu relihiinykh orhanizatsii ctanom na 1 sichnia 2021 roku* (*Report on the Network of Religious Organisations as of 1 January 2021*), report, 2022, https://dess.gov.ua/religion/ [accessed: 31.07.2024].

5 Razumkov Centre, *Ukrainske suspilstvo, derzhava i tserkva pid chas viiny. Tserkovno-relihiina hesytuatsiia v Ukraini-2023* (*Ukrainian Society, the State, and the Church in Wartime: The Situation of the Church and Religion in Ukraine in 2023*), report, 2023, 6.

of those who opposed the idea decreased (from 53 percent in 2000 to 39 percent in 2020).[6]

After the beginning of the full-scale Russian invasion, the issue of the national character of the Church led to increased division between Ukrainian Orthodox believers. Currently, the majority of OCU faithful (70 percent) believe that the Church should be nationally oriented, while a relative majority of the UOC-MP (48 percent) opposes the national orientation of the Church. Regional preferences have also changed: in the western and central regions, supporters of the national orientation of the Church make up more than half of respondents (72 percent and 57 percent, respectively); in the eastern regions, supporters are a relative majority (48 percent); and in the southern regions, a relative majority (41.5 percent) are opponents of the national orientation of the Church.[7]

At the same time, other survey data revealed that religious identity per se is much less important to Ukrainian citizens than civic or regional identity. When answering the question "Which social community do you identify yourself with in the first place?", 68 percent of respondents answered "with citizens of Ukraine", 16 percent answered "with residents of my city ([or] village)", 8 percent answered "with residents of my region", 3 percent answered "with people of the same faith as me", and only 1 percent answered "with people of the same Church to which I belong". Compared to people belonging to other churches and denominations, the faithful of the UOC-MP are most likely to identify themselves with people of the same faith as them (6 percent). For comparison, the share of such faithful among the OCU and the UGCC believers is 2 percent.[8]

In May 2017, the Pew Research Center published new data on the religious landscape of Central and Eastern Europe, including Ukraine. The survey shows that 51 percent of Ukrainians believe that being Orthodox means also being a true national representative of your country.[9] Ukrainians define their religious identity through national, cultural, and family traditions (46 percent), peculiar properties of faith (12 percent), both aforementioned elements (12 percent), and other factors (seven percent). Meanwhile, 12 percent explain being Catholic or Orthodox due to a primarily national-cultural factor. Another strong position is religious exclusivism. Generally,

6 Razumkov Centre, *Osoblyvosti relihiynoho i tserkovno-relihiynoho samovyznachennya hromadyan Ukrayiny: tendentsiyi 2000–2020 rr.* (*Specifics of the Religious and Church Self-Determination of the Citizens of Ukraine: Trends 2000–2020*), report, 2020, 7.

7 Razumkov Centre, *Ukrainske suspilstvo*, 7.

8 Razumkov Centre, *Osoblyvosti relihiynoho i tserkovno-relihiynoho samovyznachennia hromadyan Ukrainy: tendentsiyi 2000–2021 rr.* (*Specifics of the Religious and Church Self-Determination of the Citizens of Ukraine: Trends 2000–2021*], report, 2021, 6 [authors' trans.].

9 Pew Research Center, *Religious Belief and National Belonging in Central and Eastern Europe*, report, 2017, http://www.pewforum.org/2017/05/10/religious-belief-and-national-belongin g-in-central-and-eastern-europe/ [accessed: 31.07.2024].

this is declining, but 33 percent of respondents believe that only their faith paves the way to heaven. Lastly, more religious people are prone to be proud of their nationality; 48 percent of Ukrainians who are very proud of their nationality say that religion is important.

The Ukrainian Orthodox Church in Crisis

Today, the UOC-MP has found itself in perhaps the most serious crisis in its entire existence. Since 2014, the UOC-MP has been viewed by some Ukrainians as an agent of the Russian Orthodox Church (ROC) and Russia more broadly. A vivid manifestation of this was a renewal of the transfers of individual religious communities from one jurisdiction to another (in this case from the UOC-MP to the OCU). As Viktor Yelensky, head of the State Service of Ukraine for Ethnic Policy and Freedom of Conscience (DESS), said during a speech at the national TV marathon, "After receiving the *tomos*, more than 1,600 communities joined the Orthodox Church of Ukraine. This year [2023], 400 communities have joined. As of 24 February 2022, 1,000 communities have joined the Orthodox Church of Ukraine".[10] These transfers would sometimes take radical forms, resulting in the forceful seizures of church buildings. According to the UOC-MP Chancellor, Metropolitan Anthony (Pakanych), the number of raider seizures of UOC-MP parishes increased significantly in 2022. While in 2021, only seven such cases were recorded, in 2022 there were 129 cases. According to him, local governments made 74 decisions to ban the activities of religious organisations associated with the UOC-MP.[11]

Pressure from the independent OCU from the outside only exacerbated this internal crisis, with OCU leader Metropolitan Epiphany actively urging UOC-MP priests to move to the OCU. Cases of the forcible transfer of parishes have become more frequent, primarily in the western regions of Ukraine, sometimes accompanied by the abduction of UOC-MP priests.[12] On the other hand, there were repeated

10 TSN, "Novyny za 26 hrudnia 2023 roku | Novyny Ukrainy" ("News for 26 December 2023 | News from Ukraine"), YouTube video, 11:55:00, here 5:58:45–5:59:15, 26 December 2023, https://www.youtube.com/watch?v=6WG24A9K4RA [accessed: 31.07.2024] [authors' trans.].

11 Ukrainska Pravoslavna Tserkva (Ukrainian Orthodox Church), *Zvit Keruiuchoho spravamy Ukrainskoi Pravoslavnoi Tserkvy za 2022 rik* (*Report of the Chancellor of the Ukrainian Orthodox Church for 2022*), report, 2022, https://news.church.ua/2022/12/24/zvit-keruyuchogo-spravami-ukrajinskoji-pravoslavnoji-cerkvi-za-2022-rik/ [accessed: 31.07.2024].

12 Ukrainska Pravoslavna Tserkva (Ukrainian Orthodox Church), "Pid dulom avtomativ vidibraly khram, vykraly monakhiv" ("A Church Was Taken at Gunpoint, Monks Were Kidnapped], 2022, https://news.church.ua/2022/03/10/pid-dulom-avtomativ-vidibrali-xram-vikrali-monaxiv-na-verxovini-rozpravlyayutsya-z-viruyuchimi-ivano-frankivskoji-jeparxiji-upc/ [accessed: 31.07.2024].

cases of anti-Ukrainian propaganda, collaboration with the Russian military, and signs of treason on the part of some ministers of the UOC-MP. However, not all of them receive a continuation in the legal field in the form of criminal proceedings or, even more so, court cases. By his Decree No. 898/2022 from 28 December 2022, President Volodymyr Zelenskyy suspended the citizenship of a number of priests of the UOC-MP, with Ukrainian media sharing the list of 13 clergymen.[13] According to official data, in 2022, more than 40 counterintelligence and security measures were conducted in the church environment of the UOC-MP, and 61 criminal proceedings were instituted against 61 clergymen. In total, the courts have already issued seven verdicts against individual clerics. Two of them were used in exchange for Ukrainian prisoners of war. Sanctions were introduced against 17 officials of the UOC-MP, and almost 250 clerics of the ROC were banned from entering Ukraine. Also, 19 clergymen of the UOC-MP and two just initiated[14] who were citizens of Russia had their Ukrainian citizenship terminated.[15]

The Russian full-scale invasion gave the UOC-MP leadership and believers a choice: are they part of the ROC (in the canonical sense) or a Ukrainian and pro-Ukrainian church on an independent basis? As such, the head of the UOC-MP, Metropolitan Onuphryy (Berezovsky), was forced to take a clear position on the war and made an early appeal to believers in which he acknowledged Russian aggression and called for unity to protect the sovereignty and integrity of Ukraine.

Moreover, the decree of 27 May 2022 of the Unified Council, the highest UOC-MP leading structure, directly "considered issues of Church life that arose as a result of the military aggression of the Russian Federation in Ukraine".[16] In its decisions, the Council condemned the war as a violation of the commandment "thou shalt not kill" and also expressed their disagreement with the position of the Patriarch Kirill of Moscow and All Rus regarding the war in Ukraine.

However, at the beginning of the invasion, Metropolitan Onuphryy was not ready for a direct conflict with the ROC and its leader Patriarch Kirill, as our re-

---

13 Sonia Koshkina, "Prezydent Ukrainy pryzupynyv hromadianstvo 13 sviashchennykiv UPTs-MP, – dzherela" ("President of Ukraine Suspends Citizenship of 13 Priests of the UOC-MP – Sources], *Livyi Bereg* (*Left Bank*), 28 December 2023, https://lb.ua/society/2023/01/07/541773_prezident_ukraini_prizupiniv.html [accessed: 31.07.2024].

14 Initiated means to go through the procedure of becoming a priest.

15 Security Service of Ukraine, "SBU povidomyla pro pidozru mytropolytu UPTs(MP) Pavlu (video)" ("The SSU Serves Notice of Suspicion to Metropolitan Pavlo of the UOC(MP) (video)"), 2023, https://ssu.gov.ua/novyny/sbu-povidomyla-pro-pidozru-mytropolytu-upts-mp-pavlu-video [accessed: 31.07.2024].

16 Ukrainska Pravoslavna Tserkva (Ukrainian Orthodox Church), "Resolutions of the Council of the Ukrainian Orthodox Church of May 27, 2022", 28 May 2022, https://news.church.ua/2022/05/28/resolutions-council-ukrainian-orthodox-church-may-27-2022/?lang=en [accessed: 31.07.2024].

spondents mentioned. This has led to a serious crisis within the UOC-MP, with clergy reacting in three different ways: 1) some withdrew from the UOC-MP and transitioned to the OCU; 2) some maintained a pro-Moscow position, including direct support for Russia; and 3) some refused to commemorate Patriarch Kirill and called for the leadership of the UOC-MP to break the canonical connection with the ROC.

Some UOC-MP priests, shocked by the hard-line and pro-invasion position of the ROC and the deaths of some clergymen at the hands of the Russian military, seemed inclined to join the independent OCU. For example, Priest and Rector of the Holy Resurrection New Athos Monastery in Lviv, Father Job (Olshansky), who transferred with his community to the OCU in March 2022, stated, "Our delay makes us Russian collaborators. I want you and me to be just Orthodox Christians who praise God, love their state and pray for it [...] to pray for the Ukrainian Army, for the Ukrainian state and Ukrainian authorities".[17]

The main reason for this group's transition to the OCU was their unwillingness to associate themselves with the ROC, the 'murderer church', and become 'Russian collaborators', as they are called in discussions on social media. That is, here, civic identity prevailed. At the same time, unlike the communities that transferred before the start of the war, and especially in the western regions, where religious identity was largely determined by regional and ethnic characteristics, following the start of the Russo–Ukrainian War, local UOC-MP priests had a different understanding of the relationship between religious and national identity. For example, priest Andrii Ponomarenko from the village of Aleksandrovka in the Dnipropetrovsk Oblast, who joined the OCU in April 2022, stated:

> People often talk about the national idea; what it should be. The people of Ukraine are showing this idea today – personal initiative and self-organisation, decentralisation, and local responsibility add to this transparency, and we will get both a national idea and an example of a canonical Church.[18]

---

17 Dukhovna velych Lvova (The Ducal Majesty of Lviv), "Ihumen monastyrya UPTS (MP) u Lvovi pereyshov z hromadoyu do PTsU" ("Abbot of the UOC (MP) Monastery in Lviv Joins the OCU with Community"), 20 March 2022, https://velychlviv.com/igumen-monastyrya-upts-mp-u-lvovi-perejshov-z-gromadoyu-do-ptsu/ [accessed: 31.07.2024] [authors' trans.].

18 Taras Antoshevskyy, "'Potribna nova arkhitektura tserkovnoho zhyttya', — o. Andriy Ponomarenko pro sviy vykhid z UPTs-MP ta poshuk tserkovnoyi yednosti" ("'We Need a New Architecture of Church Life', Fr. Andriy Ponomarenko on His Withdrawal from the UOC-MP and the Search for Church Unity"), *Relihiyno-informatsiyna sluzhba Ukrayiny (Religious Information Service of Ukraine)*, 03 May 2022, https://risu.ua/potribna-nova-arhitektura-cerkovnogo-zhittya--o-andrij-ponomarenko-pro-svij-vihid-z-upc-mp-ta-poshuk-cerkovnoyi-yednosti_n128894 [accessed: 31.07.2024] [authors' trans.].

But in the context of the total number of communities in the UOC-MP at present, this is a very small group. From February to September 2022, less than 600 parishes transferred from the UOC-MP to the OCU, and just over a thousand since the receiving of the *tomos*. Of the communities that moved from the UOC-MP to the OCU since the beginning of the Russian invasion, those in the Khmelnytskyy, Kyiv, and Volyn Oblasts are in the lead.

The second group, which includes some of the high-ranking priests of the UOC-MP (primarily those based in Kyiv), retains a pro-Moscow orientation but has not publicly declared this. This group also includes the priests of the UOC-MP who are convicted of collaboration. Not only those from the patriotic segments of Ukrainian society but also some from within the UOC-MP itself reacted negatively to the behaviour of these priests.

At the same time, an important part of the religious identity of this category of priests (and believers) is the idea that Ukrainians and Russians are fraternal peoples connected by a common origin and faith. Antoshevsky argues: "The last drop was information about the participation of the UOC-MP clerics (priests and monks) in the pseudo-referendums on 'joining Russia' in the temporarily occupied territories and their calls for the 'unification of the brotherly people in a single country'".[19] In public spaces and on social media, as well as in expert opinions, this group is called a supporter of the concept of the 'Russian world'.[20] However, this concept is not a message of the church of the ROC, despite accusations by Ukrainian priests and activists against Patriarch Kirill of his adherence to this 'heretical teaching'. Rather, this concept was born in intellectual circles in the Russian Federation in the 1990s and was influenced by Petr Schedrovitskyy and Efim Ostrovskyy.[21]

The third group, which includes a significant number of priests, is not ready to move to the independent OCU but also does not want to remain part of the ROC. This last group is made up of those who have advocated for the convening of the Holy Council of Bishops of the UOC-MP to withdraw from their canonical subordination to the ROC.

According to Father Nikolai Danylevych, the Deputy Chairman of the Foreign Relations Department of the UOC-MP, who voiced the official position of the church,

19 Ibid.

20 *Portal Polsko-Ukrainski* (*Polish–Ukrainian Portal*), "UPTs MP – ostannii marker 'ruskoho mira' v Ukraini" – ukrainskyi relihiieznavets Andrii Yurash" ("The UOC-MP is the Last Marker of the 'Russian World' in Ukraine – Ukrainian Religious Scholar Andriy Yurash], 2023, http://www.polukr.net/uk/blog/2023/05/upcmp-ostannyj-marker-ruskovo-mira/ [accessed: 31.07.2024].

21 Denys Brylov and Tetiana Kalenychenko, "Religion and Nationalism in Post-Soviet Space: Between State, Society and Nation", in: Jayeel Cornelio, François Gauthier, Tuomas Martikainen, and Linda Woodhead (eds.), *Routledge International Handbook of Religion in Global Society*, New York: Routledge, 2021, 399–409, here 401.

> the statements and actions of Patriarch Kirill and his assessment of the Russo–Ukrainian War, the attack on Ukraine, and the open invasion of Ukraine are, to put it mildly, strange, or rather, absolutely inadequate. And his statements aroused fierce opposition. Misunderstanding, rejection, and resistance. Many priests and even bishops stopped commemorating Patriarch Kirill.[22]

On March 1, the clergy of the Sumy Diocese, supported by their bishop, Metropolitan Evlogii, refused to commemorate Kirill. Within a short time – just a few days – the number of dioceses that refused to commemorate Patriarch Kirill exceeded 15 (out of more than 50 dioceses in the UOC-MP). Even in those dioceses where there were neither collective appeals nor corresponding decisions by local bishops, some priests stopped commemorating the Patriarch individually.[23] The position of the parishioners of the UOC-MP largely explains this behaviour. As a sociological survey conducted by Sociological Group "Rating" on 8– 9 March 2022 shows, 52 percent of the parishioners of the UOC-MP supported "the idea of breaking ties with the Russian Orthodox Church" (and only 13 percent refused).[24]

Among the members of this group is Priest Andrii Pinchuk from the Dnipropetrovsk Oblast, who sent an open letter to the court of the Pentarchy (the five heads of the oldest Orthodox Churches) with a request to condemn Patriarch Kirill (to whom the UOC-MP is formally subordinate) for propagandising the 'Russian World' doctrine for years, which became the ideological basis for Russia's full-scale war against Ukraine. His appeal collected more than 400 signatures of UOC-MP priests from all over Ukraine.[25]

---

22 Krym.Realii (Crimea.Realities), "V Ukraine 15 yeparkhiy UPTs Moskovskogo patriarkhata perestali pominat patriarkha RPTS Kirilla – Danilevich" ("In Ukraine, 15 Dioceses of the UOC-MP Have Stopped Memorialising Patriarch Kirill – Danilevych"), 2022, https://ru.krymr.com/a/news-ukraina-15-eparhiy-upc-mp/31754601.html [accessed: 31.07.2024] [authors' trans.].

23 Andrii Fert, "'Nasha pastva ne zhelaet bolshe slyshat imya patriarkha Kirilla'" ("Our Flock Does Not Want to Hear the Name of Patriarch Kirill Anymore"), *OpenDemocracy*, 11 March 2022, https://www.opendemocracy.net/ru/ukraina-tserkov-voina-protest-protiv-patriarcha-fert-/ [accessed: 31.07.2024].

24 Sotsiolohichna hrupa "Reitynh" (Sociological Group "Rating") "Otsinka sytuatsii v Ukraini (8–9 bereznia 2022)" ("Evaluating situation in Ukraine (8–9 March 2022)"), 10 March 2022, https://ratinggroup.ua/research/ukraine/ocenka_situacii_v_ukraine_8-9_marta_2022.html [accessed: 31.07.2024] [authors' trans.].

25 Tetiana Kalenychenko and Denys Brylov, "'Whoever saves one life saves the world entire': Ukrainian religious denominations during the war", *Bulletin de l'Observatoire international du religieux (Bulletin of the International Observatory on Religion)*, 37, 2022, https://obsreligion.cnrs.fr/bulletin/whoever-saves-one-life-saves-the-world-entire-ukrainian-religious-denominations-during-the-war-english-version/ [accessed: 31.07.2024].

In mid-May of 2022, the Holy Synod of the UOC-MP decided to hold a meeting of bishops, clergy, monks, and laity on 27 May to discuss the challenges faced by the UOC-MP. At the meeting itself, the head of the UOC-MP, Metropolitan Onuphryy, referring to the reaction of believers, proposed to consider the issue of the autocephaly of the UOC-MP. Because only the Council of the Ukrainian Orthodox Church can decide on changing the status of the church, on May 27, Metropolitan Onuphryy initiated and successively held a meeting of the Holy Synod of the UOC-MP, the Council of Bishops of the UOC-MP, and the Council of the UOC-MP with the participation of laity, monastic members, and clergy. As a result, 95 percent of the participants of the Council of the UOC-MP voted to change the status of the Church.[26]

In its final document, the Council of the UOC-MP condemned the war in the first paragraphs, appealed to the authorities of Ukraine and Russia to continue searching for ways to stop the bloodshed, expressed disagreement with the position of Patriarch Kirill of Moscow regarding the war in Ukraine, and approved additions and amendments to the Statute on the Management of the UOC-MP, "which testify to the full independence and autonomy of the Ukrainian Orthodox Church".[27]

Despite the enormous pressure exerted by Ukrainian society, the parishioners of the UOC-MP, and the authorities of Ukraine, the leadership of the UOC-MP was not ready to violate the canonical rules (as it understands them) in favour of a patriotic pro-state position. Moreover, as one of the high-ranking priests of the UOC-MP noted, the motives of Metropolitan Onuphryy, who became the driving force behind the holding of the Council of the UOC-MP and the move to separate from the ROC, were not sociopolitical factors but religious: "For the Primate, the main thing was not that Russia attacked Ukraine. The Church thinks in centuries. Borders may change, [but] Orthodoxy remains. The main thing was that Vladyka [Onuphryy] decided that Kirill had deviated from Christian values".[28]

For a significant part of the parishioners and clergy of the UOC-MP, religious identity turned out to be more important than regional-ethnic or even national identity – even for those who are not supporters of the idea of the 'Russian World'. The results of in-depth interviews done with completely pro-Ukrainian parishioners and priests of the UOC-MP in the Volyn Oblast in Western Ukraine in the first months of the Russian invasion (when Ukrainian society actively discussed the possibility of a legislative ban on the activities of the UOC-MP) back up this view on identity. In these interviews, the interviewees expressed that in the event of a ban on the

26 #Dialog.TUT (#Dialogue.HERE), "Kak prokhodil Sobor UPTs i kakiye prinyaty resheniya" ("How the Council of the UOC Took Place and What Decisions Were Made"), 27 May 2022, https://www.dialogtut.org/kak-prohodil-sobor-upcz-i-kakie-prinyaty-resheniya/ [accessed: 31.07.2024].

27 Ukrainska Pravoslavna Tserkva, "Resolutions of the Council".

28 Interview with the authors, Kyiv, Ukraine, August 2022.

UOC-MP, parishioners and priests of the UOC-MP could go to the Orthodox Autocephalous Church of Poland (which operated on the territory of Volhyn until 1944). At the same time, they did not even consider the possibility of moving to the OCU due to canonical (essentially religious) reasons.

In their rationale for the non-canonicity of the OCU as a newly created autocephalous church, supporters of the UOC-MP largely reproduce (often without indicating the source) the explanation of the Biblical and Theological Commission of the ROC "[o]n the invalidity of the consecrations of Ukrainian schismatics and the non-canonicity of the 'Orthodox Church of Ukraine'".[29] This document emphasises, first of all, "the unilateral actions of the Patriarchate of Constantinople in Ukraine, culminating in the signing in January 2019 of the so-called *tomos* of autocephaly against the will of the episcopate, clergy, monastics, and laity of the Ukrainian Orthodox Church".[30] The main problem, according to the document, is that the Synod of the Patriarchate of Constantinople accepted into Eucharistic communion persons "without legal ordination" without the consent of the ROC. In this case, this means that a significant part of the consecrations of the episcopate of the OCU was received from Metropolitan Filaret (Denysenko) of Kyiv and All Ukraine, who was excommunicated (anathematised) by the ROC in 1997. The Biblical and Theological Commission of the ROC insists that only the ROC itself can cancel the anathematisation of Metropolitan Filaret since they are the ones who anathematised him[31]. Meanwhile, the Patriarchate of Constantinople argues that, as the 'mother church' of the UOC-MP (and through it, the ROC), they can lift the anathema of the churches descended from them and that this was not taken into account.

Thus, we can say that for a significant part of the laity and clergy of the UOC-MP, religious identity is no less significant than national identity, and sometimes, it is even more significant. Following the model of Abdelal, Herrera, Johnston, and McDermott the most important concept here is 'canonicity'. In the context of relational comparisons, it is placed in opposition to the 'non-canonicity' of the OCU. Metropolitan Klyment has commented on the impossibility of the UOC-MP joining the OCU in response to the Russian invasion and, rather, its necessity to stay in the ROC: "The option to go to the OCU is unrealistic. We will lose the most important

29 Tatyana Chaika, "ROC publishes theological clarification on non-canonicity of OCU", *Union of Orthodox Journalists*, 09 October 2019, https://spzh.news/en/news/65558-rpc-opublikovala-bogoslovskoje-razyasnenije-o-nekanonichnosti-pcu [accessed: 31.07.2024].

30 Ibid.

31 Metr. Antony, "Znyaty anafemu z Filareta mozhe til'ky RPTS" ("Only the ROC can lift anathema from Filaret"), https://ukranews.com/ua/news/586240-znyaty-anafemu-z-filareta-mozhe-tilky-rpc-mytropolit-antoniy [accessed 31.07.2024].

thing – the canonical truth of our church. And this is exactly what our congregation is looking for and what it finds in our church".[32]

Metropolitan Anthony, often considered the main lobbyist for the interests of the ROC within the UOC-MP, spoke even more sharply in his address to believers on the 1035th anniversary of the baptism of Russia by Prince Volodymyr. He declared:

> Our disagreement with "OCU" is mainly on the canonical plane. First of all, there is a question regarding the legality of the ordinations of the "clergy" of this organisation, which does not allow us to have any common prayer or Eucharistic communication both with it and with those churches that, despite church rules, have decided to recognise its "sacraments" as allegedly legal. And no dialogue with this structure will change this essence: the apostolic succession cannot be filled with anything except repentance and canonical ordination. And if the Ukrainian Orthodox Church started such communication, it would actually cease to exist as a canonical church.[33]

To understand the identity of believers, an important indicator is the relationship between a declared identity and the recognition of oneself as a member of a certain parish. One can call oneself a believer of a particular denomination without practicing one's religious beliefs. According to Sergei Bortnik, this is a common problem in Ukraine: with a stated total of 67.8 percent of people who call themselves 'believers', only 20.9 percent call themselves members of a certain parish. While a weak connection to a parish is expected from those identifying as "just Orthodox" (5 percent are parish members) and "just Christians" (7.1 percent are parish members), it is a significant problem for the leading denominations. The same source shows that "In the UOC-MP this figure is slightly higher: 36.1 percent are those who identify as members of a parish as opposed to 58.2 percent who do not consider themselves members of a specific parish. In the OCU, the numbers are only 25.8 percent of those who identify as members of a parish as opposed to 70.9 percent who are not."[34] This

---

32 Sviatoslav Khomenko, Vitalii Chervonenko, and Anastasiia Lotarieva, "'Byttia vyznachaie svidomist'. Chy pozbavylasia UPTs vid Moskovskoho patriarkhatu" ("'Being Defines Consciousness': Did the Ukrainian Orthodox Church Get Rid of the Moscow Patriarchate?"), *BBC Ukraine*, 30 May 2022, https://www.bbc.com/ukrainian/features-61625756 [accessed: 31.07.2024] [authors' trans.].

33 Metropolitan Antony (Pakanych), "Bozhe, zberezhy Tserkvu Tvoiu v istyni i yednosti!" ("God, Save Your Church in Truth and Unity!"), *Pravoslavnaia Zhyzn* (*Orthodox Life*), 28 July 2023, https://pravlife.org/uk/content/mytr-antoniy-pakanych-bozhe-zberezhy-cerkvu-tvoyu-v-istyni-i-yednosti [accessed: 31.07.2024] [authors' trans.].

34 Sergei Bortnyk, "Overestimated declared identity of the OCU faithful and unexpected tolerance of the UOC(MP) faithful: analysis of the Razumkov Center's data", *CF "Academic initiative"*, 2022, https://www.academic-initiative.org.ua/en/2022/02/16/analysis_of_razumkov/ [accessed: 31.07.2024].

means that only a quarter of the declared members of the OCU have the opportunity to or regularly attend the church services of their denomination.

Other data also testify in favour of greater involvement of parishioners of the UOC-MP in church life when compared to the OCU. Specifically, they are much more likely to attend church services: 18.9 percent of UOC-MP parishioners attend "once a week", as opposed to 10.1 percent of OCU parishioners, and 6.5 percent of UOC-MP parishioners attend "more often than once a week", as opposed to 3.4 percent of those of the OCU. Similarly, when asked the question "Have you attended church service last Sunday?" 38.5 percent of UOC-MP parishioners answered "yes" as compared to 25.1 percent from the OCU.[35]

When considering the OCU, instead of religious identity, it is more appropriate to talk about the phenomenon of 'civil religion'. On this matter, we agree with Reverend Cyril Hovorun, who states that in order to understand social and political processes in contemporary states that associate themselves with the Eastern Christian tradition (in particular Ukraine), the concept of 'civil religion' is a useful hermeneutic key. In his view, we can observe the collision of two types of civil religion in Ukraine: the Russian imperial version that is propagated as the 'Russian world' (represented partly by the UOC-MP) and a Balkan-style nationalistic one, in which a set of beliefs, symbols, and rituals constitute a quasi-religion (a superficial and not religiously based movement) of the nation (represented by the UOC-KP and later the OCU).[36] A good illustration of this "quasi-religion of the nation" is the meme "atheist of the Kyiv Patriarchate", which was coined by President Petro Poroshenko's advisor Yuri Biryukov and spread widely among the intelligentsia that positions itself as patriotic.[37] At the same time, there is no need to talk about any transformation of the identity of the followers of the OCU after the start of the Russian invasion in February 2022, since from the very beginning their identity had a more pronounced national character. Moreover, the OCU could become a special civil-religious centre of attraction (a basis for cultural identity but not real or regular religious practice) for those pro-Ukrainian citizens who are not active in their beliefs and religious affiliations. At the same time, this could be detrimental for the OCU as a religious institution – the 'Church of Christ' – that aims for confessional affiliation.

---

35 Razumkov Centre, *Osoblyvosti relihiynoho i tserkovno-relihiynoho samovyznachennia hromadyan Ukrainy: tendentsiyi 2000–2021*, 50 [authors' trans.].

36 Reverend Cyril (Hovorun), "Pravoslavnaya grazhdanskaya religiya" ("Orthodox Civil Religion"), *Relihiia v Ukraini* (*Religion in Ukraine*), 18 May 2015, https://www.religion.in.ua/main/bogoslovya/29171-pravoslavnaya-grazhdanskaya-religiya.html [accessed: 31.07.2024].

37 Denys Brylov, Tetiana Kalenychenko, and Andrii Kryshtal, *The Religious Factor in Conflict: Research on the Peacebuilding Potential of Religious Communities in Ukraine*, PAX, report, 2021, 25–26.

Division in the Ukrainian and Russian Protestant Worlds

Protestantism began to spread in Ukraine following the collapse of the Soviet Union. Congregations of every major Protestant tradition exist in contemporary Ukraine, though their numbers are still comparatively small. A 2021 study by the Razumkov Centre noted that 1.5 percent of the population identifies as Protestant.[38] However, state religious statistics show that the number of Protestant religious communities is about 30 percent of all Christian communities in Ukraine (in total, there are 10,774 Protestant communities, 5,280 Catholic communities, and 19,860 Orthodox communities).[39] However, we can challenge the state statistics for several reasons and suggest that they did not investigate the activities of existing parishes.

Catherine Wanner, who has for many years researched Protestants in post-Soviet countries, claims that Ukrainian Protestants are less oriented towards national identity than Orthodox followers because they do not belong to a 'traditional' church. "The Orthodox Church", she writes, "including Uniate 'relatives' in her midst [meaning the UGCC], considers Orthodoxy an attribute of Ukrainian nationality, that is, a Ukrainian, by definition, is Orthodox".[40] Evangelicals, on the contrary, are less inclined to think ethno-nationally. In interviews she conducted in Ukraine in 2000–2002, she notes that when faced with open questions, most Evangelicals preferred the categories 'Christian' or 'believers' to nationality (or other competing categories).[41] In the post-Soviet space, Ukraine is the country where the evangelical movement has achieved the greatest success. For example, in Ukraine, there are more than twice as many evangelical missionaries as in Russia, but the population is three times smaller.[42]

The full-scale invasion deepened earlier misunderstandings among Ukrainian and Russian Protestants[43] once they were facing issues of life and death on one side

38 Razumkov Centre, *Osoblyvosti relihiynoho i tserkovno-relihiynoho samovyznachennia hromayian Ukrainy: tendentsiyi 2000–2021*, 39.

39 DESS, *Zvit pro merezhu relihiinykh*.

40 Ibid.

41 Catherine Wanner, "Explaining the Appeal of Evangelicalism in Ukraine", in: Dominique Arel and Blair A. Ruble (eds.), *Rebounding Identities: The Politics of Identity in Russia and Ukraine*, Washington, D.C.: Woodrow Wilson Center Press, 2006, 243–272, here 243.

42 Dominique Arel, "Introduction: Theorizing the Politics of Cultural Identities in Russia and Ukraine", in: Dominique Arel and Blair A. Ruble (eds.), *Rebounding Identities: The Politics of Identity in Russia and Ukraine*, Washington, D.C.: Woodrow Wilson Center Press, 2006, 1–30, here 22.

43 Tetiana Mukhomorova, "When a Brother Doesn't Hear His Brother: Post-Maidan Problems in Relations between Ukrainian and Russian Protestants", *Religious Information Service of Ukraine*, 25 March 2014, https://risu.ua/en/when-a-brother-doesn-t-hear-his-brother-post-maidan-problems-in-relations-between-ukrainian-and-russian-protestants_n68021 [accessed: 31.07.2024].

and limitations from the state on the other. Unlike Ukrainian evangelicals,[44] Russian pastors either remained quiet in public, spoke in support of Putin, or remained neutral with "we are for peace" calls, personally urging Ukrainian pastors to remain silent about suffering and death on their side. One of the respondents from among Protestant theologians says, "I received numerous messages where I was asked not to write, to remain silent, which can be summed up very simply: please, if you die, do it silently".[45] At the official level, as early as 25 February[46] statements and appeals from the Russian Union of Christian Churches of the Evangelical Faith called for peace in "this fratricidal war, where the reasons are not important" and later responded with the same general phrases to concerns about partial mobilisation in Russia.[47] At the level of action, they were the first to enter Mariupol after the Russian military and declared that they were building their church there,[48] regardless of the destroyed churches and the statements of Ukrainian pastors from Mariupol.

Given the earlier worldview differences and the new divisions, Russian and Ukrainian Protestants will be unable to resume not only cooperation but even communication in the near future, which will affect their understanding of the relationship between power and religious organisations. However, we should pay special attention to the relationships between Protestants in Ukraine, who faced both theological and logistical crises and challenges. Some of the pastors will remain as refugees abroad, and the main seminaries are jointly thinking about what the focus of the training of future ministers should be. A recent attempt was a gathering

44 Rada Yevanhelskykh Protestantskykh Tserkov Ukrainy (Council of Evangelical Protestant Churches of Ukraine), "Spilna zaiava SIeA, YeIeA ta RIePTsU z pryvodu richnytsi rosiiskoho vtorhnennia" ("Joint Statement of the CEA, the EEA, and the REPCU on the Anniversary of the Russian Invasion"), 2023, https://repcu.org/2023/02/27/1615/ [accessed: 31.07.2024].

45 Interview with the authors, April 2022.

46 Rossiyskiy obyedinennyy Soyuz khristian very evangelskoy (pyatidesyatnikov) (ROSKhVE) (Russian United Union of Christians of Evangelical Faith (Pentecostals)), "Zayavleniye episkopa Sergeya Ryakhovskogo (ot imeni Dukhovnogo soveta ROSKhVE) po situatsii na Ukraine" ("Statement by Bishop Sergey Ryakhovsky (on Behalf of the Spiritual Council of the ROSKhVE) on the Situation in Ukraine"), 2022, https://www.cef.ru/documents/docitem/article/1640677 [accessed: 31.07.2024].

47 Rossiyskiy obyedinennyy Soyuz khristian very evangelskoy (pyatidesyatnikov) (ROSKhVE) (Russian United Union of Christians of Evangelical Faith (Pentecostals)), "Zayavleniye Dukhovnogo soveta ROSKhVE v svyazi s obyavleniyem chastichnoy mobilizatsii" ("Statement of the Spiritual Council of the ROSKhVE in Connection with the Announcement of Partial Mobilisation"), 2022, https://www.cef.ru/documents/docitem/article/1674593 [accessed: 31.07.2024].

48 Rossiyskiy obyedinennyy Soyuz khristian very evangelskoy (pyatidesyatnikov) (ROSKhVE) (Russian United Union of Christians of Evangelical Faith (Pentecostals)), "Rossiyskiye missionery sozdali tserkov v Mariupole" ("Russian Missionaries Set Up a Church in Mariupol"), 2022, https://www.cef.ru/infoblock/news/read/article/1669783 [accessed: 31.07.2024].

of pastors to discuss "Theology after Bucha",[49] where they began to look for answers to these questions. The process of the transformation of their identity remains unequivocal; within this, the civil rather than the national component comes to the fore.

Conclusions

The Russian invasion of Ukraine in February 2022 led to significant changes in public consciousness and major transformations in the identity of Ukrainians, as well as in the religious field. This especially affected supporters of the UOC-MP, which for many years was part of the ROC. The personal position of the head of the ROC, Patriarch Kirill, who justifies the invasion and appeals to the imagined community of the Russian and Ukrainian peoples within the framework of the nationalist concept of the 'Russian World', alienated many priests and laity of the UOC-MP from the ROC. At the same time, the more pronounced religious identity of the parishioners of the UOC-MP and public pressure on the church led to dramatic processes that brought the UOC-MP closer to a situation of internal schism. As our study shows, for a significant part of the laity and clergy of the UOC-MP, religious identity is no less significant than national, and sometimes even more so. Applying the methodological approach of Abdelal, Herrera, Johnston, and McDermott, we see that the relational type of identity is key among believers in the UOC-MP. The believers of the UOC-MP define their identity through the definition of what it is not: namely, it is not non-canonical, which they consider their opponents in the OCU (and earlier the UOC-KP and the UAOC) to be. Crises in the UOC-MP in 2022 and 2023 showed that even for the most pro-Ukrainian priests and laity, it is extremely difficult to overcome the perception of the OCU as a 'non-canonical' and 'graceless' structure and, accordingly, the invalidity of church sacraments in this church.

At the same time, interestingly enough, the clergy of the UOC-MP found a way out of the impossibility of maintaining close relations with the ROC, pressure from Ukrainian society and the authorities, and the request of their own flock to preserve 'canonicity' in their appeal to early 'pre-Nicaea'[50] Christianity, when bishops enjoyed wide autonomy in decision-making. Thus, point 7 of the Decree of the Council of the UOC-MP of 27 May 2022 says:

---

49 Eastern European Institute of Theology, "Ofitsiine komiunike, pryiniate uchasnykamy konsultatsii 'Bohoslovska osvita pislia Buchi'" ("Official Communique Adopted by the Participants of the Consultation 'Theological Education after Bucha'"), 15–19 August 2022, https://eeit-edu.info/theological-education-after-bucha/ [accessed: 31.07.2024].

50 The period of Christianity during its first centuries, before the Nicene Council of 325.

> During the period of conflict, when means of communication between the eparchies and the ecclesiastical centre are complicated or become absent, the Council considered it expedient to grant eparchial bishops the right to decide on certain issues of eparchial life that is usually within the competence of the Holy Synod or the Primate of the Ukrainian Orthodox Church. Subsequently, when the possibility arises and upon restoration of ties to notify the ruling hierarchs.[51]

As Metropolitan Klyment (Vecherya) said, the Council was based on the understanding that each diocese is a local church, and each bishop is the head of his local church. In his opinion, only such a nonstandard form of the further existence of the Ukrainian Orthodox Church will allow it to preserve its internal unity in the conditions of war.[52] If the question of affiliation and transparency of the activities and intentions of the UOC-MP remains a cornerstone in the public space for religious and nonreligious people, these splits in identity and changes of priorities also occur in other religious currents, in particular protestant ones. As we explained above, Protestants experienced a final split with their Russian brothers in faith who remained neutral or loyal to the Russian regime; instead, the majority of Ukrainian Protestant ministers took a proactive position and are trying to rethink the latest crisis theologically.

Considering the metamorphoses of the religious world, we can trace which parts of the identity mosaic prevail. For example, why does national identity come before religious identity for some, and for others, on the contrary, religious affiliation still dominates despite their clear civic position? Our findings from the first eleven months of the full-scale invasion of Ukraine indicate a revision of priorities regarding the components of identity: first, the national component occupies an increasingly important position; second, there are attempts to form and consolidate a religious-civil identity, which remains visible in public but almost does not touch the personal lives and spiritual practices of citizens; and third, there is a split among religious organisations, which traditionally had long-term relations in the post-Soviet space and are now losing or severing ties with Russia. Paying attention to the religious sphere adds to our understanding of the dynamics of identity because religion constitutes an existential component of identity that drives decision-making in the context of crisis. However, it is also worth considering the formation of a civil narrative on the part of religious communities as well as representatives of the authorities and opinion leaders, where the very concept of citizenship can be inclusive and does not concentrate on a certain ethnicity or religion.

51 Ukrainska Pravoslavna Tserkva, "Resolutions of the Council".

52 Khomenko, Chervonenko, and Lotarieva, "Byttia vyznachaie svidomist".

Bibliography

#Dialog.TUT (#Dialogue.HERE), "Kak prokhodil Sobor UPTs i kakiye prinyaty resheniya" ("How the Council of the UOC Took Place and What Decisions Were Made"), 27 May 2022, https://www.dialogtut.org/kak-prohodil-sobor-upcz-i-kakie-prinyaty-resheniya/ [accessed: 29.07.2024].

Abdelal, Rawi, Yoshiko M. Herrera, Alastair Iain Johnston, and Rose McDermott, "Identity as a Variable", *Perspectives on Politics* 4/4, 2006, 695–711.

Antoshevskyy, Taras, "'Potribna nova arkhitektura tserkovnoho zhyttya', — o. Andriy Ponomarenko pro sviy vykhid z UPTs-MP ta poshuk tserkovnoyi yednosti" ("'We Need a New Architecture of Church Life', Fr. Andriy Ponomarenko on His Withdrawal from the UOC-MP and the Search for Church Unity"), *Relihiyno-informatsiyna sluzhba Ukrayiny* (*Religious Information Service of Ukraine*), 03 May 2022, https://risu.ua/potribna-nova-arhitektura-cerkovnogo-zhittya--o-andrij-ponomarenko-pro-svij-vihid-z-upc-mp-ta-poshuk-cerkovnoyi-yednosti_n128894 [accessed: 29.07.2024].

Arel, Dominique, "Introduction: Theorizing the Politics of Cultural Identities in Russia and Ukraine", in: Dominique Arel and Blair A. Ruble (eds.), *Rebounding Identities: The Politics of Identity in Russia and Ukraine*, Washington, D.C.: Woodrow Wilson Center Press, 2006, 1–30, here 22.

Bortnyk, Sergei, "Overestimated declared identity of the OCU faithful and unexpected tolerance of the UOC(MP) faithful: analysis of the Razumkov Center's data", *CF "Academic initiative"*, 2022, https://www.academic-initiative.org.ua/en/2022/02/16/analysis_of_razumkov/ [accessed: 29.07.2024].

Brylov, Denys, and Tetiana Kalenychenko, "Ukrainian Religious Actors and Organizations after Russia's Invasion: The Struggle for Peace", *Berkley Center*, 27 September 2022, https://berkleycenter.georgetown.edu/events/ukrainian-religious-actors-and-organizations-after-russia-s-invasion [accessed: 29.07.2024].

Brylov, Denys, and Tetiana Kalenychenko, "Religion and Nationalism in Post-Soviet Space: Between State, Society and Nation", in: Jayeel Cornelio, François Gauthier, Tuomas Martikainen, and Linda Woodhead (eds.), *Routledge International Handbook of Religion in Global Society*, New York: Routledge, 2021, 399–409.

Brylov, Denys, Tetiana Kalenychenko, and Andrii Kryshtal, *The Religious Factor in Conflict: Research on the Peacebuilding Potential of Religious Communities in Ukraine*, PAX, report, 2021

Chaika, Tatyana, "ROC publishes theological clarification on non-canonicity of OCU", *Union of Orthodox Journalists*, 09 October 2019, https://spzh.news/en/news/65558-rpc-opublikovala-bogoslovskoje-razyasnenije-o-nekanonichnosti-pcu [accessed: 11.11.2023].

Derzhavna sluzhba Ukrainy z etnopolityky ta svobody sovisti (DESS) (State Service of Ukraine for Ethnic Policy and Freedom of Conscience), *Zvit pro merezhu reli-*

hiinykh orhanizatsii ctanom na 1 sichnia 2021 roku (*Report on the Network of Religious Organisations as of 1 January 2021*), report, 2022, https://dess.gov.ua/religion/ [accessed: 09.11.2023].

Dukhovna velych Lvova (The Ducal Majesty of Lviv), "Ihumen monastyrya UPTS (MP) u Lvovi pereyshov z hromadoyu do PTsU" ("Abbot of the UOC (MP) Monastery in Lviv Joins the OCU with Community"), 20 March 2022, https://velychlviv.com/igumen-monastyrya-upts-mp-u-lvovi-perejshov-z-gromadoyu-do-ptsu/ [accessed: 29.07.2024].

Eastern European Institute of Theology, "Ofitsiine komiunike, pryiniate uchasnykamy konsultatsii 'Bohoslovska osvita pislia Buchi'" ("Official Communique Adopted by the Participants of the Consultation 'Theological Education after Bucha'"), 15–19 August 2022, https://eeit-edu.info/theological-education-after-bucha/ [accessed: 29.07.2024].

Fert, Andrii, "'Nasha pastva ne zhelaet bolshe slyshat imya patriarkha Kirilla'" ("Our Flock Does Not Want to Hear the Name of Patriarch Kirill Anymore"), *OpenDemocracy*, 11 March 2022, https://www.opendemocracy.net/ru/ukraina-tserkov-voina-protest-protiv-patriarcha-fert-/ [accessed: 29.07.2024].

Kalenychenko, Tetiana, and Denys Brylov, "'Whoever saves one life saves the world entire': Ukrainian religious denominations during the war", *Bulletin de l'Observatoire international du religieux* (*Bulletin of the International Observatory on Religion*) 37, 2022, https://obsreligion.cnrs.fr/bulletin/whoever-saves-one-life-saves-the-world-entire-ukrainian-religious-denominations-during-the-war-english-version/ [accessed: 29.07.2024].

Khomenko, Sviatoslav, Vitalii Chervonenko, and Anastasiia Lotarieva, "'Byttia vyznachaie svidomist'. Chy pozbavylasia UPTs vid Moskovskoho patriarkhatu" ("'Being Defines Consciousness': Did the Ukrainian Orthodox Church Get Rid of the Moscow Patriarchate?"), *BBC Ukraine*, 30 May 2022, https://www.bbc.com/ukrainian/features-61625756 [accessed: 29.07.2024].

Koshkina, Sonia, "Prezydent Ukrainy pryzupynyv hromadianstvo 13 sviashchennykiv UPTs-MP, – dzherela" ("President of Ukraine Suspends Citizenship of 13 Priests of the UOC-MP – Sources], *Livyi Bereg* (*Left Bank*), 28 December 2023, https://lb.ua/society/2023/01/07/541773_prezident_ukraini_prizupiniv.html [accessed: 29.07.2024].

Krym.Realii (Crimea.Realities), "V Ukraine 15 yeparkhiy UPTs Moskovskogo patriarkhata perestali pominat patriarkha RPTS Kirilla – Danilevich" ("In Ukraine, 15 Dioceses of the UOC-MP Have Stopped Memorialising Patriarch Kirill – Danilevych"), 2022, https://ru.krymr.com/a/news-ukraina-15-eparhiy-upc-mp/31754601.html [accessed: 29.07.2024].

Metropolitan Antony (Pakanych), "Bozhe, zberezhy Tserkvu Tvoiu v istyni i yednosti!" ("God, Save Your Church in Truth and Unity!"), *Pravoslavnaia Zhyzn* (*Or-*

thodox Life), 28 July 2023, https://pravlife.org/uk/content/mytr-antoniy-pakanych-bozhe-zberezhy-cerkvu-tvoyu-v-istyni-i-yednosti [accessed: 29.07.2024].

Metropolitan Antony (Pakanych), "Znyaty anafemu z Filareta mozhe til'ky RPTS" ("Only the ROC can lift anathema from Filaret"), https://ukranews.com/ua/news/586240-znyaty-anafemu-z-filareta-mozhe-tilky-rpc-mytropolit-antoniy [accessed 29.07.2024].

Mukhomorova, Tetiana, "When a Brother Doesn't Hear His Brother: Post-Maidan Problems in Relations between Ukrainian and Russian Protestants", *Religious Information Service of Ukraine*, 25 March 2014, https://risu.ua/en/when-a-brother-doesn-t-hear-his-brother-post-maidan-problems-in-relations-between-ukrainian-and-russian-protestants_n68021 [accessed: 29.07.2024].

Pew Research Center, *Religious Belief and National Belonging in Central and Eastern Europe*, report, 2017, http://www.pewforum.org/2017/05/10/religious-belief-and-national-belonging-in-central-and-eastern-europe/ [accessed: 29.07.2024].

Portal Polsko-Ukrainski (Polish–Ukrainian Portal), "UPTs MP – ostannii marker 'ruskoho mira' v Ukraini" – ukrainskyi relihiieznavets Andrii Yurash" ("The UOC-MP is the Last Marker of the 'Russian World' in Ukraine – Ukrainian Religious Scholar Andriy Yurash], 2023, http://www.polukr.net/uk/blog/2023/05/upcmp-ostannyj-marker-ruskovo-mira/ [accessed: 29.07.2024].

Pravoslavna Tserkva Ukrainy (Orthodox Church of Ukraine), "Pravoslavna Tserkva Ukrainy: shliakh kriz viky" ("Orthodox Church of Ukraine: The Path through the Centuries"), https://www.pomisna.info/uk/tserkva/istoriya/ [accessed: 29.07.2024].

Rada Yevanhelskykh Protestantskykh Tserkov Ukrainy (Council of Evangelical Protestant Churches of Ukraine), "Spilna zaiava SIeA, YeIeA ta RIePTsU z pryvodu richnytsi rosiiskoho vtorhnennia" ("Joint Statement of the CEA, the EEA, and the REPCU on the Anniversary of the Russian Invasion"), 2023, https://repcu.org/2023/02/27/1615/ [accessed: 11.11.2023].

Razumkov Centre, *Ukrainske suspilstvo, derzhava i tserkva pid chas viiny. Tserkovno-relihiina hesytuatsiia v Ukraini-2023* (*Ukrainian Society, the State, and the Church in Wartime: The Situation of the Church and Religion in Ukraine in 2023*), report, 2023.

Razumkov Centre, *Osoblyvosti relihiynoho i tserkovno-relihiynoho samovyznachennia hromadyan Ukrainy: tendentsiyi 2000–2021 rr.* (*Specifics of the Religious and Church Self-Determination of the Citizens of Ukraine: Trends 2000–2021*], report, 2021.

Razumkov Centre, *Osoblyvosti relihiynoho i tserkovno-relihiynoho samovyznachennya hromadyan Ukrayiny: tendentsiyi 2000–2020 rr.* (*Specifics of the Religious and Church Self-Determination of the Citizens of Ukraine: Trends 2000–2020*), report, 2020.

Reverend Cyril (Hovorun), "Pravoslavnaya grazhdanskaya religiya" ("Orthodox Civil Religion"), *Relihiia v Ukraini* (*Religion in Ukraine*), 18 May 2015, https://www.religion.in.ua/main/bogoslovya/29171-pravoslavnaya-grazhdanskaya-religiya.html [accessed: 29.07.2024].

Rossiyskiy obyedinennyy Soyuz khristian very evangelskoy (pyatidesyatnikov) (ROSKhVE) (Russian United Union of Christians of Evangelical Faith (Pentecostals)), "Rossiyskiye missionery sozdali tserkov v Mariupole" ("Russian Missionaries Set Up a Church in Mariupol"), 2022, https://www.cef.ru/infoblock/news/read/article/1669783 [accessed: 29.07.2024].

Rossiyskiy obyedinennyy Soyuz khristian very evangelskoy (pyatidesyatnikov) (ROSKhVE) (Russian United Union of Christians of Evangelical Faith (Pentecostals)), "Zayavleniye Dukhovnogo soveta ROSKhVE v svyazi s obyavleniyem chastichnoy mobilizatsii" ("Statement of the Spiritual Council of the ROSKhVE in Connection with the Announcement of Partial Mobilisation"), 2022, https://www.cef.ru/documents/docitem/article/1674593 [accessed: 29.07.2024].

Rossiyskiy obyedinennyy Soyuz khristian very evangelskoy (pyatidesyatnikov) (ROSKhVE) (Russian United Union of Christians of Evangelical Faith (Pentecostals)), "Zayavleniye episkopa Sergeya Ryakhovskogo (ot imeni Dukhovnogo soveta ROSKhVE) po situatsii na Ukraine" ("Statement by Bishop Sergey Ryakhovsky (on Behalf of the Spiritual Council of the ROSKhVE) on the Situation in Ukraine"), 2022, https://www.cef.ru/documents/docitem/article/1640677 [accessed: 29.07.2024].

Security Service of Ukraine, "SBU povidomyla pro pidozru mytropolytu UPTs(MP) Pavlu (video)" ("The SSU Serves Notice of Suspicion to Metropolitan Pavlo of the UOC(MP) (video)"), 2023, https://ssu.gov.ua/novyny/sbu-povidomyla-pro-pidozru-mytropolytu-upts-mp-pavlu-video [accessed: 29.07.2024].

Sotsiolohichna hrupa "Reitynh" (Sociological Group "Rating") "Otsinka sytuatsii v Ukraini (8–9 bereznia 2022)" ("Evaluating situation in Ukraine (8–9 March 2022)"), 10 March 2022, https://ratinggroup.ua/research/ukraine/ocenka_situacii_v_ukraine_8-9_marta_2022.html [accessed: 29.07.2024].

TSN, "Novyny za 26 hrudnia 2023 roku | Novyny Ukrainy" ("News for 26 December 2023 | News from Ukraine"), YouTube video, 11:55:00, 26 December 2023, https://www.youtube.com/watch?v=6WG24A9K4RA [accessed: 29.07.2024].

Ukrainska Pravoslavna Tserkva (Ukrainian Orthodox Church), "Pid dulom avtomativ vidibraly khram, vykraly monakhiv" ("A Church Was Taken at Gunpoint, Monks Were Kidnapped], 2022, https://news.church.ua/2022/03/10/pid-dulom-avtomativ-vidibrali-xram-vikrali-monaxiv-na-verxovini-rozpravlyayutsya-z-viruyuchimi-ivano-frankivskoji-jeparxiji-upc/ [accessed: 29.07.2024].

Ukrainska Pravoslavna Tserkva (Ukrainian Orthodox Church), "Resolutions of the Council of the Ukrainian Orthodox Church of May 27, 2022", 28 May 2022, https://news.church.ua/2022/05/28/resolutions-council-ukrainian-orthodox-church-may-27-2022/?lang=en [accessed: 29.07.2024].

Ukrainska Pravoslavna Tserkva (Ukrainian Orthodox Church), *Zvit Keruiuchoho spravamy Ukrainskoi Pravoslavnoi Tserkvy za 2022 rik* (*Report of the Chancellor of the Ukrainian Orthodox Church for 2022*), report, 2022, https://news.church.ua/2022/

12/24/zvit-keruyuchogo-spravami-ukrajinskoji-pravoslavnoji-cerkvi-za-2022-rik/ [accessed: 29.07.2024].

Wanner, Catherine, "Explaining the Appeal of Evangelicalism in Ukraine", in: Dominique Arel and Blair A. Ruble (eds.), *Rebounding Identities: The Politics of Identity in Russia and Ukraine,* Washington, D.C.: Woodrow Wilson Center Press, 2006, 243–272.

From a Pilfered Nail to a Stolen Tank

The Role of a Media Event in the Consolidation of the Ukrainian Political Nation

Mykola Homanyuk and Janush Panchenko

A Ukrainian of Azerbaijani origin was awarded the title of Hero of Ukraine,[1] Pope Francis accused Buryats and Chechens of cruelty,[2] Tajiks mobilised to the Russian Army shot their commander,[3] Turkey evacuated Ukrainian Ahiska Turks[4]: from the first days of Russia's full-scale aggression against Ukraine, national (ethnic) minorities began to regularly appear in both Russian and Ukrainian news. During the war so far, actors across information spaces and those making propaganda and counter-propaganda have been actively exploiting discourses about ethnic minorities. This can influence the assessment of current events as well as both the self-perception of these ethnic groups and how they are perceived externally, forming new stereotypes, new memories, and new senses of belonging.

One of the most remarkable stories from the first days of the war was the news that some Romani people from the village of Liubymivka stole a Russian tank. On the evening of 26 February 2022, Aliona Ostistova shared an emotional post on Facebook with a link to a screenshot from a private conversation. The next day, a news report by the TV channel 1+1 made this information public. The report also clarified that the

---

1 Baku Press Klub, "Ukrainets azerbaydzhanskogo proiskhozhdeniya poluchil zvaniye geroya strany" ("A Ukrainian of Azerbaijani Descent Has Been Honoured as a Hero of the Country"), 17 May 2022, https://pressklub.az/news_ru/world_ru/ukrainecz-azerbajdzhanskogo-proishozhdeniya-poluchil-zvanie-geroya-strany/?lang=ru [accessed: 15.04.2023].

2 TASS Russian News *Agency*, "Russian ambassador protests Pope Francis' allegation", 29 November 2022, https://tass.com/society/1543159 [accessed: 29.07.2024].

3 Timur Mura, "Rasstrel na poligone v Solote – k chemu privela nasilstvennaya mobilizatsiya tadzhykov" ("Shooting at the Soloti Shooting Range – What the Forced Mobilisation of Tajiks Has Led to"), *Viral News*, 24 November 2022, https://www.caviral.com/rasstrel-na-poligone-v-soloti-k-chemu-privela-nasilnaya-mobilizacziya-tadzhikov/ [accessed: 29.07.2024].

4 Daily Sabah, "Türkiye evacuates 88 more Ahıska Turks from Ukraine's Kherson", 20 November 2022, https://www.dailysabah.com/politics/diplomacy/turkiye-evacuates-88-more-ahiska-turks-from-ukraines-kherson [accessed: 29.07.2024].

incident took place in Liubymivka, a village in the Kakhovka district of the Kherson Oblast, which is indeed home to a large community of Krymskja (Crimean) Roma, one of the sub-ethnic groups of Romani people who are distinguished by their traditional way of life.[5] On the same day, the popular Telegram channel "Huyovyi Kherson"[6] published the following message:

> The information about the tank that the Tsygane [see footnote for translation][7] supposedly hijacked in Liubymivka turned out not to be entirely true. [They] didn't hijack the tank but dismantled it to the point of inoperability. And not just the Tsygane, but also their coalition with the locals. Nearby was also a military truck, and they definitely hijacked that[8].

On 27 February, the Facebook page of the journalist Serhiy Tsyhipa also posted a text about and video of a Ukrainian farmer stealing a Russian BMP (an infantry fighting vehicle).[9] The two stories blended into one. The same day, information about the tank's theft was published on the news aggregator Meta, was shared by the TV channel 24 and other news sources, and circulated on social media around the world. The

---

5 Janush Panchenko, *Osnovnyye statisticheskiye pokazateli tsygan Khersonskoy oblasti 2016–2017 gg. (opyt etnosotsiologicheskogo issledovaniya)* (*Basic Statistical Indicators of Kherson Oblast Citizens in 2016–2017 (Experience of Ethnosociological Research)*), Dnepr: Serednyak, 2017; Janush Panchenko and Mykola Homanyuk, "Servur'a and Krym'a (Crimean Roma) as Indigenous Peoples of Ukraine", *Etnografia Polska* (*Polish Ethnography*) 67/1–2, 2023, 155–173; and Vadim Toropov, *Crimean Roma: Language and Folklore*, Ivanovo: Unona Publishing House, 2009.

6 This translates to "Fucking Kherson".

7 A note on translating the terminology: although the Ukrainian terms 'Tsyhan'/'Tsyhany' (Циган/Цигани) or the Russian 'Tsygan'/'Tsygane' (Цыган/Цыгане) can be translated as 'Gypsy'/'Gypsies' when the words come up in interviews or media sources, we decided to transliterate the words to avoid the connotations that the English terms may carry. The majority of the Roma in Eastern and Southern Ukraine do not consider the ethnonym 'Tsyhany' incorrect or offensive, and often use it as an endoethnonym along with the self-designation 'Roma'. For more, see: Natalia Zinevych, "Etnonimy romy, tsyhany v suchasnomu ukrayinskomu naukovomu dyskursi" ("Roma and Tsygan Ethnonyms in Contemporary Ukrainian Scientific Discourse"), in: K. Kozhanov, M. Oslon, and D. W. Halwachs (eds.), *Romani historija, chib taj kultura*, Graz: GLM, 2017, 484–500.

8 Telegram channel "Huyovyi Kherson", 27 February 2022, https://t.me/hueviyherson/8532 [accessed: 29.07.2024]

9 Sergiy Tsyhipa (Facebook profile), "putinski Z-yolopy na Khersonshchyni..." ("Putin's Z-morons in the Kherson Oblast..."), Facebook video, 0:07, 27 February 2022, https://www.facebook.com/tsyhipa/posts/pfbidoQyu2uPyveNZ2LPonPGZyxShhnhCdpNjSJr66AcBo3mYtzJdDDxfvHpPv9mXjKpSrl [accessed: 29.07.2024].

news went viral and even appeared on the X (formerly Twitter) page of the President of the Republic of Poland, Andrzej Duda.[10]

Later, news pieces appeared that continued this story: Romani people stole another Russian tank, seized a missile, and took an antiaircraft gun, among other things.[11] Statements also appeared that on online commercial platforms, such as OLX or eBay for instance,[12] one could find ads for military equipment and spare parts for sale. The stolen tank became the subject of patriotic songs,[13] original graphics,[14] animations,[15] merchandise,[16] humorous programmes, and plenty of jokes on social media – it even appeared on the Facebook page of the Armed Forces of Ukraine.[17] "Tsyhany stole a tank" became an internet meme.

As a result, an image of a tractor with wheels from the Roma flag towing a tank also became the background image on the landing page of the main Romani in-

10 Andrzej Duda (@AndrzejDuda), "W http://24tv.ua podają..." ("In http://24tv.ua was written...") X post, 27 February 2022, https://twitter.com/andrzejduda/status/1497899381697257475 [accessed: 29.07.2024].

11 Khabibullin 13 Khabybullyn (Facebook page), "Tsygane ukrali u rossiyan raketu..." ("Tsyhany stole a missile from the Russians..."), Facebook video, 0:12, 01 March 2022, https://www.facebook.com/watch/?v=281925007383089 [accessed: 29.07.2024].

12 Bartosz Witoszka, "Ukraińcy sprzedają przejęte rosyjskie czołgi na eBay? Wyjaśniamy" ("Are Ukrainians Selling Seized Russian Tanks on eBay? We Explain"), *Komputer Świat (Computer World)*, 03 March 2022, https://www.komputerswiat.pl/aktualnosci/bezpieczenstwo/ukraincy-sprzedaja-przejete-rosyjskie-czolgi-na-ebay-wyjasniamy/exrwzfh [accessed: 29.07.2024].

13 Oleksandr Ponomariov, "'UKRAÏNA PEREMOZHE' – O. Ponomariov, M. Khoma, T. Topolya, E. Koshovyi, Yu. Tkach, P. Chornyi, YouTube video, 19 April 2022, 3:34, screenshot from 01:25, https://www.youtube.com/watch?v=fRuiEv3JRDQ [accessed: 29.07.2024].

14 Kar, "ROMA+tank.ru=UKRAINE", 04 March 2023, http://soc.ks.ua/wp-content/uploads/2023/12/PostCard_Print.pdf [accessed: 29.07.2024].

15 Tanya Kartashova, "'Yak tsyhany tank kraly': chomu humor pid chas viyiny dopomahae pidtrymuvaty ZSU" ("'How Tsyhany Stole a Tank': Why Humour in Times of War Helps Support the Armed Forces"), *mind*, 23 March 2022, https://mind.ua/openmind/20247288-yak-cigani-tank-krali-chomu-gumor-pid-chas-vijni-dopomagae-pidtrimuvati-zsu [accessed: 29.07.2024].

16 ProstoMaiki (JustShirts), "Katalog tovariv" ("Catalogue of Goods"), 05 March 2023, https://prostomayki.com.ua/ua/tunika-s-ukrainskoy-simvolikoy/311626-tunika-tsygane-ukrali-tank.html [accessed: 29.07.2024].

17 Artem Bohomaz, "ZSU pokazaly novyi reyiting nayisylnishykh armiyi svitu pislya rosiyiskoho vtorhnennya: 'Mozhut staty reshymy, yaksho vkradut Putina'" ("The Ukrainian Armed Forces Revealed a New Ranking of the World's Strongest Armies after the Russian Invasion: 'They Can Be First if They Steal Putin'"), *Znayi.UA (Know.UA)*, 08 March 2022, https://war.znaj.ua/420822-zsu-pokazali-noviy-reyting-naysilnishih-armiy-svitu-pislya-rosiyskogo-vtorgnennya-mozhut-stati-pershimi-yakshcho-vkradut-putina [accessed: 29.07.2024].

formation and analytical agency, RomaUA (Figure 24). The graphic combines the Ukrainian flag with the Roma flag.[18]

Figure 24: Image from RomaUA, main page

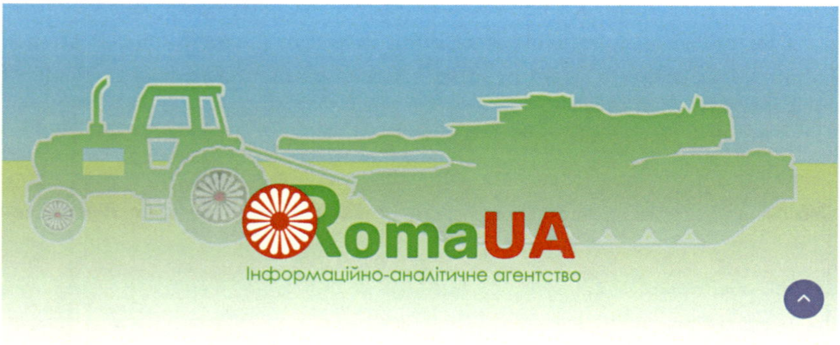

RomaUA, official website landing page, https://romaua.org.ua/ [accessed: 29.07.2024].

It is almost impossible to verify this event now. To do so, we would need to conduct an investigation, follow the traces, and look for witnesses, which, first, is impossible under the conditions of the temporary occupation of the site of the incident and, second, may endanger any people who may have been involved in some way. In addition, to us, it is not important whether the theft occurred or not, but rather the media (or communication) event around it, by which we mean an event in the information space.

Naturally, Romani people around the world actively discussed the tank theft. We conducted a series of in-depth interviews to find out the influence of this media event on the Roma in Ukraine and in other post-Soviet countries. So far, 17 Romani participants have taken part in our study. They belong to the Servurja, Vlaxurja, Krymskja (Crimean) Roma, Kishinivare Roma, and Ruska Roma sub-ethnic Roma groups. Most of the respondents are citizens of Ukraine, two are from Kazakhstan, and one is from the Russian Federation. We conducted the first part of the study from May to September 2022 with the support of the Documenting Ukraine programme initiated by the Institute for Human Sciences in Vienna.

Undoubtedly, the tank theft was the most notable event of Russia's war in Ukraine, in which the Roma were involved. The event elicited a strong emotional reaction not only among the Roma of Ukraine but also among those abroad:

18 See the landing page of: RomaUA, official website, https://romaua.org.ua/ [accessed: 29.07.2024].

> Yes, of course, at once I felt admiration (F, 55, Ukraine).

> Yes. I wish they had stolen Putin, really. I'm proud of it (F, 24, Ukraine).

> It was very exciting when I heard about it. I said: it's impossible! How can you steal a tank? Especially from under the noses of Russian soldiers. It should be impossible. But see, they managed. Those people are wonderful (M, 62, Ukraine).

> You know, I wanted this, and always thought: "If only our Tsygane would take some technical equipment from the Russian military". And exactly this happened. I just got so excited for our [people] (M, 33, Kazakhstan).

> They are just so great; I was just so happy to hear this. I really respect them for this, after all, very brave act (M, 34, Kazakhstan).

Most respondents believe in the reality of this incident. The event, which at the beginning was completely 'bare', became 'overgrown' with details, even in the dialogues with our participants:

> They hijacked this tank... and dragged it to the scrap yard. They wanted to hand it over. And the boys there were like, "guys are you crazy!?" (M, 38, Ukraine).

> They say it's all real. All of it's real. They approached these soldiers kind of slyly, proposed to drink with them, got them drunk, and they fell asleep once drunk, and they stole the tank from them (M, 62, Ukraine).

> This happened precisely in Lyubymovka. The Lyubymovka Tsygane are there. I also heard that this happened to the Lyubymovka Tsygane (M, 62, Ukraine).

> I saw facts; a video on Instagram, where the Tsygane had a tank. I think it was in a yard or somewhere behind the yard. I think they pulled it home with a tractor; that's how I remember it (M, 33, Kazakhstan).

The First Western TV channel even recorded an interview with Borys Oglou, a Crimean Romani, who testified that his relatives from the Kherson Oblast were involved in the theft of the tank: "One of the Roma, an older man, he knew how to refill it, how to start it... they refilled it, drove it home, and over the next two days took it apart for scrap metal. There were about 45 tons".[19]

According to the participants, the plausibility of this story is related to both the self-stereotypes and cultural characteristics of the Roma (according to scholarly sources, these are a tendency to adventure and risk, a sense of humour, links to a nomadic way of life, the anonymity of the protagonists, and a lower ethical threshold as compared to non-Romani people) as well as the specific economic activities of some of the Roma (e.g., collecting scrap metal is a popular way of earning money)[20]:

> At the time, I believed it 100%. It's just like that, like I saw it myself. I didn't think that it was all a lie. Knowing our people, why not believe it? And I mean the words "knowing our people" not in a bad but a good way (M, 22, Ukraine).

> I heard that they apparently took the tank apart and stole the APC [armoured personnel carrier]. It's kind of seen humorously. It's funny, really funny. But really, what was it? It's not like they stole from Tsyhany, they stole from the gadjo [non-Romani people], from the Russians. On the one hand, they could have really fucked us up with those tanks (M, 31, Ukraine).

> [Interviewer:] Did you hear that in Liubymivka Tsyhany stole a tank from the Russians?
> I heard it. Right away. Just as they took it, they said it.
> Well, what do you think? Is it true or not?
> Roma, God, they can do anything (F, 75, Ukraine).

> It's not courage, probably; it's more like dumbness, stupidity. To climb into that tank, who only knows who's sitting there, they could go ahead and shoot you (M, 31, Ukraine).

> I'm just saying, right away, it was all just really, really a lot. But later, that's what our guy said, this, what's his name... who broadcasts every evening? [Refers to Head of the Mykolaiv Oblast Administration and blogger Vitaliy Kim]. He said, "Don't steal anything anymore, don't thieve, don't throw it in

---

19 PERShYI ZAKhIDNYI (FIRST WESTERN), "Realna istoriya: yak romy vkraly tank" ("True story: How Roma stole a tank"), YouTube video, 25 May 2022, 3:15, https://www.youtube.com/watch?v=WwzMy7XwO8E [accessed: 29.07.2024].

20 Marianna Smirnova-Seslavinskaya and Georgiy Tsvetkov, *Antropologiya sotsiokulturnogo razvitiya tsyganskogo naseleniya Rossii* (*Anthropological and Cultural Development of the Tsygan Population of Russia*), Moscow: Federalnyy institut razvitiya obrazovaniya, 2011; and Oleksandr Voitenko and Mykhailo Tyahlyi, *Romy: mify i fakty. Navchalno-metodichnyi posibnyk dlya vchytelya z protydii romofobii* (*Roma: Myths and Facts, Teachers' Guide to Combating Roma-Phobia*), Kyiv: Ukrainskyi tsentr vyvchennia istorii Holokostu, 2018.

> the cellar, because it will even be punishable". Because it could blow up, something else could happen to it. And no one will accept it as [scrap] metal (F, 24, Ukraine).

These assessments of the event can be used to determine the self-stereotypes, cultural characteristics, and values of the Roma participants. That is, they show how they see themselves through the prism of the tank theft.

They also explained the theft through the fact that the Russian military was notorious for its negligence and ineptitude, especially at the beginning of the war, which itself brought this theft on them. This explanation fits perfectly with the general tone of the news coverage of the war in the first weeks of its course:

> When you heard about the tank theft, what general emotions did it evoke in you?
> Well, that the Russians are clowns. You can even steal a tank from them. That there isn't any professionalism. Even their army is weak. That from them [the tank] was snatched away like candy from a baby. And it's, somehow, like very patriotic. In a Tsygan way (M, 33, Kazakhstan).

> Do you think it's a true story, that this tank was stolen?
> There's a proverb: "If an axe lies under a bench, why not use it?" (M, 62, Ukraine).

Meanwhile, Russian media accused Ukrainians of fabricating the stolen tank story. They even claimed that the Russian Roma were involved in spreading this fake. But even this did not shake confidence in the reality of the famous abduction:

> Do you know why? On the one hand, there are pluses. [The Russians] can justify themselves this way. Well, let's say they are sure that they will gain everything from this. And, kind of, so that there will be no accusations against Tsyhany, they want to exonerate the Tsyhany; they will tell this to the Tsyhany later (M, 31, Ukraine).

> In terms of the information, well, some shared it like humour, some shared it and called it a fake, and after all, people are scared; people don't want that the Tsygane somehow get involved in all this (M, 34, Kazakhstan).

A Russian-language website also attempted to promote the news that a similar event occurred in Romania, where Romanian Roma stole an American tank during

NATO exercises.[21] Nonetheless, this information did not generate any organic interest from audiences.

There were, however, also alternative interpretations or doubts about the objectivity of the tank theft story:

> On the contrary, let both Ukrainians and Russians know that the Tsygan [man] doesn't want any harm, but he makes clear that we are against war, that we are capable... If you take [our] people into consideration, that means you understand that we Tsygane are also, as it were... that we have our own Tsygan weapons (M, 60, Ukraine).

> Well, it's hard to talk about objectivity. I saw a video where that guy recorded himself once again and said, "Here, I did this", and behind him, there's a tank. I forget how he said it. So, many said to him that "You weren't there, that you didn't do anything, didn't steal anything", and he decided to show that here, definitely, here am I, and here's the tank (M, 34, Kazakhstan).

Assessing the aftermath of the event, respondents noted both positive and negative moments. Among the positives is the fact that, because of the spread of information about this theft, there have been changes in the images of the Roma, and that this is a small but sincere contribution of the Ukrainian Roma to the defence of Ukraine:

> I don't know to which extent this is true, to which not, but some people with whom I communicate tell me, "This is all bullshit; this is just Tsygane promoting themselves", and something else like this. "Yeah, no. They're like that. The kind of people who could do anything". They stole it, turned it in as scrap metal and there you go; they got rich. Some out there say that, yeah, "Well they stole and turned it in as scrap metal and split the money, and that's all". And I think, "God, this is so nice". Sure, Tsygane aren't fighting, yes, but at least they did something, entered history, yes. This has entered history; that the Tsygane stole a tank (F, 24, Ukraine).

> This is a very positive moment here. How can you steal an entire tank from under the nose of an enemy – an enemy. Not everyone can manage this. This is very positive, very. They basically deprived the combatants of the Russian Federation of one combat unit. They deprived them of one combat unit (M, 62, Ukraine).

---

21 Vitaliy Mann, "Na ucheniyakh NATO v Rumynii tsygane ugnali tank i sdali ego v metallolom" ("At a NATO Exercise in Romania, Roma Stole a Tank and Scrapped It"), *Panorama: satiricheskoe izdanie* (*Panorama: A Satirical Publication*), 24 June 2022, https://panorama.pub/news/na-uceniah-nato-v-rumynii [accessed: 29.07.2024].

The stolen tank became a Romani news story that went far beyond the borders of Ukraine. The news especially gained popularity in Poland, Slovakia, Romania, and Moldova. Such coverage gave the impression that this was a global news story:

> The whole world already knows about it" (M, 31, Ukraine).
>
> In Kakhovka, everyone was buzzing about it. Everyone. Even the President of France once mentioned it in some interview (F, 28, Ukraine).
>
> Well, you saw how it spread everywhere and on television [...]. Even the president of Poland, Andrzej Duda, made a post on his page about the Roma (M, 37, Ukraine).

This story was discussed in different countries, and many posts related to it appeared on social media. For example, there was a popular altered image about the 'reconstruction' of a monument dedicated to the Second World War in Estonia, which was called in the comments "the monument to the Tsyhany Tractor Division"[22] (Figure 25).

The internet meme "Tsyhany stole a tank" also brought attention to the history of the Roma. For example, some Roma discovered the legendary story (likely a work of fiction) of the scout 'Yashka the Tsyhan', who single-handedly captured a German tank during World War II.[23]

22 Arkadyi Babchenko (@StarshinaZapasa), "Govoryat, proklyatye estobanderovtsy v Narve..." ("They say that the damned Esto-Banderites in Narva..."), X post, 07 April 2022, https://twitter.com/StarshinaZapasa/status/1512098167529091074/photo/1 [accessed: 29.07.2024].

23 Chtoby pomnili (So they remember), "Kak tsygan nemetskiyi tank ugnal, kak 3 tanka KV-1 razbili nemetskuyu tankovuyu rotu" ("How a gypsy stole a German tank, how 3 Kv-1 tanks defeated a German tank company"), YouTube video, 15 February 2019, 10:33, https://www.youtube.com/watch?v=iselUBiHSn8 [accessed: 29.07.2024].

Figure 25: Image from Arkadyi Babchenko, "Govoryat, proklyatye estobanderovtsy v Narve..." ("They say that the damned Esto-Banderites in Narva...")

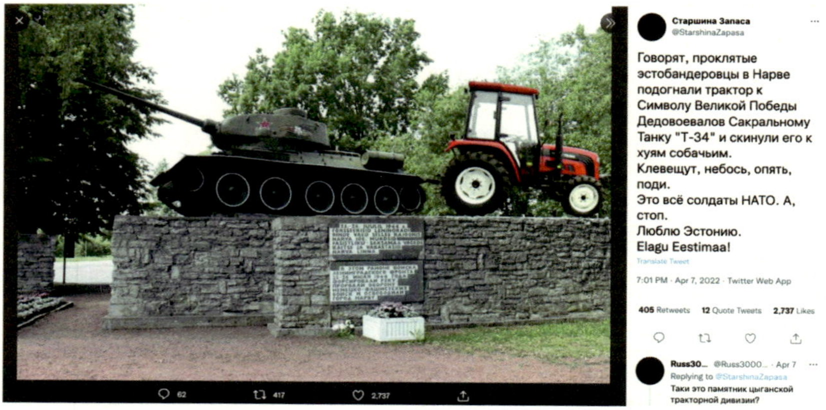

Arkadyi Babchenko (@StarshinaZapasa), "Govoryat, proklyatye estobanderovtsy v Narve..." ("They say that the damned Esto-Banderites in Narva..."), X post, 07 April 2022, https://twitter.com/StarshinaZapasa/status/1512098167529091074/photo/1 [accessed: 29.07.2024].

Parallels with the Second World War also arose during the interviews. Here is a fragment of an interview that speaks to this as well as to the idea that the Russian Army could be perceived as the army of Nazi Germany:

> Have you heard that when the war first started, they said that the Roma stole a Russian tank?
> I heard that the Roma stole a German tank – well done, well done.
>
> Not German, but Russian.
> Ah, Russian! I'm telling you, all kinds of things are mixing in my head (F, 63, Ukraine).

Thus, the tank became the point, perhaps at first accidentally and later deliberately, from which a new external and internal Roma discourse began to form, in which the Roma were integrated into the Ukrainian political nation, and the Ukrainian people themselves were consolidated on a civic rather than ethnic level:

> Tsyhany are the kind of people who live on their own. Well, that's the biggest thing; that it's funny in this regard, with nationality [or ethnic origin]. They [Ukrainians] even write, "Even the Tsyhany are fucking with you [Russians]". Tsyhany, they're always somewhere on the sidelines, and then they emerged and started stealing tanks (M, 31, Ukraine).

> There is a kind of pride there, like with the gadjo there: "Oh, there, our people snatched a tank". "Oh, well done" – gadjo are like that, basically. There is a kind of pride here, to be honest. So basically, well, the Tsyhany, it's good, on the contrary, I think, so others won't say, "Oh, the Tsyhany were sitting around; they didn't do anything". Oh no, fuck, the Tsyhany snatched a fucking tank (M, 31, Ukraine).

> And what's interesting, this is probably the first time in my life that I've seen the whole nation [of Ukraine] admire the Tsygane like this. To have them say that our Tsygane are simply stunning. Just stunning. "We're very proud of them, and we're all unified now. We're all united. We're all one nation". I'm surprised. I'm just generally surprised by this kind of unity and this kind of attitude towards Tsygane as a whole (M, 34, Kazakhstan).

The integration of the Roma into the Ukrainian political nation, even at the level of the media, seemed like a fantasy before the war. The Roma were one of the ethnic groups against which the highest level of xenophobia has long been recorded in Ukraine. According to the Kyiv International Institute of Sociology, shortly before the war (November 2021), Ukrainian attitudes towards the Roma scored 5.34 points on the Emory Bogardus social distance scale.[24] In September 2022, this figure decreased to 5.08 (-0.25) and the Roma moved up two places in the Bogardus scale, overtaking Russians living in Russia (6.39) and Belarusians living in Belarus (5.34) (as opposed to Russians or Belarusians living in Ukraine or holding Ukrainian citizenship, or Ukrainians of Russian or Belarusian origin), who previously were among those closest to Ukrainian groups.[25] This means that although a broad majority of Ukrainian citizens continue to maintain a significant sociocultural distance towards the Roma (they do not want to see them as colleagues, neighbours, or close friends or relatives), the vast majority of Ukrainians have already overcome the political barrier between them. That is, they do not see cohabitating in the same country as the Roma as an issue, despite them previously being one of the main groups for this problem.

The theft of the tank by the Roma is an important event that gave momentum to a more positive perception of Roma. And this was immediately felt in the Romani community:

---

24 The Bogardus scale is a 7-point scale measuring social distance. On it, 1 equates to accepting one as a member of one's family and 7 to not allowing members of this group inside one's country. Accordingly, the higher the mean value, the stronger the social distance.

25 Volodymyr Paniotto, *Mizhetrichni uperedzhennya v Ukraini* (*Interethnic Prejudice in Ukraine*), Kyiv International Institute of Sociology, report, September 2022, https://www.kiis.com.ua/?lang=ukr&cat=reports&id=1150&page=1 [accessed: 29.07.2024].

> Have you heard of any situations where the Roma were discriminated against during the war?
> During the war? I don't hear it right now. The fact that the Roma stole a tank had a great influence on this. This gave some idea to all the non-Roma, to other people; that the Roma also do these kinds of things, and after that all the non-Roma instead said, "well done to Tsygane, you're also on our side" – and so, it had a great impact towards us, in a positive way (M, 37, Ukraine).

The media event of the tank theft has become a notable phenomenon, both in the lives of the Roma community in Ukraine and for the entire Ukrainian population. Stories about the participation of representatives of different ethnic groups in the war are not uncommon in the information space of Ukraine. For example, attention is drawn to the Korean origin of Vitaliy Kim, and pieces are published about servicemembers representing national minorities in the Armed Forces – including those of Azerbaijani, Crimean Tatar, and Ahiska Turk origin – who have been participating in the Russo–Ukrainian War since 2014. Other ethnic groups, such as Georgians, Belarusians, and Chechens, among others, are also present in the information space. Yet, they appear more often as volunteers in the Ukrainian Army, who are thus fighting not only for Ukraine but also for the futures of their own countries. However, the Roma have become the ethnic group that has demonstrated and continues to demonstrate the consolidation of the Ukrainian political nation after the full-scale Russian invasion on a broad media level. The tank theft was the starting point. Subsequently, the Roma have been appearing in the information space of Ukraine as defenders of the country – as military and police officers with specific names and concrete accomplishments. The stolen tank is a kind of modern retelling of the popular legend about the nail stolen by a Tsyhan man from the Roman legionnaires, which they were going to use to nail the head of Christ[26]:

> Tsygane and stealing was always… it was always news. If they said "Armenians stole", or someone else stole, this wouldn't be interesting. But "Tsygane stole"… You know, it's like the silver nail that [the Tsygane] stole from Jesus Christ. Here you have Tsygane and stealing – that's all. This was always interesting for people. If they said that some other nationality stole something, this news would survive for two or three days. But if the Tsygane stole, this will be… well, even the war will end, but they'll speak about this (M, 34, Ukraine).

It is difficult to disagree that this story will live on for a long time. It is worth adding that we are aware that the way to overcome negative stereotypes cannot be easy and fast, especially if they are so deeply rooted as with the Roma. And one media event

26 Nadezhda Demeter, Nikolay Bessonov, and Valdemar Kutenkov, *Istoria tsygan: Novyi vzgliad (The History of Tsygani: A New View)*, Voronezh: IPF Voronezh, 2000.

will not remove all stereotypes and discriminatory practices towards the Roma; it may even strengthen them in some ways. But we hope that this vivid case will contribute to the creation of a new basis for rethinking the sense of belonging of the Ukrainian Roma to Ukrainian society and the Ukrainian nation, and vice versa, because Ukrainians of different ethnic origins will consider the Roma as an integral part of a multiethnic Ukraine.

War and displacement created a new dynamic in Ukrainian society and intensified its citizens' reflections on their attitudes towards minority groups living on its territory. Some of these groups have become more visible. They are positioned and recognised as those who belong to the Ukrainian political nation.

Bibliography

Babchenko, Arkadyi, (@StarshinaZapasa), "Govoryat, proklyatye estobanderovtsy v Narve..." ("They say that the damned Esto-Banderites in Narva..."), X post, 07 April 2022, https://twitter.com/StarshinaZapasa/status/1512098167529091074/photo/1 [accessed: 31.07.2024].

Baku Press Klub, "Ukrainets azerbaydzhanskogo proiskhozhdeniya poluchil zvaniye geroya strany" ("A Ukrainian of Azerbaijani Descent Has Been Honoured as a Hero of the Country"), 17 May 2022, https://pressklub.az/news_ru/world_ru/ukrainecz-azerbajdzhanskogo-proishozhdeniya-poluchil-zvanie-geroya-strany/?lang=ru [accessed: 15.04.2024].

Bohomaz, Artem, "ZSU pokazaly novyyi reyiting nayisylnishykh armiyi svitu pislya rosiyiskoho vtorhnennya: 'Mozhut staty reshymy, yaksho vkradut Putina'" ("The Ukrainian Armed Forces Revealed a New Ranking of the World's Strongest Armies after the Russian Invasion: 'They Can Be First if They Steal Putin'"), *Znayi.UA* (*Know.UA*), 08 March 2022, https://war.znaj.ua/420822-zsu-pokazali-noviy-reyting-naysilnishih-armiy-svitu-pislya-rosiyskogo-vtorgnennya-mozhut-stati-pershimi-yakshcho-vkradut-putina [accessed: 15.04.2024].

Chtoby pomnili (So they remember), "Kak tsygan nemetskiyi tank ugnal, kak 3 tanka KV-1 razbili nemetskuyu tankovuyu rotu" ("How a gypsy stole a German tank, how 3 Kv-1 tanks defeated a German tank company"), YouTube video, 15 February 2019, 10:33, https://www.youtube.com/watch?v=iselUBiHSn8 [accessed: 31.07.2024].

Daily Sabah, "Türkiye evacuates 88 more Ahıska Turks from Ukraine's Kherson", 20 November 2022, https://www.dailysabah.com/politics/diplomacy/turkiye-evacuates-88-more-ahiska-turks-from-ukraines-kherson [accessed: 31.07.2024].

Demeter, Nadezhda, Nikolay Bessonov, and Valdemar Kutenkov, *Istoria tsygan: Novyi vzgliad* (*The History of Tsygani: A New View*), Voronezh: IPF Voronezh, 2000.

Duda, Andrzej, (@AndrzejDuda), "W http://24tv.ua podają..." ("In http://24tv.ua was written...") X post, 27 February 2022, https://twitter.com/andrzejduda/status/1497899381697257475 [accessed: 31.07.2024].

"Huyovyi Kherson" (Telegram channel), 27 February 2022, https://t.me/hueviyherson/8532 [accessed: 31.07.2024].

Kar (Facebook page), "ROMA+tank.ru=UKRAINE", 04 March 2023, https://m.facebook.com/story.php?story_fbid=pfbid05CYJ5wD89zSj58DByc4KtSRKjMBu73zqT2sMPHFSFJQMLsKkJNj3tCQywCxhomq2l&id=100013509630593&mibextid=Nif5oz [accessed: 31.07.2024].

Khabibullin 13 Khabybullyn (Facebook page), "Tsygane ukrali u rossiyan raketu..." ("Tsyhany stole a missile from the Russians..."), Facebook video, 0:12, 01 March 2022, https://www.facebook.com/watch/?v=281925007383089 [accessed: 31.07.2024].

Tanya Kartashova, "'Yak tsyhany tank kraly': chomu humor pid chas viyiny dopomahae pidtrymuvaty ZSU" ("'How Tsyhany Stole a Tank': Why Humour in Times of War Helps Support the Armed Forces"), *mind*, 23 March 2022, https://mind.ua/openmind/20247288-yak-cigani-tank-krali-chomu-gumor-pid-chas-vijni-dopomagae-pidtrimuvati-zsu [accessed: 31.07.2024].

Khabibullin 13 Khabybullyn (Facebook page), "Tsygane ukrali u rossiyan raketu..." ("Tsyhany stole a missile from the Russians..."), Facebook video, 0:12, 01 March 2022, https://www.facebook.com/watch/?v=281925007383089 [accessed: 31.07.2024].

Mann, Vitaliy, "Na ucheniyakh NATO v Rumynii tsygane ugnali tank i sdali ego v metallolom" ("At a NATO Exercise in Romania, Roma Stole a Tank and Scrapped It"), *Panorama: satiricheskoe izdanie* (*Panorama: A Satirical Publication*), 24 June 2022, https://panorama.pub/news/na-uceniah-nato-v-rumynii [accessed: 31.07.2024].

Mura, Timur, "Rasstrel na poligone v Solote – k chemu privela nasil'stvennaya mobilizatsiya tadzhykov" ("Shooting at the Soloti Shooting Range – What the Forced Mobilisation of Tajiks Has Led to"), *Viral News*, 24 November 2022, https://www.caviral.com/rasstrel-na-poligone-v-soloti-k-chemu-privela-nasilnaya-mobilizacziya-tadzhikov/ [accessed: 31.07.2024].

Panchenko, Janush, *Osnovnyye statisticheskiye pokazateli tsygan Khersonskoy oblasti 2016–2017 gg. (opyt etnosotsiologicheskogo issledovaniya)* (*Basic Statistical Indicators of Kherson Oblast Citizens in 2016–2017 (Experience of Ethnosociological Research)*), Dnepr: Serednyak, 2017.

Panchenko, Janush, and Mykola Homanyuk, "Servur'a and Krym'a (Crimean Roma) as Indigenous Peoples of Ukraine", *Etnografia Polska* (*Polish Ethnography*) 67/1–2, 2023, 155–173.

Paniotto, Volodymyr, *Mizhetnichni uperedzhennya v Ukraini* (*Interethnic Prejudice in Ukraine*), Kyiv International Institute of Sociology, report, September

2022, https://www.kiis.com.ua/?lang=ukr&cat=reports&id=1150&page=1 [accessed: 31.07.2024].

PERShYI ZAKhIDNYI (FIRST WESTERN), "Realna istoriya: yak romy vkraly tank" ("True story: How Roma stole a tank"), YouTube video, 25 May 2022, 3:15, https://www.youtube.com/watch?v=WwzMy7XwO8E [accessed: 31.07.2024].

Oleksandr Ponomariov, "'UKRAÏNA PEREMOZHE' – O. Ponomariov, M. Khoma, T. Topolya, E. Koshovyi, Yu. Tkach, P. Chornyi, YouTube video, 19 April 2022, 3:34, screenshot from 01:25, https://www.youtube.com/watch?v=fRuiEv3JRDQ [accessed: 31.07.2024].

ProstoMaiki (JustShirts), "Katalog tovariv" ("Catalogue of Goods"), 05 March 2023, https://prostomayki.com.ua/ua/tunika-s-ukrainskoy-simvolikoy/311626-tunika-tsygane-ukrali-tank.html [accessed: 31.07.2024].

RomaUA, official website, https://romaua.org.ua/ [accessed: 31.07.2024].

Smirnova-Seslavinskaya, Marianna, and Georgiy Tsvetkov, *Antropologiya sotsiokulturnogo razvitiya tsyganskogo naseleniya Rossii* (*Anthropological and Cultural Development of the Tsygan Population of Russia*), Moscow: Federalnyy institut razvitiya obrazovaniya, 2011.

TASS Russian News Agency, "Russian ambassador protests Pope Francis' allegation", 29 November 2022, https://tass.com/society/1543159 [accessed: 31.07.2024].

Tetiana Chasnyk, "'UKRAÏNA PEREMOZHE' – O Ponomarov M Khoma T Topolya E Koshoviy Yu Tkach P Chornii. Plyus dlya rozuchuvannya" ("'UKRAINE WILL WIN' – O Ponomarev M Khoma T Topolya E Koshevyi Y Tkach P Chornyi. Plus for learning"), YouTube video, 19 April 2022, 3:34, https://www.youtube.com/watch?v=XXkGZoSQno4&t=6s [accessed: 31.07.2024].

Toropov, Vadim, *Crimean Roma: Language and Folklore*, Ivanovo: Unona Publishing House, 2009.

Tsyhipa, Sergiy (Facebook profile), "putinski Z-yolopy na Khersonshchyni..." ("Putin's Z-men in the Kherson Oblast..."), Facebook video, 0:07, 27 February 2022, https://www.facebook.com/tsyhipa/posts/pfbid0Qyu2uPyveNZ2LPonPGZyxShhnhCdpNjSJr66AcBo3mYtzJdDDxfvHpPv9mXjKpSrl [accessed: 31.07.2024].

Voitenko, Oleksandr, and Mykhailo Tyahlyi, *Romy: mify i fakty. Navchalno-metodichnyi posibnyk dlya vchytelya z protydii romofobii* (*Roma: Myths and Facts, Teachers' Guide to Combating Roma-Phobia*), Kyiv: Ukrainskyi tsentr vyvchennia istorii Holokostu, 2018.

Witoszka, Bartosz, "Ukraińcy sprzedają przejęte rosyjskie czołgi na eBay? Wyjaśniamy" ("Are Ukrainians Selling Seized Russian Tanks on eBay? We Explain"), *Komputer Świat* (*Computer World*), 03 March 2022, https://www.komputerswiat.pl/aktualnosci/bezpieczenstwo/ukraincy-sprzedaja-przejete-rosyjskie-czolgi-na-ebay-wyjasniamy/exrwzfh [accessed: 31.07.2024].

Zinevych, Natalia, "Etnonimy romy, tsyhany v suchasnomu ukrayinskomu naukovomu dyskursi" ("Roma and Tsygan Ethnonyms in Contemporary

Ukrainian Scientific Discourse"), in: K. Kozhanov, M. Oslon, and D. W. Halwachs (eds.), *Romani historija, chib taj kultura*, Graz: GLM, 2017, 484–500.

Reclaiming the History of Crimea and the Crimean Tatars through One Family Story

Emine Ziyatdinova

This personal essay presents stories told by three generations of Crimean Tatar women – my grandmother, my mother, and myself – about our evolving relationship with Crimea and its history from 1937 to 2022. Denied the right to know or remember tragic events, such as my great-grandfather's arrest and execution in 1937–1938 and the deportation of Crimean Tatars in 1944, my grandmother was only able to reclaim her history after the collapse of the Soviet Union and our return to Crimea from Uzbekistan in 1990. This essay is based on my personal experiences living and working in Crimea and incorporates several in-depth biographical interviews that I recorded between 2008 and 2022 with my family members.

I interviewed my grandmother and mother on multiple occasions. The story became more complex as I was able to return and ask more questions about events and as I was considered mature enough to hear some of the answers. Personal memories often mix with and differ from the historical narratives that exist in society. They are not structured as linear narratives but rather as kaleidoscopic bits and descriptions of experience intertwined with collective memory. But these personal memories have the power to tell the story of a place more intimately and honestly, especially when historical narratives are twisted and rewritten for political purposes.

Historical Background

Crimean Tatars are an Indigenous, Turkic-speaking Muslim ethnic group with an estimated current population of 250,000 in Ukraine,[1] primarily on the Crimean Peninsula. Before the annexation of Crimea by the Russian Empire under the leadership of Catherine II in 1783, following the Russo–Ottoman Wars, Crimean

1 Derzhavnyi komitet statistyky Ukrainy (State Statistics Committee of Ukraine), "Vseukrainskii perepys naselennia 2001" ("The All-Ukrainian Population Census of 2001"), http://2001.ukrcensus.gov.ua/eng/results/general/nationality/ [accessed: 29.07.2024].

Tatars constituted the demographic majority in Crimea.[2] Before the annexation, Crimean Tatars lived under a state structure called the Crimean Khanate, which was under Ottoman rule. With the arrival of imperial Russia and its administrative and governance structures, Crimean Tatars lost their effective self-rule. Moreover, the demographic situation on the Crimean Peninsula also changed. First, there were several waves of emigration by the Crimean Tatars, primarily to Turkey. Second, the Russian Empire implemented policies of Russian immigration to Crimea.[3] By the early 20th century, when the Russian Empire collapsed and the Soviet Union superseded it, Crimean Tatars were no longer a demographic majority on the peninsula.

In 1944, the entire Crimean Tatar population was deported by the Stalin regime from Crimea, mainly to Central Asia. This was justified by false accusations of Crimean Tatar collaboration with Nazi Germany in the Second World War. Within a three-year period, more than one-third of the population died.[4] These two events – the annexation of Crimea by Catherine II in 1783 and the deportation of the Crimean Tatars by Stalin in 1944 – defined the Russian and Soviet historical narratives of Crimea and the role of Crimean Tatars in them. The intention was to justify Russian dominance on the peninsula and the inhumane deportation of an entire nation. These narratives therefore deemphasised the Crimean Tatar population and the culture and institutions that preceded Russian colonial rule. Instead, the narrative strove to establish the Russian ethnic and cultural presence on the peninsula. Additionally, many historical Crimean Tatar documents were destroyed,[5] lost, or became widely inaccessible due to language (Crimean Khanate documents were in the Crimean Tatar language but written in Arabic script, and there are not many researchers in Ukraine who can read and research them). Overall, this contributed to the reinforcement of Slavic and Russian dominance in the Crimean historical narrative and the absence of Crimean Tatar voices.

---

2 O. M. Gladun, O. P. Rudnytskyi, and N. V. Kulyk, "Otsinka demografichnykh vtrat krymskotatarskoho narody vnaslidok deportatsii 1944 roku" ("Assessment of the Demographic Losses of the Crimean Tatar People as a Result of the 1944 Deportation"), *Demografiia ta sotsialna ekonomika* (*Demographics and the Social Economy*) 30/2, 2017, 11–28, https://dse.org.ua/arhcive/30/1.pdf [accessed: 29.07.2024].

3 Alan W. Fisher, "Emigration of Muslims from the Russian Empire in the Years After the Crimean War", Jahrbücher für Geschichte Osteuropas (*Yearbooks for the History of Eastern Europe*) 35/3, 1987, 356–371, https://www.jstor.org/stable/41047947 [accessed: 29.07.2024].

4 Brian Glyn Williams, "Hidden ethnocide in the Soviet Muslim borderlands: The ethnic cleansing of the Crimean Tatars", *Journal of Genocide Research* 4/3, 2002, 357–373, http://dx.doi.org/10.1080/14623520220151952 [accessed: 29.07.2024].

5 Aurélie Campana, "Sürgün: The Crimean Tatars' Deportation and Exile", *SciencesPo*, 16 June 2008, https://www.sciencespo.fr/mass-violence-war-massacre-resistance/fr/document/suerguen-crimean-tatars-deportation-and-exile.html [accessed: 29.07.2024].

As depicted in various historical and media narratives of the Soviet period, Crimean Tatars first became an 'exotic Other' and champions of ethnic diversity, before being recast as traitors and deported by the Soviets. Soviet authorities allowed Crimean Tatars to legally return to and settle in Crimea only in 1989, where they soon became a largely ignored minority by the government and society of independent Ukraine. With the 2014 annexation of Crimea by the Russian Federation, many Ukrainian citizens have embraced a new perspective of Crimean Tatars as Ukraine's vulnerable Indigenous group and the most important cultural and ethnic minority. Yet, despite perceiving them as allies in the war against Russia since 2014, most of the Ukrainian population still considers Crimean Tatars as 'Others' and would struggle to integrate their history and identity into the larger Ukrainian historical narrative and identity. At the same time, on the other side of the Russian–Ukrainian border, the Russian regime portrays Crimean Tatars as extremist enemies of the state on the one hand and as lucky 'beneficiaries' of Russian largesse on the other.[6]

Beyond this, the historical narratives – as well as media representations – around Crimean Tatars are extremely politicised. Each time the group is mentioned, questions arise: To whom does Crimea belong? Is it Russian, Ukrainian, or Crimean Tatar? Is Crimea Slavic or Turkic? And is it part of the Muslim or Christian world? In these narratives, the voices, stories, and perspectives of the very people who experienced the historical events are often under- or misrepresented. As a journalist covering the 2014 Russian annexation of Crimea, I witnessed how this politicised narrative became propaganda and was about to turn violent.

The challenges of understanding the historical place and experience of Crimean Tatars in Crimea are further exacerbated by the efforts of the occupying Russian state to erase or override the 'post-Soviet Ukrainian' presence on the peninsula. This occurs in many ways, and one of them is the choreographed and ideologically informed narrative of Russian–Crimean unity and a shared historical destiny. The Russian government's current measures to improve local infrastructure in some areas of rural Crimea serve the same strategic purpose: to function as another reminder of how important reunification is for the Crimeans.

---

6 Andrew Wilson, "Imagining Crimean Tatar History since 2014: Indigenous Rights, Russian Recolonisation and the New Ukrainian Narrative of Cooperation", *Europe–Asia Studies* 73/5, 2021, 837–868, https://www.tandfonline.com/doi/full/10.1080/09668136.2020.1867709 [accessed: 29.07.2024].

Emine Ziyatdinova (Author), Born in 1987 on the Lenina Collective Farm in Uzbekistan

My family moved from Central Asia to Crimea in October 1990. I was three years old. I have no memories from before that, nor do I feel any connection to my place of birth, even though the words "Lenina, Uzbekistan" travel with me around the world and continue to define who I am – at least to border control staff. My paternal grandmother was forcefully deported to the Lenina Collective Farm from Crimea in 1944. It is the same collective farm where my parents held their wedding celebration, and where my brother and I spent our early childhood. It is also in the same village from which my family moved back to our homeland on the brink of the Soviet Union's collapse. We packed 46 years of life into a 20-tonne container and shipped it to the village of Berezovka in northern Crimea. Some relatives arranged a small temporary house for us to stay in for free.

"Otmekmen may", I demanded, asking for "bread with butter" for breakfast at the new house. My grandmother spread a layer of butter over bread, topped it with honey, and cut it into cubes for me. I followed my brother to play in the street with the neighbouring kids. I spoke to them in a mix of Crimean Tatar and Uzbek, while they shouted back in Russian.

It was relatively easy for repatriates to find a job doing manual labour on a collective farm, but my parents were both dentists and didn't want to give up their profession. It took a relative's Crimean Tatar friend, that friend's Russian coworker, the coworker's husband, and a 500-ruble bribe to the head of the district hospital (which came from the 5,000 rubles that my parents had saved for their move) to secure their jobs. The head of the district hospital even drove my parents to meet the heads of two collective farms and asked for their approval.

The following September, the collective farm that employed my dad as a dentist provided us with a vacant house in the neighbouring village of Serebryanka, which was an upgrade. My mom often repeated that she always dreamt of having a "spacious living room" like the one in our new house, where she could host guests. Waves of relatives would pass through that living room, sleeping on thin mattresses on the floor. Some who had just moved from Uzbekistan stayed with us, while others simply came to visit and spent the night, and some already living in Crimea needed the occasional dental treatment.

We would set a small table and serve coffee with refined sugar, followed by green tea and sweets. I was taught to pay respect to older folks by performing the 'k'ol almaga' ritual, which involved kissing an elder's hand and pressing it to my forehead. Older kids taught me how to cheat by moving the hand close enough to my lips but skipping the kiss and going straight to the forehead. This was especially useful during 'duvas', when many older people would come to pray and celebrate new beginnings or mourn the dead. During holidays like Kurban Bayram and Oraza Bayram, performing the k'ol almaga was quite rewarding, as people would usually give candies or chocolates. My grandmother would also give us some money, and if not too many kids came to our house, I could hope for an extra Lion chocolate bar.

By 10 o'clock in the morning, my grandmother Ayriye would finish her household chores, which included feeding the dogs, cats, chickens, and other animals. My parents would be at work, and my brother would be at school. She would then prepare coffee in a jezve, the Turkish-style coffee pot with a long handle, and sit by the window in the kitchen, enjoying her quiet time by reading her magazines, newspapers, and the Turkish translation of the Koran. She had three subscriptions: a local newspaper in Russian called *Crimean News* (*Krymskiye Izvestiya*), a Crimean Tatar newspaper called *New World* (*Yani Dyunya*), and a Crimean Tatar magazine called *The Star* (*Yildiz*). Through them, she rediscovered the history, culture, and Islamic stories of Crimea.

At over 80 years old, she read an article about how the Italian scientist Guglielmo Marconi, not Alexander Popov, invented the radio. She recalled how every year she taught her high school students about Popov, the Russian physicist who was supposedly the first in the world to invent this technology. She laughed and said that it turned out that she had not only told lies about the radio to children, but she was also the "best propagandist" in the district for teaching "scientific atheism", which was part of Communist ideology. But she emphasised that she had never said directly that Allah does not exist.

I was excited to start school. I was able to read and count to 100. I was the child who rang the first bell of the school year of 1994 at the celebratory gathering on 1 September. One of the school graduates carried me on his shoulders while I swung the heavy metal bell with a red bow tied around it for the whole school. I was proud, thinking I must have been the smartest kid in class to be chosen for this important task. In reality, the school director was our neighbour, and my mom was friends with her. I was also friends with her son Maxim, whom I would call "achpit" ("greedy guts") behind his back because he ate more than me even though he was younger by a year.

My parents decided that I should join the 1-A class taught by Valentina Dmitriyevna. Everyone in the village respected her and thought she was better than Gulnara Ibragimovna, the 1-B class teacher. Ibragimovna was a newly hired Crimean Tatar teacher who arrived from Uzbekistan, just like us. In the eyes of the villagers, she wasn't equal to the local teachers. They never questioned their superiority and sometimes commented on Crimean Tatars' qualifications, including those of my parents, saying that their diplomas "were bought for a sheep" in Central Asia. On top of this, for the first time, Dmitriyevna taught Ukrainian as a second language to children in first grade; this was part of the changing curriculum in Ukrainian Crimea in 1994. My mom was convinced that I should learn Ukrainian right away, as we lived in Ukraine and it would be important for my future. "If you live with wolves, you will have to howl like one", my mom repeated many times over the years.

I was the only Crimean Tatar child in the class. Ayshe, Lemara, Evelina, Elvina, Aider, and the others were in 1-B. They had Crimean Tatar as a second language. I have always been a fast learner, so Russian, Ukrainian, and English came quite naturally to me at different stages of my life. But my mother tongue was lost somewhere in the village of Serebryanka, between our house on Gorkogo Street and elementary school. Whenever I try to say something in Crimean Tatar, the words do not come to mind. When I remember the words, they do not form into sentences. And if the sentence is made, I have trouble pronouncing it, and it sounds foreign even to me.

One summer day in the late '90s, my grandmother and I attended an event in Buyuk As, the village from which my great-grandmother came. It was only 20 kilometres away from Serebryanka. The sun was strong, and it was hot outside. I walked with my grandmother from a nearby settlement into the field. The landscape was too familiar, with a flat horizon interrupted by a thin line of trees that protected the road from the wind. Brownish thistle stems and drying tumbleweed, mixed with patches of faded green, covered the ground. Some cars were parked, and families were greeting each other. There was no shade to hide in, and the steppe wind carried the smell of plov, a traditional meal made on a fire several kilometres away. The only thing left of the village were the remains of one of several wells that used to serve the 70 families who lived there before their deportation in 1944. My grandmother had briefly lived here with her relatives during the Nazi occupation. My great-grandmother, Adjire, left the village at the age of 17 in 1913, when she was married off to someone in the village of Eski Burnaq, which was 40–50 kilometres away.

My Paternal Grandmother Ayriye, Born in 1932 in the Village of Eski Burnaq, Crimea[7]

When I was 5, in 1937, our house was searched at night. I needed to pee, so my mom and I went out into the corridor, where I sat on the potty. There was a small kerosene lamp barely burning. My mom said to me, "Don't cry, my dear daughter. Look, Sheikh Babai is also here". I looked over, and in the corner, an old man was sitting with a beard and a turban on his head. It turned out to be Sheikh Babai from the mosque. They searched our entire closet and everything in the bedroom. I was crying and afraid. When I finished, my mother put me to bed, and I fell asleep again. They took my father away [that night]. I remember it very well.

7 The text here and in the following section is an edited transcription of interviews that I conducted in Russian and Crimean Tatar. Additional information is provided in square brackets where necessary.

[According to the records of the State Archives of Ukraine, the Crimean branch of the People's Commissariat for Internal Affairs (NKVD) arrested Sheikh Mefa Abkerim[8] (born 1872) and my great-grandfather Emir Veli Abdul Kerim[9] (born 1889) on 6 November in Eski Burnaq. They were accused of anti-Soviet propaganda and sabotage. The files also mention that Sheikh Mefa conducted religious gatherings and that Emir Veli was a 'kulak' and used hired labour. Both were sentenced to death by an NKVD troika and executed in early 1938. My grandmother found out about her father's fate only after the Soviet Union collapsed.]

Our belongings were also taken away – the new duvet, the sheets – and sold to poorer people. If something cost three rubles in the shop, they [the authorities] sold it for one and a half rubles. Our uncle helped us run away from Eski Burnaq to Yevpatoria, so they wouldn't touch us. My mother and uncle were worried that my older brother would be taken as well. [Her older brother Shaib was mobilised to the Red Army in 1941].

[During the Nazi occupation of Crimea from 1941 to 1944], we were evacuated from Yevpatoria to Kenegez, which was a Jewish village with two streets. Our uncle Ismail lived in the middle of the street, we were at the top, and there was a kind woman down the street. She was the only one left there, and she baked very tasty gingerbread every day until she died. When you put it in your mouth, it melted. My mother talked to her a lot, and they became friends. My mother tried to convince her to stay with us, as we were in a big empty house. "Stay with us. Leave your windows and doors open; let them take everything. Put on my old clothes, throw away all your own, and cover your head with a scarf like this. Throw away all your documents, and I'll protect you". However, the Jewish woman refused, saying, "You have two children. They will bury them in the same pit as me. I'd rather go myself". So they took her alone and put her in the pit, where all the Jews were buried. The Germans did it, not the Soviet Union. Whomever the Soviet Union did not kill, the Germans did.

[By the end of 1945, the population of Crimea had drastically changed from the Holocaust carried out by the Nazi regime and the forced deportation of Crimean Tatars – as well as Italians, Armenians, and Greeks, among others – by the Soviets. In the 1939 census, the population of Crimea was about 19.4 percent Crimean Tatar and 5.8 percent Jewish.]

[After the deportations of 18 May 1944], people already began to starve on the way [to Central Asia]. The starving people started dying after a few months in Uzbek-

8 National Archival Service of Ukraine, digital copies of the Mentric books of the National Archive of the Autonomic Republic of Crimea, Fund N6 (R), Case N28 – Protocol 23 of the Crimean Autonomic Social Soviet Republic's NKVD Troika session from 02.12.1937, slide 99, https://tsdea.archives.gov.ua/metric-books/?arch_id=39&fund_id=88&affair_id=6663#lg=1 [accessed: 29.07.2024].

9 Ibid., slide 98.

istan. But my mother did not sit still – she went around the village to the Uzbek neighbours and talked to the old ladies. She sewed up everything for them, not leaving a single garment torn. They fed her and even gave her pieces of flatbread, flour, or corn so that we children wouldn't die. They [the local Uzbeks] were also hungry; they didn't have it [food] either, but among them, there were those who gave this much [she shows her palm]. And she [her mother] ate half herself – and half, hidden, she brought to us. Then I made soup.

I found grass, horse sorrel, and onions, mixed them with flour, and made porridge. Not porridge, but rather a thin soup. We ate, and my mother gave me a few more spoonfuls in a separate, very little bowl: "Go, there is a girl who is dying of hunger. You stand next to her; feed this girl. But don't show your brother!" Of course, my brother was already a teenager and was protecting us: "We ourselves are dying of hunger. Do not give to others!" I hid the bowl under an apron, fed [her] and gave [her] water. Then my mother went to bury those who died. She used any old sheets and rags that she could find to wrap their bodies before burying them.

She also had several strings of pearls. In Uzbekistan, she divided them into pieces and sold them to wealthier Uzbeks. Clothes, scarves, whatever she had – she sold everything. There was no bed, either. We cut reeds ourselves, then made a bed. The satin duvet, which my father probably brought from Turkey, my mother reused in Uzbekistan. She took its satin, sewed an Uzbek dress, and sold it. And we made ourselves a cover – a simple cover from my mother's old dresses. And the three of us slept under one cover. And so, we survived.

As a child, I didn't know that this was a deportation. How could I know? We continued living, and I told everyone at school in Uzbekistan that we weren't deported; there was a war going on, and we were evacuated in 1944.

Throughout my childhood, my mother lived with the hope that my father would turn up one day and my brother would return from the Soviet Army. She claimed that many people were sent to Samarkand in 1938 and that some pilgrims had even spotted my father there. Whenever she acquired some jam or sugar, she would split it in half, saving one half in case my father or brother came back.

Every day, they prayed to return to Crimea. They cursed Stalin and said, "Allah boynini ursun onin [let God punish him on the neck]". When the older women gathered in our house, they used to say: "Soon, we will be going back to Crimea. Somebody saw that the wagons had already come. It was a mistake that they brought us here to Uzbekistan". I heard that.

My mother and Aunt Zylha were always whispering together and crying. Whenever I approached them, they would stop. I would ask, "Why is that?" My mother replied, "If you know everything, they'll kick you out of school. You won't go to school!" That's how we lived; they didn't tell me anything.

In 1953, Stalin died. I was in tenth grade. We attended the march and cried and cried that our leader had died. But then we went around the corner and laughed and laughed, wiping our eyes.

My Mother Katibe, Born in 1961 in Syrdarya, Uzbekistan

It was a known fact that the deportation had happened. In Uzbekistan, the Tatars were always called traitors. Even when I was a kid, other children would say things like "go back to your Crimea".

But, you see, we were brought up in a Soviet manner, so I thought it didn't include us. We believed we were all Soviets. We were always taught that we should love our motherland, that we were all so happy, that we had the happiest childhood, that the state cared for the children, and that we were building communism and all that. Develop socialism first, and then we would move on to communism.

19 May was Pioneer Day, so every year, a big fire was made in the school courtyard. There were marching and singing contests, and each class had to prepare a slogan for the marches. "Look who is marching in one line – a young Lenin-followers troop. Look who is marching all at the same time – give the way to the pioneers". There was music [and] singing, and everyone was running around the fire. It was fun for us.

During school, we were sent to pick cotton. You get tired and want to sit down after working the whole day. They don't let you. And if you didn't collect the standard quota, which was 50 kilogrammes a day, or if you went to the toilet more than two or three times, they would say it was an "apolitical protest"; that you did not support society. I was in ninth grade when the Komsomol committee called me and scolded me because my friends and I took a break for more than 10 minutes, and they said it was an apolitical protest. I came home crying. I still remember the teacher scolding me because we didn't harvest enough cotton.

I already knew something about our ethnicity and deportation. My mother always blamed Stalin and said that all our misfortunes were his fault. She said that he deported the Crimean Tatars to Uzbekistan. My mother used to listen to Crimean Tatar concerts on the radio. They were only [played] on certain dates and on certain radio stations. At weddings, they used to play "Alushtadan Esken Yeller" ("The Winds Blown from Alushta"). People must have felt nostalgic.

I remember the first time someone from our family tried to move back to Crimea. My mother's aunt, Ayshe-anay, and her husband left. We all took a bus to see them off from the railway station in Syrdarya. It must have been 1967. I remember they cried and said goodbye. But something didn't work out because they came back within a few months. Ayshe-anay never made it back to Crimea and was buried in Uzbekistan. In those years, the Tatars were trying to go back but were not allowed to settle in Crimea. Many ended up in the Kherson Oblast of Ukraine or Krasnodar Krai in Russia.

The first time we went to Crimea for vacation, I was in ninth grade, in 1977. We were shocked because everything was [available] in the shops there. Everything was cheap. Borscht with chicken at the diner cost 36 kopecks. Cheap cherries were sold everywhere. In Uzbekistan, cherries were expensive and in short supply. We could buy a whole wheel of cheese. Eating cheese with bread every morning was a luxury we couldn't afford in Uzbekistan. Probably, Crimea was supplied differently because it was a resort destination.

We went to Bakhchisarai, and it was the beginning of June. Everything was in bloom. The lavender fields and poppy fields were beautiful. My mother said, "Look how beautiful it is; the Tatars lived here. They took everything away from us".

When we went on excursions, my mother always got mad. The guides always said that Turkic people and Greeks lived here, but they never mentioned Crimean Tatars at any point. Of course, that made her angry. But she didn't argue with them; it was not acceptable then. She told us her ancestors had lived there, that we Crimean Tatars had always lived there, and that what they said wasn't true.

We decided to move back to Crimea in 1990. At the time, everyone was going, and the events with the Meskhetian Turks in 1989 provided an additional push. The neighbours living on either side of my mother-in-law were Meskhetian Turks. Their wives used to make flatbread in a tandir [a special oven], while my son played with their kids. In the spring of 1989, there were events in Namangan – local disputes and fights between Uzbeks and Meskhetian Turks. Then the Uzbeks started to kick out the Meshetian Turks deliberately and set their houses on fire.

In our village [in Uzbekistan], the Uzbeks filled a whole truck with stones, and someone pointed out where the Turks lived. They drove slowly down the street and started to throw stones at the Turks' houses. There was a loud banging. They threw stones at the windows and roof shingles, and I woke up from the loud noise. I was scared. My husband Bakhtiyar grabbed a knife, which he had under the pillow. I told him, "Please don't go". Of course, everyone was afraid for their own life. I think he didn't leave the courtyard. When they drove to the next house to throw the stones, someone [in it] had a shotgun and fired it, killing one of the Uzbeks. The next day, the whole village was cordoned off by the police and internal troops.

They all knew each other, and Bakhtiyar knew all of them: the one who was killed and the one who shot the gun. They all lived together for many years and went to the same school. And they had done it anyway. By human standards, I don't even know what to call it. It was a stab in the back. Our neighbours had to leave and had to hide at their relatives' places first. Many years later, they came to visit us here in Crimea. Some of them immigrated to the USA, some settled in the Krasnodar Krai, and some settled in Kherson – [they ended up] all over the world.

We thought that it could happen to Crimean Tatars as well, because we, too, were a minority. If they started to kick out the Turks, then they could do the same to the Tatars. That's why the following year, in autumn, we moved.

We weren't the first to move, and we weren't going to an empty place. We knew that there was already a house in Berezovka that we would move into. We sent a container there, and our relatives had already been living there for almost a year.

Emine Ziyatdinova (Author)

I had always thought of Crimea as a place to recharge and return to when things got tough, but in 2014, that all changed within just one month. The ground beneath my feet felt like it was cracking, and it took me years to redefine what home meant for me.

As a journalist, I covered the annexation of Crimea by the Russian Federation in 2014. On the evening of 16 March, my Danish colleagues and I were stationed at Lenin Square in Simferopol, where the local pro-Russian government organised a concert and celebration for the upcoming illegitimate polling result, which they called a 'referendum'. There were no sane people in the square; those who had never believed they could change anything played their roles in the Russian performance and were rewarded with entitlement.

We finished the final live broadcast at 11 o'clock in the evening. A barely standing, intoxicated woman with straight blonde hair and a sense of privilege wanted to be on camera. The crowd chanted, "Crimea – Russia – Forever!" I had to deal with her, explaining that we were finished with work and that the reporters did not speak Russian. She shouted at me and pushed me. As the Danish reporters packed up their cameras, they didn't pay any attention to me. I looked at our driver, Misha, the husband of my dear childhood friend, who was leaning against the bumper of the car and watching the whole scene with a slight smile on his face. I felt alone and surrounded by a hostile world.

I grabbed the driver's arm and said, "Misha, we're paying you. Get her away from me", and then I hid behind him. I was exhausted and ready to cry. They announced the 96.77 percent vote for joining Russia, and even though I knew this fraudulent result was coming, I was still not ready to hear it. I saw Jenya, a photographer from Kyiv and a friend, in the crowd. I wailed on his shoulder for a while, grieving the loss of my homeland.

Eight years later, in March 2022, Jenya was trapped in Mariupol as the city was being erased by Russian forces. I didn't find the strength to text him; instead, I prayed that he had someone to lean on.

Around the same time, my relatives in Crimea gathered to pray for my grandmother's soul to find peace a year after her death. It was the first day of Ramadan and over a month since the full-scale Russian invasion of Ukraine.

My mom entered the room and saw that people were talking in loud and agitated voices. The imam from the local mosque asked for donations to support wounded Russian soldiers, and one of my aunts gave a pack of pasta. My other aunt Zekie's two sons were in Kyiv living under threat of Russian missile attacks. She was angry, saying, "Why should you be giving it? I hope your children experience the same as mine".

Someone from my street in Serebryanka, whom I remember from when he was a small boy, was killed near Energodar. He probably should have known better than to sign a contract with the Russian Army. I felt sorry for his mother and grandmother. He was the only son and the only grandchild.

My Crimean Tatar neighbour, who lived across from my backyard, was taken during a raid for Russian Army mobilisation in September. He openly supported Ukraine before they forced him to join the Russian Army. The Russian Federal Security Service (FSB) had already searched his house several times before that. The last I heard from him was that he was wounded in a Russian hospital.

My brother decided to leave for Poland with his family, leaving their life behind. After five days on the road, they arrived in Warsaw, where I met them. I hugged the kids. They hadn't been told what was going on.

"Mom, we're not going back home because they could take away Dad, right?" my nephew asked.

I embraced the identity of being a 'Ukrainian Crimean Tatar' in 2004, when I was 16. That year, I moved from my home in Crimea to the Lviv Oblast to pursue my studies. Many around the university had a hard time understanding how Crimean Tatars could be 'truly' Ukrainian. Crimean Tatars can speak Ukrainian, but many thought that Muslims with Asian features did not make the cut to share the Ukrainian national identity. Back in Crimea, many believed that adopting a Ukrainian identity meant assimilation, a concept my people had resisted for years. A significant shift in perception occurred around 2014 due to the political turmoil in the country and the need to redefine Ukraine and Ukrainian identity in the face of external threats from Russia.

In 2014, the Ukrainian government finally recognised Crimean Tatars as an ethnic group indigenous to Ukraine and Crimea, after three decades of efforts by the Crimean Tatar movement to achieve this. This incorporation of our ethnic group into the macro-political discourse of the nation and statehood is an illustrative example of a shift towards perceiving Ukraine as a multicultural, multiethnic, and secular state (in contrast to the history of excluding rather than including ethnic and religious minorities). This process has become even more pronounced since the full-scale Russian invasion in 2022. The increased media representation of the Roma (as discussed in the chapter of this volume by Mykola Homanyuk and Janush Panchenko) and other ethnic and minority groups in the war effort serves a clear campaigning purpose while simultaneously legitimising, on a larger scale, the belonging of these groups to the political nation. The government's efforts to recognise the contributions of fighting the aggressor go beyond verbal statements on an individual or community level and extend to legislation, state recognitions, and making various religious services, including Muslim, Orthodox, and Protestant ones, available.

It appears that my adapted identity has now become viable and easily understood by most people around me. My friends in Kyiv and Lviv no longer question it, and it is now generally accepted in the community of Crimean Tatars displaced since 2014. However, the gap in the perception and experience of Crimean Tatars living in government-controlled Ukraine and those continuing to live under Russian occupation grows larger as the years pass. Holding a Russian passport and working for various state institutions — from schools and hospitals to government administrations and the military (including due to forced conscription) — are some survival strategies often perceived as unacceptable collaboration. The majority of Crimean Tatars still live in Crimea, and their reality is vastly different and distant from Kyiv politics.

All these processes depend on government policies. The inclusion of ethnic and other minority groups into the idea of Ukrainian statehood could potentially become fragile with changes in government policies. Additionally, there is the risk that the positive dynamics of recent years could reverse when these groups no longer play a role that the state and society perceive as contributing to the war effort and national unity. The question of whether these groups have invested enough in the national cause and Ukrainian identity could arise once again.

Bibliography

Aurélie, Campana, "Sürgün: The Crimean Tatars' Deportation and Exile", *SciencesPo*, 16 June 2008, https://www.sciencespo.fr/mass-violence-war-massacre-resistance/fr/document/suerguen-crimean-tatars-deportation-and-exile.html [accessed: 31.07.2024].

Derzhavnyi komitet statistyky Ukrainy (State Statistics Committee of Ukraine), "Vseukrainskii perepys naselennia 2001" ("The All-Ukrainian Population Census of 2001"), http://2001.ukrcensus.gov.ua/eng/results/general/nationality/ [accessed: 31.07.2024].

Fisher, Alan W., "Emigration of Muslims from the Russian Empire in the Years After the Crimean War", Jahrbücher für Geschichte Osteuropas (*Yearbooks for the His-*

tory of Eastern Europe) 35/3, 1987, 356–371, https://www.jstor.org/stable/41047947 [accessed: 31.07.2024].

Gladun, O. M., O. P. Rudnytskyi, and N. V. Kulyk, "Otsinka demografichnykh vtrat krymskotatarskoho narody vnaslidok deportatsii 1944 roku" ("Assessment of the Demographic Losses of the Crimean Tatar People as a Result of the 1944 Deportation"), *Demografiia ta sotsialna ekonomika* (*Demographics and the Social Economy*) 30/2, 2017, 11–28, https://dse.org.ua/arhcive/30/1.pdf [accessed: 31.07.2024].

National Archival Service of Ukraine, Fund N6 (R), Case N28 – Protocol 23 of the Crimean Autonomic Social Soviet Republic's NKVD Troika session from 02.12.1937, https://tsdea.archives.gov.ua/metric- books/?arch_id=39&fund_id=88&affair_id=6663#lg=1 [accessed: 31.07.2024].

Williams, Brian Glyn, "Hidden ethnocide in the Soviet Muslim borderlands: The ethnic cleansing of the Crimean Tatars", *Journal of Genocide Research* 4/3, 2002, 357–373, http://dx.doi.org/10.1080/14623520220151952 [accessed: 31.07.2024].

Wilson, Andrew, "Imagining Crimean Tatar History since 2014: Indigenous Rights, Russian Recolonisation and the New Ukrainian Narrative of Cooperation", *Europe–Asia Studies* 73/5, 2021, 837–868, https://www.tandfonline.com/doi/full/10.1080/09668136.2020.1867709 [accessed: 31.07.2024].

Militarised Cancer

People with a Diagnosis and the War in Ukraine

Olha Labur

War is an extraordinary and powerful event in a person's life. It changes destinies, evokes feelings of helplessness and doom, and brings suffering and death. War militarises lives, languages, and everyday experiences – even disease becomes a metaphorical image for war. When we talk about something dangerous or threatening, we often use such metaphors. Metaphors of war have also long penetrated the world of cancer, for instance with the so-called 'war on cancer'. The term's history closely intertwines with a speech given by American President Richard Nixon in 1971.[1] For the first time, a war on cancer was declared on an official level and a law was passed to create a network of research centres to investigate the disease. The aim was to turn cancer into an illness from which one was able to recover. The efforts of many researchers and government support led to positive results. Mortality from the disease decreased, but in public discourse, the term 'war on cancer' remained. The militarised vocabulary of the struggle and battle for life refers to those who 'won' or 'lost' against the disease, whether they are celebrities or ordinary people. A quick Google search for 'war on cancer' leads to many articles about the medical and social aspects of this 'war', a discourse on 'winners' or 'losers', and the 'battles' of doctors and patients against the sickness.[2] There are also calls from treating doctors to abandon the use of 'war on cancer' and apply the more neutral expression 'recovery from cancer', or to say that "we are 'living with cancer' for as long and as well as we can".[3]

---

1 National Cancer Institute, U.S. National Institute of Health, "Milestone (1971). National Cancer Act of 1971", https://dtp.cancer.gov/timeline/noflash/milestones/m4_nixon.htm [accessed: 29.07.2024].

2 Jonathan M. Chestnut et al., "Waging War on War Metaphors in Cancer and COVID-19", *JCO Oncology Practice* 16/10, 2020, 627–628, https://ascopubs.org/doi/full/10.1200/OP.20.00542 [accessed: 29.07.2024]; and Vincent T. DeVita Jr., "The 'War on Cancer' and its impact", *Nature Clinical Practice Oncology* 1/55, 2004, 55, https://doi.org/10.1038/ncponc0036 [accessed: 13.04.2024].

3 Young-Joon Surh, "The 50-Year War on Cancer Revisited: Should We Continue to Fight the Enemy Within?", *Journal of Cancer Prevention* 26(4), 2021, 219–223, here 221,

However, what happens to this militarised language during a real war? To offer one answer to this question, I look at Ukraine's experience since 24 February 2022, when Russia began the invasion of its territory. Tracking the connection between the 'real war' and the 'war on cancer' in digital media can help us see certain trends that have been emerging since the first days of the war. Militarised language in connection to cancer was not widely represented in the media or broader public discussions in Ukraine before the war and only appeared during it. At least, I could not find any earlier articles that used the words 'war', 'fight', 'confrontation', or 'battle'. Up until 2022, articles described the current treatment situation,[4] the state of international clinical trials, and the plan for National Cancer Control Strategy.[5] With the outbreak of the war, however, the situation began to change, and both vocabularies (of the war itself and the war on cancer) began to resonate and grow in the media. Meanwhile, since 24 February 2022, the physical destruction of medical infrastructure and the disruption of the usual system of cancer care have become real battles for survival.

This research aims to identify the changes and new processes that have been taking place in the oncological system of Ukraine since the Russian invasion on 24 February 2022. The focus is on large-scale phenomena such as the militarisation of mass media language in the spheres of oncology, the military experiences of patients and doctors, and the exodus of female cancer patients to other countries. 24 February 2022 created a considerable chasm in the lives and treatment of patients before and after this date, and became a point of complication in the provision of medical services to cancer patients; it also caused tectonic rifts in the entire oncological sphere of Ukraine. To understand how the situation changed and by what margin, I have conducted 'desk research'.[6] I collected, organised, and analysed data available on open information sources (e.g., online media, open Facebook pages, Telegram channels, etc.).

As a result, I identified numerous cases of using military/war-related markers in stories about cancer treatment during the war, showing that militarisation of language occurred in discussions of cancer. In this militarisation process, war subtly invades society and relations between people, enters culture, and forms militarised

---

doi: 10.15430/JCP.2021.26.4.219. https://www.ncbi.nlm.nih.gov/pmc/articles/PMC8749321/ [accessed 29.07.2024].

4 Apteka.ua (Pharmacy.ua), "Onkolohiya–2021: sohodennia ta perspektyvy rozvytku" ("Oncology – 2021: The Present and Prospects for Development"), no. 5 (1276), 08 February 2021, https://www.apteka.ua/article/582977 [accessed: 29.07.2024].

5 A.P. Beznosenko, "Onkologiya v Ukraine: itogi 2021 goda" ("Oncology in Ukraine: The Results of 2021"), *Health.ua.com*, 20 June 2022, https://health-ua.com/article/69965-onkologya-vukran-pdsumki-2021roku [accessed: 29.07.2024].

6 Midas PR Group, "Desk Research: How It Works and Why It's Your Key to Success", 30 October 2018, https://www.midas-pr.com/desk-research-works-key-success/ [access: 13.04.2024].

behaviours, thoughts, and values.[7] An important point in my research was the fact that the militarisation of language in the media was not necessarily related to official governmental or corporate policies but manifested in society in a spontaneous and uncontrolled way. This was to be expected because of the everyday survival needs and complications of opportunities for further treatment that the full-scale war brought with it. The struggle for life at this point became more important for cancer patients and required more efforts and actions on their part to receive treatment and find new hospitals and doctors. The war created new challenges for them and pushed them to take decisive steps in finding safe places and evaluating available treatment methods.

A previously unknown tendency also started to form: cancer patients left Ukraine to seek new and more effective treatment. The scale and significance of this process allow it to be characterised as an unprecedented practice. Waves of medical refugees formed, and, rather than the former isolated cases of travelling abroad for treatment, this became a mass phenomenon and included the involvement of governmental agencies (in particular, in the medical evacuation of patients that started in the summer of 2022). This process does not have an endpoint and continues as long as the war lasts. To understand the reasons, nuances, and depth of this medical exodus, I conducted individual interviews with women who have cancer. Through these interviews, I collected the first testimonies from cancer patients who decided to seek treatment abroad without relying on anyone's help in the first months of the full-scale invasion of Ukraine. Later, this information started to emerge on social media, where refugee women were exchanging experiences concerning treatment abroad in different European countries. Thus, an opportunity to extend the research coverage by studying new information sources appeared. For this, I used the methods of data organisation and logical comparative analysis of data in a historical context.

Still, it is necessary to emphasise the limitations that manifested themselves in this research. To a considerable degree, this study depends on the length and outcome of the war. Additionally, to understand the situation of the refugees, extended interviews need to be conducted with a larger number of respondents. New facts that might be uncovered this way could identify a broader spectrum of the cancer patient exodus, the phenomenon of cancer refugees, and the positive and negative nuances and consequences of these processes. However, the incompleteness of this research should be an incentive to continue and extend the circle of researchers, rep-

7 Roberto J. González, *Militarizing Culture: Essays on the Warfare State*, New York: Routledge, 2010; and Richard H. Kohn, "Using the Military at Home: Yesterday, Today, and Tomorrow", *Chicago Journal of International Law* 4/1, 2003, 165–192, https://chicagounbound.uchicago.edu/cjil/vol4/iss1/12 [accessed: 29.07.2024].

resentatives of the patient community, and other parties who are interested and engaged.

The Conditions of Oncological Treatment in Ukraine on the Eve of the War

The scale of the destruction and the critical state of Ukraine's cancer system in the first months of the war become clear when compared to the prewar period. Up until 24 February 2022, there were 1.3 million cancer patients in Ukraine, a country with a population of 44 million. Over the past 10 years, the incidence rate has increased by almost 35. Every year, there are about 160,000–180,000 new cases. Moreover, more than half of them are residents of Eastern Ukraine,[8] where fighting is now actively underway.[9] The last two pandemic years slowed down the usual rhythm of cancer detection and treatment. The number of newly discovered cases and deaths decreased. Doctors expected a boom of newly diagnosed patients in the post pandemic years (2022–2023), with most of them in the last stages of the disease.[10] Many doctors and managers were ready to implement changes that would improve the cancer situation. In particular, the agenda included an increase in funding for the medical guarantees programme and a transition to a new prevention and treatment practice. To modernise healthcare, the construction of a new oncology centre with the latest technologies was planned in Kharkiv for 2022.[11] It would have been a stronghold for aiding several eastern regions simultaneously.

---

8 Denis Krasnikov and Victoria Martyniuk, "Skhidna Ukraina poterpaie vid raku bilshe, nizh Zakhidna, i zavody – ne holovnyi faktor. Shcho kazhe statystyka" ("Eastern Ukraine Suffers from Cancer More Than Western Ukraine, and Factories Are Not the Main Factor: What the Statistics Say"), *Forbes*, 05 November 2021, https://forbes.ua/lifestyle/vostochnaya-ukraina-stradaet-ot-raka-bolshe-zapadnoy-i-zavody-ne-glavnyy-faktor-chto-govorit-statistika-05112021-2729 [accessed: 29.07.2024].

9 Ukrainian Ministry of Health, "Shist bezoplatnykh doslidzhen dlia rannoho vyiavlennia onkolohii" ("Six Free Tests for Early Detection of Cancer"), 08 June 2022, https://moz.gov.ua/article/news/shist-bezoplatnih-doslidzhen-dlja-rannogo-vijavlennja-onkologii [accessed: 29.07.2024].

10 Priamyi (Direct), "V Ukraini diiut shist obstezhen dlia vyiavlennia onkolohichnykh zakhvoriuvan – MOZ" ("Six Examinations for Detecting Cancer in Ukraine – Ministry of Health"), 08 June 2022, https://prm.ua/v-ukraini-diiut-shist-obstezhen-dlia-vyiavlennia-onkolohichnykh-zakhvoriuvan-moz/ [accessed: 29.07.2024].

11 UNIAN: Informatsiine ahenstvo (UNIAN: Information Agency), "'Velyke budivnytstvo': u Kharkovi ziavytsia novyi onkotsentr na pivtysiachi lizhok" ("'Big Construction': A New Oncology Centre with Five Hundred Beds to Be Built in Kharkiv"), 07 February 2022, https://www.unian.ua/health/velike-budivnictvo-u-harkovi-z-yavitsya-noviy-onkocentr-na-piv-tisyachi-lizhok-novini-harkova-11696071.html [accessed: 29.07.2024].

The COVID-19 pandemic and various quarantine events coincided with the second stage of the medical reform. The plan was to shift the entire secondary chain of medical institutions, including oncological ones, to being financed by the National Health Service of Ukraine, but the pandemic prevented it. According to this plan, each oncological communal institution was supposed to receive several times higher funds for the treatment of patients compared to what they had been allocated through subventions from 2018 to 2020.[12] From 2020 to 2022, the total financing almost tripled.[13] This meant better access to free medication and early diagnostics of cancer. Additionally, there were international randomised controlled trials, grants, partnership programmes, and projects. In Ternopil, for example, owing to the Together for Ukraine Foundation and Radiologists without Borders – US charity organisations connected to the Ukrainian diaspora – a free modern mammalogy office was opened. Women now had the opportunity to undergo a free examination using the Selenia Dimensions Mammography System, powerful and innovative digital equipment.[14] Initiated by the company MSD, the first immune-oncology medication in Ukraine was registered.[15] The words of the Director of the Sumy Oncological Dispensary, Volodymyr Shevchenko, seem fair: "[T]his is not just new equipment, this is a new epoch in treatment".[16]

12 Anna Levchenko, "Dytyacha onkolohiya ta patsiyenty z vazhkymy suputnimy patolohiyamy dosi ye prerohatyvoyu derzhavnykh klinik – holovnyy likar NIR" ("Paediatric Oncology and Patients with Severe Comorbidities Are Still the Prerogative of State Clinics – Chief Medical Officer of the NIR"), *Interfax-Ukraina: Informatsiine ahenstvo (Interfax-Ukraine: Information Agency)*, 04 February 22, https://interfax.com.ua/news/interview/796147.html [accessed: 29.07.2024].

13 Daria Kolomiets, "Kinsha Daria. Yak likuyut onkologiu v Ukraini ta skilky na tse vydiliaye hroshey derzhava — vdipovidaie MOZ" ("How Oncology Is Treated in Ukraine and How Much Money the State Allocates for It – The Ministry of Health Answers"), *Suspilne novyny (Public News)*, 04 February 2022, https://suspilne.media/203940-ak-likuut-onkologicni-zahvoruvanna-v-ukraini-ta-skilki-na-ce-vidilae-grosej-derzava/ [accessed: 29.07.2024].

14 Nataliia Burlaku, "Rak u zhinok. Shcho povinna robiti kozhna z nas, aby zhiti?" ("Cancer In Women: What Should Each of Us Do to Live?"), *20 Khvylyn, Ternopil (20 Minutes, Ternopil)*, 04 February 2023, https://te.20minut.ua/Zdorovya/kozhna-z-nas-mozhe-zahvoriti-yak-u-ternopoli-pid-chas-viyni-likuyut-ra-11691867.html [accessed: 29.07.2024].

15 Iryna Bondarchuk, "Nova era likuvannya raku vzhe v Ukrayini" ("A New Era of Cancer Treatment Is Already in Ukraine"), *Ukrayinskiiy medichniiy zhurnal* 1/117, 2017, https://www.umj.com.ua/article/105350/nova-era-likuvannya-raku-vzhe-v-ukrayini [accessed: 29.07.2024].

16 Nataliia Kalinichenko, "'Popry viynu, onkokhvori mayut otrimaty yakisnu medychnu dopomohu'" ("'Despite the war, cancer patients should receive quality medical care'"), *Uryadoviiy kuryer (Government Courier)*, 23 July 2022, https://ukurier.gov.ua/uk/articles/popri-vijnu-onkohvori-mayut-otrimuvati-yakisnu-med/ [accessed: 29.07.2024] [author's trans.].

Oncology in Ukraine had a practice of diagnosing and treating oncological diseases, was integrated into international programmes and standards, and, on the eve of the war, was on the brink of medical reform. However, compared to other European countries, the Ukrainian oncological service had worse base indexes for cancer diagnostics and treatment. Based on the data from the European Federation of Pharmaceutical Industries and Associations (EFPIA), they were 2–2.5 times lower.[17] Ukraine required further reform and changes in the diagnostics and treatment of cancer. But the war nullified these plans, as well as the general availability of timely treatment and assistance. Many people had to stop cancer treatment and care. There are thousands of such cases, and each person faces the decision of what to do instead.

The New Reality: An Outside Perspective

Russia's invasion of Ukraine on 24 February 2022 drew the attention of many people internationally, including oncologists. With the participation of the European Cancer Organisation and the American Society of Clinical Oncology (ASCO), the Special Network on the Impact of the War in Ukraine on Cancer was created. It incorporated 300 organisations and five general meetings were conducted in 2022.[18] At the first meeting, on 10 May 2022, it was declared that "Ukrainian cancer patients, and their care, have been drastically impacted by Russia's invasion".[19] Among the identified key points were bombardments, destruction of critical infrastructure, mass relocations of patients, and other factors. This network's main tasks are now monitoring and analysing the situation in Ukraine, and creating effective assistance mechanisms. The United Nations, EFPIA, and other medical organisations around the world also expressed deep concern and condemnation.[20]

Analytical articles about the increasing rate of threatening phenomena in the oncology of Ukraine also began to emerge. One of the first was a study by an anony-

---

17 European Federation of Pharmaceutical Industries and Associations (EFPIA), *The Impact of the War in Ukraine on Oncology Patients: Overview and recommendations for European and Ukrainian health authorities and policymakers*, report, 2022, https://www.efpia.eu/media/677256/the-impact-of-the-war-in-ukraine-on-oncology-patients.pdf [accessed: 29.07.2024].

18 European Cancer Organisation, "ECO-ASCO Special Network: Impact of the War in Ukraine on Cancer", 04 June 2022, https://www.europeancancer.org/topic-networks/20:impact-war-in-ukraine-on-cancer.html [accessed: 29.07.2024].

19 European Cancer Organisation, "ECO Statements on Ukraine", 10 May 2022, https://www.europeancancer.org/resources/246:eco-statement-of-support-for-ukraine.html [accessed: 29.07.2024].

20 European Federation of Pharmaceutical Industries and Associations (EFPIA), *The Impact of the War in Ukraine on Oncology Patients.*

mous author, "Russia's war in Ukraine is killing cancer care in both countries". It was published in English by the online media outlet of the peer-reviewed medical magazine *The BMJ* and details the rapid militarisation of the oncological community. The author writes that "the prognosis for cancer patients and survivors is getting darker by the day".[21] The article's title presents a figurative and associative comparison of the oncological system with the combat space. Both have frontlines with killing, casualties, the wounded, and an enemy that brings destruction and extermination. That is, through metaphors of war, the anonymous author identified threats to and casualties among cancer patients and doctors, as well as the destruction of hospitals and violations of procedures and treatment systems.[22] Reading it, I understood the author's motives for anonymity. I assume they were familiar with oncology, especially in Russia. With the possibility of prosecution (or punishment) for using the words "Russia's war in Ukraine" and "killing cancer care", the author was forced to remain anonymous. Nonetheless, they tried to be objective in the text and assess the situation in the oncological system in Ukraine. Notably, this article appeared on 23 March 2022, less than a month after the full-scale invasion of Ukraine. It was a prompt response to the dangers that the field of oncology in Ukraine has been facing. It is worth noting that the anonymous author themself used militarised language to explain the current situation.

A representative of the Royal College of London, Richard Sullivan, went even further in his assessment of the situation of oncological services in Ukraine. He suggested that the situation with cancer care is more complicated than in previous wars in Syria, Afghanistan, or Palestine: "One of these differences is the sheer volume of cancer care required for the Ukrainian population".[23] Sullivan was convinced that before the war, Ukraine had a well-developed system of cancer treatment, unlike many other countries affected by conflicts. For this reason, the quick destruction of infrastructure, including hospitals, and dangerous travels for patients and medics became a serious challenge during the war. He wrote that the oncology system can become a de facto 'second front' of the war, one terrible and dangerous, which will require emergency measures and considerable efforts.

Opinions like this are also developed in the article "The War in Ukraine and Cancer Patients: Early Experiences from the Frontline" by Peter McIntyre, written by

21 Anonymous, "Russia's war in Ukraine is killing cancer care in both countries", *The BMJ*, 23 March 2022, https://doi.org/10.1136/bmj.o701 [accessed: 29.07.2024].

22 Ibid.

23 Richard Sullivan, "What impact does war have on Ukrainian cancer care?", *King's College London*, 29 April 2022, https://www.kcl.ac.uk/what-impact-does-war-have-on-ukrainian-cancer-care [accessed: 29.07.2024].

the independent journalist with support from Richard Sullivan.[24] This report details how the cancer community responded to the challenges of delivering cancer care in the first three to four months of the Russian invasion. Drawing on witness testimonies, the author sought to capture the lived reality. He pointed out that people living with cancer were thrown into a state of great anxiety, separated from their clinical teams and even their medical records. According to the estimates of experts, in the first two months of the war, the number of cancer patients in Ukraine receiving surgery, chemotherapy, or radiotherapy was halved. People living with cancer felt that lifesaving treatments and care were available only at great risk. Some warehouses with medications were captured along with the occupied territories, medicine procurement logistics were disrupted, and the threat of the destruction or looting of those warehouses became real. Over 1 million people diagnosed with cancer found themselves in an extremely complicated survival situation.

Such assessments by foreign specialists coincided with the declaration of Ukrainian President Volodymyr Zelenskyy about the "complete stoppage of cancer patient treatment"[25] in the first months of the war. 'Complete stoppage' meant the disruption of the entire cycle and system of providing cancer treatment and care, with hospitals standing, partially or completely destroyed, without patients and doctors. This is the reality of war: when everything is being shelled, patients and doctors are evacuated, and all planned operations are cancelled. A considerable number of patients moved to Western Ukraine and to neighbouring European countries. The scale and urgency of the situation in the oncological sphere in Ukraine after 24 February 2022 caused a global feeling of concern in the European and international oncological community, creating a need for an effective and rapid response and the consolidation of efforts. To guarantee the uninterrupted treatment of Ukrainian children with cancer, they were evacuated to neighbouring European countries, and starting in the summer of 2022, an intergovernmental programme to evacuate adult patients began as well. Within this framework of supporting Ukrainian refugees, free oncological help was also provided. To the extent that it was possible, technical and legal barriers to patient transfers to a new host country were eliminated.

---

24 Peter McIntyre, "The war in Ukraine and cancer patients: Early experiences from the frontline", *eCancer*, 22 September 2022, https://ecancer.org/en/news/22234-the-war-in-ukraine-and-cancer-patients-early-experiences-from-the-frontline [accessed: 29.07.2024].

25 Olha Demianchuk, "V Ukraini prypyneno likuvannia khvorykh n arak – Zelenskyi" ("Zelenskyy: Treatment of Cancer Patients Stopped in Ukraine"), *Korespondent.Net* (*Correspondent.Net*), 06 May 2022, https://ua.korrespondent.net/ukraine/4475561-v-ukraini-prypyneno-likuvannia-khvorykh-na-rak-zelenskyi [accessed: 29.07.2024] [author's trans.].

Two Wars, Two Fronts: The Militarisation of the Cancer-Related Media Space of Ukraine

The first Ukrainian publications comparing war and cancer appeared in March 2022, less than a month after the start of the war. *BBC News Ukraine* published an article about children with cancer.[26] One of the subheadings read, "They [the young patients] are fighting two wars". The author of the article quotes paediatric oncologist Roman Kazym, who is "very angry about what happened [with Russia's attack on Ukraine]" and regrets that "now these children fight two wars – one with cancer, the other with Russia".[27] Another article appeared in *The Village*, in which the author talks about the experiences of different people who are "fighting cancer during the war".[28] She relates the experiences of 17 people who already had or learnt about a cancer diagnosis on the eve of the war. These are short stories, and each describes treatment in the new reality. The article presents the war as an event that complicated treatment and made the 'fight' more difficult. The words of one of the authors – that the war deprived her of "a chance to fight the disease" – sound like a verdict for many people in Ukraine who were diagnosed with cancer.[29]

The Ukrainian information space reacted quickly to the situation of the oncology system after the invasion on 24 February 2022. Articles about war and cancer began to appear sporadically at first and then regularly, and the platforms ranged from local and regional media to national and official newspapers. These digital publications of differing status, purpose, and scope of distribution raise the issue of cancer in their discussion of the war. The only component that unites them is the use of military vocabulary and cancer. Frequently, they use phrases such as 'second war', 'second front', 'war squared', and 'two wars'. Eventually, journalists themselves began to acknowledge that "the media often call cancer the second front of the war".[30]

26 Filippa Roksbi, "Yak riatuiut vid viiny khvorykh na rak ukrainskykh ditei" ("How Ukrainian Children with Cancer Are Being Saved from War"), *BBC News Ukraine*, 26 March 2022, https://www.bbc.com/ukrainian/features-60880184 [accessed: 29.07.2024].

27 Ibid. [author's trans.].

28 Viktoriia Kudryashova, "Tse liudy, iaki boriutsia z rakom pid chas viiny" ("These Are People Who Are Fighting Cancer During the War"), *The Village*, 3 June 2022, https://www.the-village.com.ua/village/knowledge/practice/326609-rak-i-viyna [accessed: 29.07.2024] [author's trans.].

29 Ibid.

30 Maryna Stepanenko, "Dumaty pro maibutnie zaraz: ekspert MOZ Ukrainy pro zapobihannia epidemii raku psilia viyny" ("Thinking about the Future Now: Expert of the Ministry of Health of Ukraine on Preventing the Epidemic of Brain Cancer"), *RFI-Ukraina*, 30 March 2023, https://www.rfi.fr/uk/%D1%83%D0%BA%D1%80%D0%B0%D1%97%D0%BD% 0%B0/20230330 [accessed: 15.04.2024] [author's trans.].

That is, for more than a year, war metaphors in cancer news were organic and unchanged.

Terribly, in the current Russo–Ukrainian War there have also been unexpected losses of doctors. This occurred not just on battlefields, where doctors were mobilised to the Armed Forces of Ukraine (AFU), but also from the Russian bombing and shelling of peaceful Ukrainian cities. These losses became a tragic part of the newly created information space about cancer and war. For example, during the shelling of Kyiv, Oksana Leontieva died on the way to the Okhmatdyt hospital, where she worked in the bone marrow transplant department for 11 years and treated children with blood cancer.[31] Taras Gavrilenko, an oncological surgeon at the Zaporizhzhia Regional Antitumor Center, was killed during rocket attacks on Zaporizhzhia.[32] The same fate befell Yevhenii Lutsenko, a young and promising oncological-thoracic surgeon at the Chernihiv Medical Center of Modern Oncology.[33] All this brings to mind the words of Hryhoriy Klymniuk, a children's oncologist at the National Cancer Institute: "[O]vercoming cancer in military conditions is almost a [death] sentence".[34] This is difficult to read, considering that every oncologist saves hundreds and thousands of lives, especially when knowing that thousands of people who are ill in Ukraine still hope to recover. The scale of the disaster, as stressed by Sullivan when he writes of "the huge amount of cancer care that Ukrainians need",[35] is evident.

---

31 Marina Petik, "Vid udaru rosiiskoi rakety ii mashyna spalakhnula, iak sirnyk: y Kyevi zahynula likara Okhmatdytu, sin zalyshvsia syrotoiu" ("A Russian Missile Hit Her Car Like a Match: A Doctor From the Kyiv Regional Medical Centre Was Killed and Her Son Was Left an Orphan"), *Obozrevatel* (*Observer*), 12 October 2022, https://news.obozrevatel.com/ukr/society/vid-udaru-rosijskoi-raketi-ii-mashina-spalahnula-yak-sirnik-u-kievi-zaginula-likar-ohmatdita.html [accessed: 15.04.2024].

32 Alyona Katashinska, "Zhertoviu raketnoho udaru u Zaporizhzhi stav vidmoii khirurg-onkolog" ("Famous Oncological Surgeon Becomes Victim of Missile Attack in Zaporizhzhia"), *Komsomolskaia Pravda in Ukraine*, 13 October 2022, https://kp.ua/ua/incidents/a657652-zhertvoju-raketnoho-udaru-u-zaporizhzhi-stav-vidomij-khirurh-onkoloh [accessed: 29.07.2024].

33 Galina King, "Likari Chernihova: Evhenii Lutsenko ikhav u mikroavtobusi, iakii obstriliali rosiis'ki neliudi" ("Doctors in Chernihiv: Yevheniy Lutsenko Was in a Minibus When It Was Fired Upon by Russian Proxies"), *Chernihiv.City*, 19 September 2022, https://chernihiv.city/articles/234585/yevgenij-lucenko-3-misyaci-vvazhavsya-bezvisti-zniklim [accessed: 15.04.2024].

34 Nataliia Buzhinetska, "Dolatu rak u voennykh umovakh – maizhe vyrok: istorii evakuatsii onkokhvorikh ditei z Ukrainy" ("Overcoming Cancer in Wartime Is Almost a Sentence: Stories of the Evacuation of Children with Cancer from Ukraine"), *Ukrayinska Pravda* (*Ukrainian Truth*), 08 April 2022, https://life.pravda.com.ua/health/2022/04/8/248153/ [accessed: 29.07.2024] [author's trans.].

35 Sullivan, "What impact does war have on Ukrainian cancer care?".

There have also been changes in the rhetoric of the patients themselves, who described their stories to journalists. They began to talk about undergoing treatment during the war as a heroic deed, about medical personnel as heroes, and about themselves as 'winners' in the war. They used metaphors of 'heroism' to describe the process of undergoing chemotherapy: "heroic" eight hours of waiting in line for an appointment or hunting for medicine and medical instruments.[36] From the occupied territories, patients added to the theme of 'heroism' descriptions of how they managed to get to and inside medical institutions: "[we] stood under the scorching sun for four hours", "it was necessary to sail by boat to get treatment", or "I will never forget how we drove under shelling and how [they] inserted a catheter for 30 minutes, also under fire".[37] Journalists also contributed to this idea of heroism in their comments: "They are used to fighting, but now they are forced to battle on two fronts".[38] This use of the military metaphors 'fighting' and 'two fronts' emphasises and enhances the importance of survival, turning the healing process into a frontline of war. War and cancer treatment become close in their significance and semantic content. Sometimes, patients and their loved ones took the stress of war as an incentive for recovery: "Due to an emergency, patients recovered 3–4 times faster".[39]

The articles are set in a combat space where there are literal and metaphorical enemies, defence forces, and military tasks. For example, one article includes the phrases "I stood in line for chemotherapy for seven hours" and "the only chance to survive is to go abroad".[40] These words point to 'winning' under circumstances and difficulties that arose in the war. In addition, for successful conduct during the war, new military tactics, methods, and circumstances of treatment are needed. Even doctors and organisations that support cancer patients have switched to military rhetoric: "One war [was] with cancer, the second – in Ukraine. It was sheer despair", recalls Olena Semenyuk, coordinator of the support programme of the Tabletochki

36 Kudryashova, "Tse liudy, iaki boriutsia z rakom pid chas viiny".

37 Ibid.

38 Anastasia Loza, "'Rak ne chekae na zaverwhennia viiny', – iak boriutsa za zhyttia onkokhvori z Chernihivshchyny" ("'Cancer Does Not Wait for the End of the War' – How Cancer Patients from the Chernihiv Oblast Fight for Their Lives"), *Suspilne novyny* (*Public News*), 03 April 2022, https://suspilne.media/224627-rak-ne-cekae-na-zaversenna-vijni-ak-borutsa-za-zitta-onkohvori-z-cernigivsini/ [accessed: 29.07.2024] [author's trans.].

39 Tetyana Venglinska, "Fighting Disease During the War: A Story of a Cancer Patient", *UkraineWorld*, 12 September 2022, https://ukraineworld.org/articles/stories/story-cancer-patient [accessed: 29.07.2024] [author's trans.].

40 Inesa Matyushenko and Olga Syrotyuk, "Viina v kvadrati: shansy dlia onkopatsientiv na vyzhyvannia" ("War Squared: Chances for Cancer Patients to Survive"), *Hromadske*, 02 October 2022, https://hromadske.ua/posts/vijna-v-kvadrati-shansi-dlya-onkopaciyentiv-na-vizhivannya [accessed: 29.07.2024] [author's trans.].

Charitable Foundation, about the first months of the war.[41] Readers get the impression that new operational bases are formed from patient communities and charities, which seem to take command of the 'oncological front'. Moreover, the use of military vocabulary appears naturally. In times of war, militarised metaphors are part of everyday life. People start to compare the world around them to war and use military metaphors.

Nevertheless, their stories carry despair, fatalism, and a feeling of helplessness. Patients talked about going to places where there are doctors, hospitals, medicine, and equipment as their only chance of being saved – that is, either to Western Ukraine or abroad. They described their search for treatment as more difficult, exhausting, and destructive now: "[My] panic attacks started from fear about where and how to be treated now, and [I] lost six kilogrammes in a week because of this".[42] Others believed that the only chance to survive was to travel abroad.[43] People were frightened by an uncertain future, the fate of abandoned homes, and the difficult pursuit of survival. By telling such stories, they reinforced the devastating aspects of the war, showing themselves as its unjust victims. Only later, when they managed to improve their situation, they felt calmer about themselves, their lives, and their experiences.[44] The hope for survival is full of references to treatment abroad. Nevertheless, there are few such statements among the patient stories in Ukrainian online publications. The life experiences of those going abroad are mostly represented on social networks.

Articles about the initiatives of some patients, charitable organisations, and volunteers are unexpected and inspiring. They allowed cancer patients to navigate extremely difficult conditions and helped them make important decisions. Above all, the activities of two Ukrainian organisations aided cancer patients even before the war. These are the charitable foundation Inspiration Family and the patient organisation Athena: Women Against Cancer. Both were created by people who themselves once faced this disease. The war greatly changed their activities, forced them to respond quickly to challenges, and turned them into important agents of influence. In

---

41 Lina Krivoruchko, "Rak ne znae, shcho die velyka vijina: istorii medykiv ta volonteriv, iaki boriutsia za zhyttia onkokhvorykh ditei" ("Cancer Does not Know That There is a Great War: Stories of Doctors and Volunteers Fighting for the Lives of Children with Cancer), *Ukrayinska Pravda* (*Ukrainian Truth*), 03 September 2022, https: life.pravda.com.ua/health/2022/09/3/250299/ [accessed: 15.04.2024] [author's trans.].

42 Vita Sakhnik, "Koly u tebe dvi viiny. Iak onkokhvori znakhodiat prykhystok na Volyni" ("When You Have Two Wars: How Cancer Patients Find Refuge In Volyn"), *Pershii Kanal Sotsialnykh Novyn* (*First Social News Channel*), 12 March 2022, https://pershyj.com/p-koli-u-tebe-dvi-viini-yak-onkohvori-znahodyat-prihistok-na-volini-56128 [accessed: 29.07.2024] [author's trans.].

43 Matyushenko and Syrotyuk, "Viina v kvadrati".

44 Venglinska, "Fighting Disease During the War".

the first three months of the war, they received more than 3,000 appeals from cancer patients. According to Anna Uzlova, the head of Inspiration Family, "[T]he first week was psychological hell. I just sat at the computer and kept answering questions. The number of requests was tearing me apart".[45] The members of the organisation say that many people turned to them for help with finding doctors, medication, and money. Later, they organised a network of free online consultations with oncologists and created Telegram groups, Facebook pages, and Instagram posts. They provided information about the Contact Centre of the Ministry of Health of Ukraine, the possibility of obtaining treatment and residence in Western Ukraine, and the availability of oncological drugs. A new feature of their information campaigns was the possibility of treatment abroad. There was information about free assistance for Ukrainians through the Regina Maria Health Network in Romania, the National Cancer Institute in Lithuania, and the OmeaLife Foundation in Poland, among others. Another important area of work was collecting information about the required medication that had run out and writing letters of request for humanitarian aid to foreign manufacturers.[46]

Cancer Medicine Shortages and Refugees with Cancer

Medicine shortages are one of the most painful issues of the war. Almost half of the media reports I consulted are related to problems regarding access to medications. In the first year of the full-scale war, there was no procurement of at least 22 types of medication, the majority of which were for cancer treatment. Sometimes, there were waiting periods of two to four months for the necessary medication.[47] In an interview, Iryna Koshkina, the representative of the charity foundation Svoi, said that starting in the autumn of 2022, shortages of necessary first-line medications for chemotherapy began. According to Koshkina, these medications were out of stock in oncology centres and pharmacies. She emphasised that she had never before had

45 Nastia Ivantsiv, "'Rosiia vbyvae ne lyshe bombamy'. Iak onkopatsienty zhyvut i pomyraiut pid cahs viiny" ("'Russia Kills Not Only with Bombs': How Cancer Patients Live and Die During the War"), *LB.ua*, 20 May 2022, https://lb.ua/society/2022/05/20/517366_rosiya_vbivaie_lishe_bombami_yak.html [accessed: 29.07.2024] [author's trans.].

46 BF Inspiration family support, "Anketa na ridkisni abo spetsyfichni liky..." ("Form for rare or specific medicines"), Telegram post, 28 February 2022, https://t.me/onkosupportua/21 [accessed: 29.07.2024].

47 Natalya Helij, "Pid chas tryvog boyimosya perepadiv napruhy, bo todi mozhe vyity z ladu medychne obladnannya" ("During Alarms, We Are Afraid of Power Surges, Because then Medical Equipment Can Break Down – Oleh Duda"), *Espreso.Zahid* (*Espreso.West*), 05 February, 2023, https://zahid.espreso.tv/pid-chas-trivog-boimosya-perepadiv-naprugi-bo-todi-mozhe-viyti-z-ladu-medichne-obladnannya-oleg-duda [accessed: 29.07.2024].

to face a situation like this: "[T]he oncology chat was simply bursting with the same questions: When will it be delivered?"[48] Almost every other day, there were messages about medication (shortages, deliveries, delays) in the Telegram chats. Based on the evaluation of the patient organisation Athena, the majority of calls (amounting to 2,424 in six months) to Patients Have a Right, a cancer patient information support hotline, were about free medication and the possibility of medical evacuation abroad.

Personal stories collected on the Facebook spaces of this community also talk about the lack of medication. The Facebook page of Athena declared May 2023 'Cancer Awareness Month'. In the same post, they told the story of Nadia from the Chernihiv Oblast, who searched for medication while her area was occupied. She owes her rescue to her brother, who went through several Russian checkpoints to get the medication Nadia and another woman needed at the Chernihiv Center of Modern Oncology. She said that what he did was "unbelievable"; he risked his life to be "able to do this" under those conditions.[49] Her labelling her brother's actions as heroic is no exaggeration. At that time, Russian occupation forces besieged Chernihiv, and it remained under siege for almost 40 days. During this period, Russians killed 658 civilian residents of the oblast's capital and injured over 1,000 others.[50] Put differently, the occupiers killed 16 civilians a day. Nadia's brother's search for medicine was a dangerous quest with numerous life-threatening encounters.

Patients in the Kherson Oblast, who were occupied for a long time, also reported complications getting medication. According to their testimonies, the pharmacies had almost no medication left, so they had to get them from Kharkiv, which remained under the control of the Ukrainian government. As a result, cancer patients had to wait two months to receive medication, which is extremely dangerous for such patients. Leaving the occupied territories was even harder. For example, it took

---

48 Alla Kotliar, "Rak I viyna. Chomu v Ukrayini nemaye bazovih onkopreparativ, I koly vony zyavlyansya" ("Cancer and War: Why There Are No Basic Oncological Drugs in Ukraine, and When They Will Appear"), *ZN.UA*, 28 January 2023, https://zn.ua/ukr/HEALTH/rak-i-vijna-chomu-v-ukrajini-nemaje-bazovikh-onkopreparativ-i-koli-voni-zjavljatsja.html [accessed: 29.07.2024] [author's trans.].

49 Afina. Zhinky protiv raku (Athena: Women Against Cancer) (Facebook page), "Traven ye misiatsem obiznanosti pro melanoma…" ("May is Melanoma Awareness Month…"), Facebook post, 17 May 2023, https://m.facebook.com/story.php?story_fbid=pfbidoc5dUTg7H3w4G8HwRPrXzCWfb3AUjLyWapg3huCptvKNfFvWD2L3Xzq2jjUXwDUa1l&id=386590811758587 [accessed: 29.07.2024] [author's trans.].

50 Dobrota Valentyna, "Chernihivtsi za rik pislya okupatsiyi pyshayutsya perehodom na ukrayinsku movu i vzhe hotuyutsya do myru" ("A Year After the Occupation, the Residents of Chernihiv Are Proud to Switch to the Ukrainian Language and Are Preparing for Peace"), *TSN*, 03 April 2023, https://tsn.ua/exclusive/chernigivci-za-rik-pislya-okupaciyi-pishayutsya-perehodom-na-ukrayinsku-movu-i-vzhe-gotuyutsya-do-miru-2299600.htm [accessed: 15.04.2024].

Khrystyna from Kherson five difficult days to get to Bremen, Germany, through Crimea.[51] It took Olena from occupied Berdiansk almost the same amount of time to get to Kyiv. Olena writes that she had to get through 15 Russian checkpoints before she got to territory controlled by Ukraine.[52] Each story like this is the tale of a small victory over the complications with treatment that were caused by the Russian aggression towards Ukrainians, especially those who have cancer.

Another courageous story is that of the Head of the Cherkasy Oblast Oncological Dispensary, Viktor Paramonov, and his driver. Viktoria Romaniuk, co-founder of Athena, told this story to the information agency *UkrInform*. Risking their lives, Paramonov and his driver brought medication to their oncological centre from the occupied Kyiv Oblast – specifically, from the warehouse of the national agency Medical Procurement of Ukraine in the Kyiv Oblast, where all medicine for public procurement is stored.[53] Paramonov said, "[O]nly a truly concerned individual could do a thing like this, considering the danger that existed then".[54] And there were many other such examples in the first months of the war. Andriy Bezsonenko, an oncologist from Kyiv, did not exaggerate when he said that the "conscience and courage of Ukrainian oncologists will be recorded in world history".[55]

The medics in their interviews often emphasised that from the very start of the war, there were problems with medicine, and not only in the occupied territories. There are many stories about complications with medicine procurement in Western Ukraine, where patients and doctors from the eastern regions were evacuated. For

51 Viktoriya Melnyk, "Rak ta vijna: yak dovodytsya zhyty onkohvorym na tymchasovo okupovanyh terytoriyah" ("Cancer and War: How Cancer Patients Live in the Temporarily Occupied Territories"), *Vikna* (*Windows*), 18 September 2022, https://vikna.tv/styl-zhyttya/likuvannya-onkologiyi-na-okupovanyh-terytoriyah/ [accessed: 29.07.2024].

52 Inna Lebedenko, "Onkohvori ukrayintsi po kilka dib vybyrayutsya iz okupovanyh terytorij, schob otrymaty likuvannya, ta chasto chas vtracheno" ("Ukrainians with Cancer Take Several Days to Get Out of the Occupied Territories to Receive Treatment, But Often the Clock is Ticking"), *TSN*, 11 September 2022, https://tsn.ua/exclusive/onkohvori-ukrayinci-po-kilka-dib-vibirayutsya-iz-okupovanih-teritoriy-schob-otrimati-likuvannya-ta-chasto-chas-vtracheno-2132317.html [accessed: 29.07.2024].

53 Since 24 February 2022, many settlements in the north and west of Kyiv Oblast have been occupied. On 2 April, the Ukrainian military completely liberated the area from Russian soldiers.

54 Lyubov Baziv, "Viktoriia Romaniuk, spivzasnovnytsia HO 'Afina. Zhinky proty raku'" ("Victoria Romaniuk, Cofounder of the NGO 'Athena: Women Against Cancer'"), *Ukrinform*, 04 February 2023, https://www.ukrinform.ua/rubric-society/3665315-viktoria-romanuk-spivzasnovnica-go-afina-zinki-proti-raku.html [accessed: 29.07.2024] [author's trans.].

55 Taras Zozulynskyj, "Yak voyuyut ukrayinski onkologhy" ("How Ukrainian Oncologists are Fighting"), *Detectives. Byuro zhurnalistskih rozsliduvan* (*Detectives: Office of Journalistic Investigations*), 11 November 2022, https://detectives.org.ua/publications/iak-voiuiut-ukra-ns-k-onkologi/ [accessed: 29.07.2024] [author's trans.].

example, an oncologist from Lviv, Andriy Moskva, when recalling his experience of the first four months, admitted that "the local hospital was not prepared for such a stream of patients [increased by several times], first and foremost, due to a lack of medication". Yet the doctor has an optimistic view on resolving this problem: "Just like we have had success in reconquering each centimetre of our land, we are also constantly fighting for the lives of our people".[56] That is, the doctor compared the combat victories of the AFU to overcoming the problems that emerged in the cancer treatment system due to Russian aggression. This remark is very important in understanding the militarisation of cancer in the Russo–Ukrainian War. It shows how, during the war, the media space of oncology became full of military images. Even though the interview was published a year and a half after the start of the war in Ukraine, the military metaphors continued to maintain their associative link with cancer. A crucial feature of this comparison is not general war terminology (like enemy, battle, front, victory, weapons, violence, etc.), but a specific army, the AFU.

The well-known Ukrainian journalist Yana Osadcha, meanwhile, compared cancer with 'the second [Russian] army of the world'[57] (based on the rating of the international organisation Global Firepower[58]). In her address to Ukrainians, she emphasised that "cancer is like 'the second army of the world': only scary when

56 Diana Pidtserkovna, "Vplyv viyny na onkolohichni zakhvoryuvannya v Ukrayini: vazhlyvist profilaktychnoho ohlyadu" ("The Impact of the War on Cancer in Ukraine: The Importance of Preventive Examinations"), *Sykhiv.Media*, 25 May 2023, https://sykhiv.media/vplyv-vijny-na-zahvoryuvanist-na-rak-v-ukrayini/ [accessed: 29.07.2024] [author's trans.].

57 In the Ukrainian media, social media posts, and conversations after 24 February 2022, the phrase 'the second [Russian] army of the world' is often used. It is frequently put in quotation marks in texts or emphasised through a sarcastic tone of voice. Through this, Ukrainians convey that this expression is false. Even before the Russian invasion on 24 February, Russian media spread narratives about the strength of the Russian Army. They compared it to the US Army and identified it as one of the best. And on the eve of the invasion, another propaganda message was spread alongside this one: "reaching Kyiv in three days". However, it was not possible to do so, and as a result, the inflated grandeur of the Russian Army collapsed. Even some Russian media acknowledged the inadequacy of the praise. Since then, the phrase 'the second [Russian] army of the world' has been placed in quotation marks, highlighting its falsity and injustice. Also see: Anton Pecherskyi, "'Druha armiia svitu': chy varto nazyvaty tak viisko rashystiv" ("'The Second Army of the World': Should We Call the Ruscist Army This Way?"), *ArmiiaInform (ArmyInformation)*, 21 June 2022, https://armyinform.com.ua/2022/06/21/druga-armiya-svitu-chy-varto-nazyvaty-tak-vijsko-rashystiv/ [accessed: 29.07.2024].

58 Slovo i Dilo (Word and Deed), "Reytyng najsylnishykh armiy svitu: yake mistse posilyi Ukrayina ta rosiya" ("Ranking of the World's Strongest Armies: Where Ukraine and Russia Stand"), 06 January 2023, https://www.slovoidilo.ua/2023/01/06/novyna/svit/rejtynh-najsylnishyx-armij-svitu-yake-misce-posily-ukrayina-ta-rosiya [accessed: 29.07.2024].

unknown, and when you start to resist it, it deflates".[59] She presents a clear connection to destroying the myth of the invincibility of 'the second [Russian] army of the world', which was done by the AFU in the autumn of 2022. As Kyrylo Budanov, Head of the Main Directorate of Intelligence of the Ministry of Defence of Ukraine, said in his interview with the Polish media outlet *Virtual Poland* (*Wirtualna Polska*), Ukrainians "helped the world to bust the stories about the 'invincible Russian Army'".[60] Correspondingly, the 'incurability' of cancer can also be viewed as a myth that can be busted. Given a proper diagnosis and treatment, cancer becomes controllable and curable. Such comparisons and associations influence emotional memory, and its modulating effects are focused on victory both in the war and the struggle against cancer.

The lack of medicine, as well as their high prices, became key factors in Ukrainian cancer patients becoming refugees. In their stories, interviews, and comments, they sadly described their misadventures in search of vital and affordable medication. The Ukrainian state, based on their perceptions, was unable to help, and they could not afford such medication themselves, so going abroad became the only salvation for them. For example, Tetiana Ushakova, in a Facebook group created by Athena, called "Athena. Women against cancer – a group of mutual support for cancer patients", recalled her own quest for medication: "I needed a targeted medication. There was only one option to get it and try it – to leave. The price of it was too high for our family. Germany gave me this opportunity".[61] In their discussions in this Facebook group, women actively shared their experiences in resolving issues with medicine and treatment in Germany, Italy, Greece, Latvia, and other countries of the EU. They supported each other and advised others "to go abroad as refugees".[62] Bohdana Melnyk summarised this discussion perfectly: "[P]eople who write to you

59 Maksym Rozenko, "'Rak – vin, yak "druha armiya svitu": strashnyi, poky nevidomyi', – Osadcha pro vlasnu bitvu z Onko" ("'Cancer Is Like the "Second Army of the World": Scary, Yet Unknown' – Osadcha about Her Own Battle with Cancer"), *Radio Trek* (*Radio Track*), 05 June 2023, https://radiotrek.rv.ua/news/rak-vin-yak-druga-armiya-svitu-strashniy-lishe-poki---nevidomiy---osadcha-pro-vlasnu-bitvu-z-onko_309310.html [accessed: 29.07.2024] [author's trans.].

60 Łukasz Maziewski, "Szef wywiadu wojskowego Ukrainy: Dostrzegamy istotne zmiany wewnątrz Rosji" ("Head of Ukraine's Military Intelligence: We See Significant Changes Inside Russia"), *Wirtualna Polska: wiadomości* (*Virtual Poland: News*), 29 January 2023, https://wiadomosci.wp.pl/szef-wywiadu-wojskowego-ukrainy-dostrzegamy-istotne-zmiany-wewnatrz-rosji-6860053735013056a [accessed: 31.07.2024] [author's trans.].

61 Athena. Women against cancer, https://t.me/athena_womenagainstcancer [accessed: 31.07.2024].

62 Nataliia Chupakhina (Facebook profile), "Chy ye shche yakes likuvannia?..." ("Are there any other treatments?..."), post in Facebook group "Athena. Women against cancer – a group of mutual support for cancer patients", 08 June 2023, https://www.facebook.com/groups/247646882376950/user/100013805553987/ [accessed: 15.04.2024] [author's trans.].

are correct: we have calm, safety, and all medications are available".[63] The author singled out three key things cancer patients receive abroad: refuge from the war, undisturbed treatment, and free medication. For them, war becomes something to set aside temporarily. For this reason, their language is not saturated with military metaphors or associations with and correlations to the war, as 'the second front' is reduced to a minimum.

Unexpectedly, for cancer patients, the war became 'a window of opportunity' to access vital medication and the most modern and innovative treatments. Interviews that I conducted as part of the research group War, Migration and Memory of the Prisma Ukraïna Research Network at the Forum Transregionale Studien demonstrated how women with cancer saw this opportunity. They took it and tried to make use of it. For example, Natalia from Mykolaiv admitted that right before the war she heard from doctors that, in her case, only an expensive kind of treatment could help. Her family did not have money for this, and the government was not able to pay for her treatment. She saw treatment abroad under the status of temporary protection (based on the Temporary Protection Directive of the EU[64] and Paragraph 24[65] in Germany) as an opportunity, if not for remission, then at least for prolonging her life.[66] Similarly, Olena from Kyiv believed in better treatment conditions. She remembered that she and her husband decided that she needed to become a refugee to find treatment opportunities in Germany, in the hope that this treatment could help her enter

63 Darya Vladimirovna (Facebook profile), "U mene pytannya hto likuyetsya v Germaniyi..." ("I have a question about treatment in Germany..."), post in Facebook group "Athena. Women against cancer – a group of mutual support for cancer patients", 12 June 2023, https://www.facebook.com/groups/247646882376950/search/?q=%D0%91%D1%96%D0%B6%D0%B5%D0%BD%D1%86%D1%96 [accessed: 15.04.2024] [author's trans.].

64 European Commission, "Temporary protection", https://home-affairs.ec.europa.eu/policies/migration-and-asylum/common-european-asylum-system/temporary-protection_en [accessed: 31.07.2024].

65 During the war, refugees from Ukraine are entitled to temporary protection in the EU under the Temporary Protection Directive. Their rights include a residence permit, access to the labour market and housing, medical care, and access to education for children. In Germany, the status of Ukrainian refugees is regulated by § 24 of the Foreigners' Legal Status Act. On the basis of this section, refugees receive a temporary residence permit called an *Aufenthaltstitel*. See: Yelnveta Kamenieva, "Parahraf 24 v Nimechchyni dlia ukraintsiv v 2023 r. ta prodovzhennia statusu" ("Paragraph 24 in Germany for Ukrainians in 2023 and Extension of Status"), *Ukrainian in Germany*, 23 October 2023, https://ukrainianingermany.de/uk/legalisation-for-ukrainians-in-eu-uk/ [accessed: 31.07.2024].

66 Natalya, woman, 48 years old, Berlin, interview with author in the context of the Prisma Ukraïna War, Migration and Memory project.

remission. She also mentioned the high price of treatment in Ukraine as compared to free treatment in Berlin. [67]

Another factor that made people decide to go abroad was the complicated situation with access to innovative medication in Ukraine. In an interview, Uzlova from Inspiration Family shared that a patient she supported from Kharkiv was, before the war, being treated with an innovative medication that cost 80,000 UAH (about 1,903.12 euros per treatment). She bought the first dose herself, pooling charity funds and support from her family. The second dose was provided as humanitarian aid from the pharmaceutical company in the first months of the war. After that, the patient decided to use the medical evacuation programme[68] and currently receives medication and the necessary care in Norway.[69]

Some women went abroad to continue treatment with experimental medication that they started to take in Ukraine. For example, Yulia from Odesa took part in the randomised (arbitrarily controlled) study of an experimental medication before the war. The Russian aggression interrupted this study and her access to the medication. Wanting to continue the research, she went to Germany with her family. In Berlin, she continued to receive the medication, but, unfortunately, it did not provide the expected results.[70] The case of Yulia demonstrates that the window of opportunity

67 Olena, woman, 46 years old, Berlin, interview with author in the context of the Prisma Ukraïna War, Migration and Memory project.

68 Since April 2022, the Ministry of Health of Ukraine, in cooperation with the European Commission, has been coordinating the referral and transportation of Ukrainian citizens for further treatment abroad. The medical evacuation of affected Ukrainians is carried out with the help of international partners, including the Government of the Republic of Poland, the World Health Organization, Médecins Sans Frontières (Doctors Without Borders), the Medical Mission Foundation, and paramedic transport teams from Poland, Germany, and other countries. Children and adults with complex mine-blast wounds and burn injuries, children and adults with cancer, and people with diseases requiring complex specialised treatment are transported to foreign clinics. The transportation and treatment of Ukrainian citizens in the medical evacuation programme are funded by international organisations and host countries. See: Ministry of Health of Ukraine, "MOZ: Yak podaty zaiavku na Prohramu medychnoi evakuatsii tym, khto postrazhdav vid viiny" ("Ministry of Health: How to Apply for the Medical Evacuation Programme for Those Affected by War"), 25 July 2022: https://www.kmu.gov.ua/news/moz-iak-podaty-zaiavku-na-prohramu-medychnoi-evakuatsii-tym-khto-postrazhdav-vid-viiny [accessed: 31.07.2024].

69 Antonina Adriychuk, "Problems of cancer patients: how they survive under conditions of war and deficit of medications", *Radio Svoboda* (*Radio Freedom*), 18 March 2023, https://www.radiosvoboda.org/a/onkokhvori-defitsyt-likiv-dostup-medychni-posluhy-viyna/32310626.html [accessed: 31.07.2024].

70 Uliia, woman, 42 years old, Berlin, interview with author in the context of the Prisma Ukraïna War, Migration and Memory project.

did not give everyone a chance for remission or recovery. Rather, it was an opportunity to prolong their lives, which was unavailable to them in Ukraine under the conditions of war, daily air-raid sirens, blackouts, problems with the water supply, and missile strikes.

As I analysed social media content, it became obvious how fleeting the window of opportunity is. The first wave of Ukrainians fleeing abroad was from February to July 2022. Once abroad, many women tried to go to EU countries and find hospitals and doctors by themselves. As foreign oncologists recalled, during the "first meetings the cancer patients from Ukraine demonstrated strong stress".[71] Sometimes, the situation was so bad that they did not have money to pay for a taxi to take them to the cancer centre.[72] Starting in August, the Ukrainian Ministry of Health initiated medical evacuations for cancer patients, but not everyone was approved for it. According to Uzlova, the selection criteria were based on how complicated a case was and whether a foreign hospital agreed to accept the patient.[73] For this reason, cancer patients continued to become refugees. Based on data from a survey by the Global Medical Knowledge Alliance, conducted in April 2023 with Ukrainian cancer patients on social media, about 20 percent of patients left the country.[74] This is an approximate percentage, yet it gives an initial idea about the movement of cancer patients and their treatment options during the war. The survey concludes that a considerable part of those surveyed paid for treatment in Ukraine themselves, which can be considered an added stimulus to decide to go abroad for treatment. For example, Valeria Kharchenko, in the Facebook group "Ukrainians in Munich", described her friend's situation and asked for advice on resolving the issue of going abroad for treatment. According to her post, treatment in Ukraine costs about 100,000 UAH (about 2,377.83 euros), and the family does not have this money. For this reason, she assumes that the only chance for treatment is a trip to Germany. In response, the participants of the group shared their experiences and advised the friend to seek temporary protection for treatment. They argued that this would provide medical

71 Peter McIntyre, "The war in Ukraine and cancer patients".

72 Ibid.

73 Anna Uzlova, "Fond pidtrymki doroslykh onkopatsiyentiv Inspiration family: dosvid medychnoyi evakuatsiyi ukrayinskykh onkopatsiyentiv" ("Inspiration Family Foundation to Support Adult Cancer Patients: The Experience of the Medical Evacuation of Ukrainian Cancer Patients"), *Health.ua.com*, 03 March 2023, https://health-ua.com/article/72140-fond-pdtrimki-doroslih-onkopatcntv-Inspiration-family-dosvd-medichno-evakua [accessed: 29.07.2024].

74 Global Medical Knowledge Alliance, "Patient experience with cancer care before and after the war in Ukraine – Abstract", 01 June 2023, https://gmka.org/news/patient-experience-with-cancer-care-before-and-after-the-war-in-ukraine-abstract/ [accessed: 31.07.2024].

insurance, which allows treatment with minimal expenses and temporary protection status.[75] An interesting feature of this discussion was the references to official websites, which informed Ukrainian patients on how to act and where to seek medical help for cancer patients. That is, there were rapidly formed information resources that instructed on the procedures for actions, coordination of treatment, regional particularities, and terms of acceptance. A majority of patients were accepted by countries that have an administrative border with Ukraine, yet there was also considerable inflow to Germany, Italy, Latvia, Lithuania, and Estonia.[76]

Most of these patients were women; there were much fewer men. This is due to limitations imposed on men travelling abroad during the current war. As a result, Western doctors who specialised in forms of cancer that are more prevalent in women received the largest surplus loads. Accordingly, women used the window of opportunity to go abroad for treatment to a greater extent. In conventional and on social media, they shared their experiences and their perceptions of European oncology and its positive and negative features and compared them with their previous experiences of treatment in Ukraine. For example, Albina from Bakhmut compared Ukrainian and European oncology systems as follows: "[E]verything that is outer space for me is routine for them". And, like most Ukrainian refugees with cancer, she concluded that "Ukraine should adopt European practices after the war" and that "the personal experience of each refugee" will add to achieving this common cause.[77]

Nonetheless, the situation with cancer patients is still in an undefined, temporary state. It is not known what will happen to them in the future: will they return to Ukraine, or will they remain in the country that they are in now? Regardless of the answer, it is obvious that the oncology situation in Ukraine is complicated, even though doctors say that oncological services were able to regroup and continue to work.[78] Even in the first half year of the war, expert opinions warned

---

75 Valeriya Harchenko (Facebook profile), "Sklalas neprosta situaciya. Dopomozhit z poradoyu..." ("A difficult situation happened. Help with advice...", post in the Facebook group "Ukraintsi v Miunkheni / Ukrainer in München / Ukrainians In Munich", 22 October 2022, https://m.facebook.com/groups/1688306774761735/permalink/3562473980678329/ [accessed: 31.07.2024].

76 O. O. Kovaliov and K.O. Kovaliov. "Yak naslidky viyny mozhut vplyvaty na zakhvoryuvanist na rak v Ukrayini ta krayinah Yevrosoyuzu" ("How the Effects of War Can Affect Cancer Incidence in Ukraine and the EU"), *Health.ua.com*, 14 January 2023, https://health-ua.com/article/71485-yak-nasldki-vjni-mozhut-vplivati-nazahvoryuvanst-narak-vukran-takranah-vros [accessed: 31.07.2024].

77 Tetiana Semakovska, "Yak likuyut rak v Nimechchyni: dosvid bakhmutyanky" ("How Cancer Is Treated in Germany: The Experience of a Bakhmut Woman"), *Bahmut.in.ua*, 13 February 2023, https://bahmut.in.ua/62-korysnee/4287-yak-likuyut-rak-v-nimechchini-dosvid-bakhmutyanki [accessed: 31.07.2024] [author's trans.].

78 Oleksiy Yaremenko et al., "Naymasshtabnisha podiya vitchyznyanoyi onkolohiyi – UpToDate 3.0. Congress" ("The Largest Event in National Oncology – Uptodate 3.0

of an echo of the war through cancer morbidity after the war's end. For example, the Head of the Ukrainian Ministry of Health, Viktor Liashko, forecasts growth in the number of cancer patients in the next 5–10 years.[79] Oleksiy Kovaliov, an oncologist and Ministry of Health expert, agrees with him. Based on the example of previous wars in Vietnam, Iraq, and Afghanistan, he also forecasts an increase in cases of the disease among both the military and civilians. The causes of this are chemicals used in bombardments, shelling, and missile strikes, the use of prohibited weapons, and constant stress.[80] In her annotation, the journalist Maria Stepanenko, who interviewed Kovaliov, used an interesting comparison of "how war metastasises the nation's health and what to do about this".[81] That is, here there is a reversal of metaphors: she views war through cancer-related terminology, where metastases (remote manifestations of a pathological process) are used to describe the predicted growth of cancer cases after the war, and the war itself is seen as a pathological tumour.

Conclusions

The militarisation of the oncological sphere has been evident since the start of the war. In online publications of various fields and types, the number of articles on cancer expressed in the language of war or comparing cancer to it has increased significantly. These articles heroise or victimise cancer patients, doctors, patient organisations, and charitable foundations. The language of military metaphors makes these stories visible and accessible, and allows the reader to see a reflection of their lived reality. The 'second war' and the 'war squared' are the most common militarised metaphors, which emotionally colour the experiences of those connected to cancer and reveal the depth of the humanitarian crisis caused by the war. The militarisation of the oncological sphere during the war is not only a prompt reaction to new situations in the Russo–Ukrainian War but also impacts and transforms them. More than before, the voices of people who are marginalised and made taboo because of the disease, have a wider reach. They are recognised as more involved in socially important processes, and their stories become valuable to society.

Congress"), *Health.ua.com*, 13 January 2023, https://health-ua.com/article/71478-najmasshtabnsha-podya-vtchiznyano-onkolog-kongres-UpToDate30 [accessed: 31.07.2024].

79 *Slovo i dilo* (*Word and Deed*), "Lyashko rozpoviv, yak viyna vplyne na zdorov'ya ukrayintsiv u dovhostrokoviy perspektyvi" ("Lyashko Explains How the War Will Affect the Health of Ukrainians in the Long Term"), 18 August 2022, https://www.slovoidilo.ua/2022/08/18/novyna/suspilstvo/lyashko-rozpoviv-yak-vijna-vplyne-zdorovya-ukrayinicziv-dovhostrokovij-perspektyvi [accessed: 31.07.2024].

80 Stepanenko, "Dumaty pro maybutnie zaraz".

81 Ibid.

Strikingly, their rhetoric, their descriptions of the events, and the words they used to express their feelings have changed since the start of the war. "Russia doesn't only kill with bombs"[82] is how they define their experience and the reality they faced in the first months. The destruction of the established system of cancer care led to numerous invisible victims of the war. Many patients could not get help in time and died. Getting to a hospital was heroism, a courageous act. Because of the war, patients and doctors began to express their thoughts and experience events through militarised metaphors and to describe the world in which they sought cancer treatment through the language of war, fighting, and combat.

People perceive treatment as something more complicated when they use war metaphors compared to other terms and descriptions. A sharp increase in the prevalence of such metaphors shows the scale and depth of the humanitarian crisis that emerged in the Ukrainian oncology sphere. And the more we compare the language of people who stayed in Ukraine for treatment to that of those who left the country, the more obvious the difference in their preference for war-related metaphors. In the information space of Ukraine, after a year of war, military associations and comparisons remain widely used. In some cases, they become a reflection of real victories and defeats in the Russo–Ukrainian War. Conversely, refugees with cancer use words connected to hope, possibility, prospects, calmness, and safety. For them, treatment abroad is a 'window of opportunity' to access better European medical care and its innovative methods and medication. Even if treatment turns out to be ineffective, they see it as a chance to extend the time of their lives. An unprecedented practice of 'treatment abroad' emerged as a form of temporary protection. The international community of cancer patients and international healthcare organisations played a positive role in this. Yet this status is temporary – that is, for now, we do not have any effective control, and there are no prospects for a prolonged stay in EU countries for these patients. Many unresolved issues remain.

There is also a need to coordinate efforts and conduct new research to help overcome the consequences of the Russian armed aggression for oncology in Ukraine. I support the position of the oncologists of Ukraine, voiced at the oncology congress *UpToDate 3.0* on 24–25 November 2022: "And today it is possible that the full-scale war can cause an increase in cancer mortality and incidence rate, compared to the indicators expected in times of peace. For this reason, it is important to create a separate programme to study the consequences of war on the incidence of cancer in Ukraine".[83] It is important to apply maximum efforts to mitigate the adverse consequences of the war in Ukraine, including in the sphere of oncology. And here, it is important to work in all areas – with patients and their communities, oncologists, and international oncological organisations.

82 Ivantsiv, "'Rosiia vbyvae ne lyshe bombamy'".

83 Yaremenko, "Naymasshtabnisha podiya vitchyznyanoyi onkolohiyi" [author's trans.].

Bibliography

Adriychuk, Antonina, "Problems of cancer patients: how they survive under conditions of war and deficit of medications", *Radio Svoboda* (*Radio Freedom*), 18 March 2023. https://www.radiosvoboda.org/a/onkokhvori-defitsyt-likiv-dostup-medychni-posluhy-viyna/32310626.html [accessed: 31.07.2024].

Afina. Zhinky protiv raku (Athena: Women against Cancer) (Facebook page), "Traven ye misiatsem obiznanosti

pro melanoma..." ("May is Melanoma Awareness Month..."), Facebook post, 17 May 2023 https://m.facebook.com/story.php?story_fbid=pfbid0c5dUTg7H3w4G8HwRPrXzCWfb3AUjLyWapg3huCptvKNfFvWD2L3Xzq2jjUXwDUa1l&id=386590811758587 [accessed: 31.07.2024].

Anonymous, "Russia's war in Ukraine is killing cancer care in both countries", *The BMJ*, 23 March 2022, https://doi.org/10.1136/bmj.o701 [accessed: 31.07.2024].

Apteka.ua (Pharmacy.ua), "Onkolohiya–2021: sohodennia ta perspektyvy rozvytku" ("Oncology – 2021: The Present and Prospects for Development"), no. 5 (1276), 08 February 2021, https://www.apteka.ua/article/582977 [accessed: 31.07.2024].

Baziv, Lyubov, "Viktoriia Romaniuk, spivzasnovnytsia HO 'Afina. Zhinky proty raku'" ("Victoria Romaniuk, Cofounder of the NGO 'Athena: Women Against Cancer'"), *Ukrinform*, 04 February 2023, https://www.ukrinform.ua/rubric-society/3665315-viktoria-romanuk-spivzasnovnica-go-afina-zinki-proti-raku.html [accessed: 31.07.2024].

Beznosenko, A.P., "Onkologiya v Ukraine: itogi 2021 goda" ("Oncology in Ukraine: The Results of 2021"), *Health.ua.com*, 20 June 2022, https://health-ua.com/article/69965-onkologya-vukran-pdsumki-2021roku [accessed: 31.07.2024].

BF Inspiration family support, "Anketa na ridkisni abo spetsyfichni liky..." ("Form for rare or specific medicines"), Telegram post, 28 February 2022, https://t.me/onkosupportua/21 [accessed: 31.07.2024].

Bondarchuk, Iryna, "Nova era likuvannya raku vzhe v Ukrayini" ("A New Era of Cancer Treatment Is Already in Ukraine"), *Ukrayinskiiy medichniiy zhurnal* 1/117, 2017, https://www.umj.com.ua/article/105350/nova-era-likuvannya-raku-vzhe-v-ukrayini [accessed: 31.07.2024].

Burlaku, Nataliia, "Rak u zhinok. Shcho povinna robiti kozhna z nas, aby zhiti?" ("Cancer In Women: What Should Each of Us Do to Live?"), *20 Khvylyn, Ternopil (20 Minutes, Ternopil)*, 04 February 2023, https://te.20minut.ua/Zdorovya/kozhna-z-nas-mozhe-zahvoriti-yak-u-ternopoli-pid-chas-viyni-likuyut-ra-11691867.html [accessed: 31.07.2024].

Buzhinetska, Nataliia, "Dolatu rak u voennykh umovakh – maizhe vyrok: istorii evakuatsii onkokhvorikh ditei z Ukrainy" ("Overcoming Cancer in Wartime Is Almost a Sentence: Stories of the Evacuation of Children with Cancer from

Ukraine"), *Ukrayinska Pravda* (*Ukrainian Truth*), 08 April 2022, https://life.pravda.com.ua/health/2022/04/8/248153/ [accessed: 31.07.2024].

Chestnut, Jonathan M., et al., "Waging War on War Metaphors in Cancer and COVID-19", *JCO Oncology Practice* 16/10 2020, 627–628, https://ascopubs.org/doi/full/10.1200/OP.20.00542 [accessed: 31.07.2024].

Chupakhina, Nataliia, (Facebook profile), "Chy ye shche yakes likuvannia?..." ("Are there any other treatments?..."), post in Facebook group "Athena. Women against cancer – a group of mutual support for cancer patients", 08 June 2023, https://www.facebook.com/groups/247646882376950/user/100013805553987/ [accessed: 15.04.2024].

Demianchuk, Olha, "V Ukraini prypyneno likuvannia khvorykh n arak – Zelenskyi" ("Zelenskyy: Treatment of Cancer Patients Stopped in Ukraine"), *Korespondent.Net* (*Correspondent.Net*), 06 May 2022, https://ua.korrespondent.net/ukraine/4475561-v-ukraini-prypyneno-likuvannia-khvorykh-na-rak-zelenskyi [accessed: 31.07.2024].

DeVita Jr., Vincent T., "The 'War on Cancer' and its impact", *Nature Clinical Practice Oncology* 1/55, 2004, 55, https://doi.org/10.1038/ncponc0036 [accessed: 31.07.2024].

Dobrota, Valentyna, "Chernihivtsi za rik pislya okupatsiyi pyshayutsya perehodom na ukrayinsku movu i vzhe hotuyutsya do myru" ("A Year After the Occupation, the Residents of Chernihiv Are Proud to Switch to the Ukrainian Language and Are Preparing for Peace"), *TSN*, 03 April 2023, https://tsn.ua/exclusive/chernigivci-za-rik-pislya-okupaciyi-pishayutsya-perehodom-na-ukrayinsku-movu-i-vzhe-gotuyutsya-do-miru-2299600.html [accessed: 31.07.2024].

European Cancer Organisation, "ECO-ASCO Special Network: Impact of the War in Ukraine on Cancer", 04 June 2022, https://www.europeancancer.org/topic-networks/20:impact-war-in-ukraine-on-cancer.html [accessed: 31.07.2024].

European Cancer Organisation, "ECO Statements on Ukraine", 10 May 2022, https://www.europeancancer.org/resources/246:eco-statement-of-support-for-ukraine.html [accessed: 31.07.2024].

European Commission, "Temporary protection", https://home-affairs.ec.europa.eu/policies/migration-and-asylum/common-european-asylum-system/temporary-protection_en [accessed: 31.07.2024].

European Federation of Pharmaceutical Industries and Associations (EFPIA), *The Impact of the War in Ukraine on Oncology Patients: Overview and recommendations for European and Ukrainian health authorities and policymakers*, report, 2022, https://www.efpia.eu/media/677256/the-impact-of-the-war-in-ukraine-on-oncology-patients.pdf [accessed: 31.07.2024].

Global Medical Knowledge Alliance, "Patient experience with cancer care before and after the war in Ukraine – Abstract", 01 June 2023, https://gmka.org/news/patient-experience-with-cancer-care-before-and-after-the-war-in-ukraine-abstract/ [accessed: 31.07.2024].

González, Roberto J., *Militarizing Culture: Essays on the Warfare State*, New York: Routledge, 2010.

Harchenko, Valeriya, (Facebook profile), "Sklalas neprosta situaciya. Dopomozhit z poradoyu..." ("A difficult situation happened. Help with advice...", post in the Facebook group "Ukraintsi v Miunkheni / Ukrainer in München / Ukrainians In Munich", 22 October 2022, https://m.facebook.com/groups/1688306774761735/permalink/3562473980678329/ [accessed: 31.07.2024].

Helij, Natalya, "Pid chas tryvog boyimosya perepadiv napruhy, bo todi mozhe vyity z ladu medychne obladnannya" ("During Alarms, We Are Afraid of Power Surges, Because then Medical Equipment Can Break Down – Oleh Duda"), *Espreso.Zahid* (*Espreso.West*), 05 February, 2023, https://zahid.espreso.tv/pid-chas-trivog-boimosya-perepadiv-naprugi-bo-todi-mozhe-viyti-z-ladu-medichne-obladnannya-oleg-duda [accessed: 31.07.2024].

Ivantsiv, Nastia, "'Rosiia vbyvae ne lyshe bombamy'. Iak onkopatsienty zhyvut i pomyraiut pid cahs viiny" ("'Russia Kills Not Only with Bombs': How Cancer Patients Live and Die During the War"), *LB.ua*, 20 May 2022, https://lb.ua/society/2022/05/20/517366_rosiya_vbivaie_lishe_bombami_yak.html [accessed: 31.07.2024].

Kalinichenko, Nataliia, "'Popry viynu, onkokhvori mayut otrimaty yakisnu medychnu dopomohu'" ("'Despite the war, cancer patients should receive quality medical care'"), *Uryadoviiy kuryer* (*Government Courier*), 23 July 2022, https://ukurier.gov.ua/uk/articles/popri-vijnu-onkohvori-mayut-otrimuvati-yakisnu-med/ [accessed: 31.07.2024].

Kamenieva, Yelizaveta, "Parahraf 24 v Nimechchyni dlia ukraintsiv v 2023 r. ta prodovzhennia statusu" ("Paragraph 24 in Germany for Ukrainians in 2023 and Extension of Status"), *Ukrainian in Germany*, 23 October 2023, https://ukrainianingermany.de/uk/legalisation-for-ukrainians-in-eu-uk/ [accessed: 31.07.2024].

Katashinska, Alyona, "Zhertoviu raketnoho udaru u Zaporizhzhi stav vidmoii khirurg-onkolog" ("Famous Oncological Surgeon Becomes Victim of Missile Attack in Zaporizhzhia"), *Komsomolskaia Pravda in Ukraine*, 13 October 2022, https://kp.ua/ua/incidents/a657652-zhertvoju-raketnoho-udaru-u-zaporizhzhi-stav-vidomij-khirurh-onkoloh [accessed: 31.07.2024].

King, Galina, "Likari Chernihova: Evhenii Lutsenko ikhav u mikroavtobusi, iakii obstriliali rosiis'ki neliudi" ("Doctors in Chernihiv: Yevheniy Lutsenko Was in a Minibus When It Was Fired Upon by Russian Proxies"), *Chernihiv.City*, 19 September 2022, https://chernihiv.city/articles/234585/yevgenij-lucenko-3-misyaci-vvazhavsya-bezvisti-zniklim [accessed: 15.04.2024].

Kohn, Richard H., "Using the Military at Home: Yesterday, Today, and Tomorrow", *Chicago Journal of International Law* 4/1, 2003, 165–192, https://chicagounbound.uchicago.edu/cjil/vol4/iss1/12 [accessed: 31.07.2024].

Kolomiets, Daria, "Kinsha Daria. Yak likuyut onkologiu v Ukraini ta skilky na tse vydiliaye hroshey derzhava — vdipovidaie MOZ" ("How Oncology Is Treated in Ukraine and How Much Money the State Allocates for It – The Ministry of Health Answers"), *Suspilne novyny* (*Public News*), 04 February 2022, https://suspilne.media/203940-ak-likuut-onkologicni-zahvoruvanna-v-ukraini-ta-skilki-na-ce-vidilae-grosej-derzava/ [accessed: 31.07.2024].

Kotliar, Alla, "Rak I viyna. Chomu v Ukrayini nemaye bazovih onkopreparativ, I koly vony zyavlyansya" ("Cancer and War: Why There Are No Basic Oncological Drugs in Ukraine, and When They Will Appear"), *ZN.UA*, 28 January 2023, https://zn.ua/ukr/HEALTH/rak-i-vijna-chomu-v-ukrajini-nemaje-bazovikh-onkopreparativ-i-koli-voni-zjavljatsja.html [accessed: 31.07.2024].

Kovaliov, O. O., and K.O. Kovaliov. "Yak naslidky viyny mozhut vplyvaty na zakhvoryuvanist na rak v Ukrayini ta krayinah Yevrosoyuzu" ("How the Effects of War Can Affect Cancer Incidence in Ukraine and the EU"), *Health.ua.com*, 14 January 2023, https://health-ua.com/article/71485-yak-nasldki-vjni-mozhut-vplivati-nazahvoryuvanst-narak-vukran-takranah-vros [accessed: 31.07.2024].

Krasnikov, Denis, and Victoria Martyniuk, "Skhidna Ukraina poterpaie vid raku bilshe, nizh Zakhidna, i zavody – ne holovnyi faktor. Shcho kazhe statystyka" ("Eastern Ukraine Suffers from Cancer More Than Western Ukraine, and Factories Are Not the Main Factor: What the Statistics Say"), *Forbes*, 05 November 2021, https://forbes.ua/lifestyle/vostochnaya-ukraina-stradaet-ot-raka-bolshe-zapadnoy-i-zavody-ne-glavnyy-faktor-chto-govorit-statistika-05112021-2729 [accessed: 31.07.2024].

Krivoruchko, Lina, "Rak ne znae, shcho die velyka vijina: istorii medykiv ta volonteriv, iaki boriutsia za zhyttia onkokhvorykh ditei" ("Cancer Does not Know That There is a Great War: Stories of Doctors and Volunteers Fighting for the Lives of Children with Cancer), *Ukrayinska Pravda* (*Ukrainian Truth*), 03 September 2022, https://life.pravda.com.ua/health/2022/09/3/250299/ [accessed: 31.07.2024].

Kudryashova, Viktoriia, "Tse liudy, iaki boriutsia z rakom pid chas viiny" ("These Are People Who Are Fighting Cancer During the War"), *The Village*, 3 June 2022, https://www.the-village.com.ua/village/knowledge/practice/326609-rak-i-viyna [accessed: 29.07.2024].

Lebedenko, Inna, "Onkohvori ukrayintsi po kilka dib vybyrayutsya iz okupovanyh terytorij, schob otrymaty likuvannya, ta chasto chas vtracheno" ("Ukrainians with Cancer Take Several Days to Get Out of the Occupied Territories to Receive Treatment, But Often the Clock is Ticking"), *TSN*, 11 September 2022, https://tsn.ua/exclusive/onkohvori-ukrayinci-po-kilka-dib-vibirayutsya-iz-okupovanih-teritoriy-schob-otrimati-likuvannya-ta-chasto-chas-vtracheno-2132317.html [accessed: 29.07.2024].

Levchenko, Anna, "Dytyacha onkolohiya ta patsiyenty z vazhkymy suputnimy patolohiyamy dosi ye prerohatyvoyu derzhavnykh klinik – holovnyy likar NIR"

("Paediatric Oncology and Patients with Severe Comorbidities Are Still the Prerogative of State Clinics – Chief Medical Officer of the NIR"), *Interfax-Ukraina: Informatsiine ahenstvo* (*Interfax-Ukraine: Information Agency*), 04 February 22, https://interfax.com.ua/news/interview/796147.html [accessed: 31.07.2024].

Loza, Anastasia, "'Rak ne chekae na zaverwhennia viiny', – iak boriutsa za zhyttia onkokhvori z Chernihivshchyny" ("'Cancer Does Not Wait for the End of the War' – How Cancer Patients from the Chernihiv Oblast Fight for Their Lives"), *Suspilne novyny* (*Public News*), 03 April 2022, https://suspilne.media/224627-rak-ne-cekae-na-zaversenna-vijni-ak-borutsa-za-zitta-onkohvori-z-cernigivsini/ [accessed: 31.07.2024].

Matyushenko, Inesa, and Olga Syrotyuk, "Viina v kvadrati: shansy dlia onkopatsientiv na vyzhyvannia" ("War Squared: Chances for Cancer Patients to Survive"), *Hromadske,* 02 October 2022, https://hromadske.ua/posts/vijna-v-kvadrati-shansi-dlya-onkopaciyentiv-na-vizhivannya [accessed: 31.07.2024].

Maziewski, Łukasz, "Szef wywiadu wojskowego Ukrainy: Dostrzegamy istotne zmiany wewnątrz Rosji" ("Head of Ukraine's Military Intelligence: We See Significant Changes Inside Russia"), *Wirtualna Polska: wiadomości* (*Virtual Poland: News*), 29 January 2023, https://wiadomosci.wp.pl/szef-wywiadu-wojskowego-ukrainy-dostrzegamy-istotne-zmiany-wewnatrz-rosji-6860053735013056a [accessed: 31.07.2024].

McIntyre, Peter, "The war in Ukraine and cancer patients: Early experiences from the frontline", *eCancer,* 22 September 2022, https://ecancer.org/en/news/22234-the-war-in-ukraine-and-cancer-patients-early-experiences-from-the-frontline [accessed: 31.07.2024].

Melnyk, Viktoriya, "Rak ta vijna: yak dovodytsya zhyty onkohvorym na tymchasovo okupovanyh terytoriyah" ("Cancer and War: How Cancer Patients Live in the Temporarily Occupied Territories"), *Vikna* (*Windows*), 18 September 2022, https://vikna.tv/styl-zhyttya/likuvannya-onkologiyi-na-okupovanyh-terytoriyah/ [accessed: 31.07.2024].

Midas PR Group, "Desk Research: How it Works and Why It's Your Key to Success", 30 October 2018, https://www.midas-pr.com/desk-research-works-key-success/ [access: 31.07.2024].

Ministry of Health of Ukraine, "MOZ: Yak podaty zaiavku na Prohramu medychnoi evakuatsii tym, khto postrazhdav vid viiny" ("Ministry of Health: How to Apply for the Medical Evacuation Programme for Those Affected by War"), 25 July 2022: https://www.kmu.gov.ua/news/moz-iak-podaty-zaiavku-na-prohramu-medychnoi-evakuatsii-tym-khto-postrazhdav-vid-viiny [accessed: 31.07.2024].

National Cancer Institute, U.S. National Institute of Health, "Milestone (1971). National Cancer Act of 1971", https://dtp.cancer.gov/timeline/noflash/milestones/m4_nixon.htm [accessed: 31.07.2024].

Pecherskyi, Anton, "'Druha armiia svitu': chy varto nazyvaty tak viisko rashystiv" ("'The Second Army of the World': Should We Call the Ruscist Army This Way?"), *ArmiiaInform* (*ArmyInformation*), 21 June 2022, https://armyinform.com.ua/2022/06/21/druga-armiya-svitu-chy-varto-nazyvaty-tak-vijsko-rashystiv/ [accessed: 31.07.2024].

Petik, Marina, "Vid udaru rosiiskoi rakety ii mashyna spalakhnula, iak sirnyk: y Kyevi zahynula likara Okhmatdytu, sin zalyshvsia syrotoiu" ("A Russian Missile Hit Her Car Like a Match: A Doctor From the Kyiv Regional Medical Centre Was Killed and Her Son Was Left an Orphan"), *Obozrevatel* (*Observer*), 12 October 2022, https://news.obozrevatel.com/ukr/society/vid-udaru-rosijskoi-raketi-ii-mashina-spalahnula-yak-sirnik-u-kievi-zaginula-likar-ohmatdita.html [accessed: 15.04.2024].

Pidtserkovna, Diana, "Vplyv viyny na onkolohichni zakhvoryuvannya v Ukrayini: vazhlyvist profilaktychnoho ohlyadu" ("The Impact of the War on Cancer in Ukraine: The Importance of Preventive Examinations"), *Sykhiv.Media*, 25 May 2023, https://sykhiv.media/vplyv-vijny-na-zahvoryuvanist-na-rak-v-ukrayini/ [accessed: 31.07.2024].

Priamyi (Direct), "V Ukraini diiut shist obstezhen dlia vyiavlennia onkolohichnykh zakhvoriuvan – MOZ" ("Six Examinations for Detecting Cancer in Ukraine – Ministry of Health"), 08 June 2022, https://prm.ua/v-ukraini-diiut-shist-obstezhen-dlia-vyiavlennia-onkolohichnykh-zakhvoriuvan-moz/ [accessed: 31.07.2024].

Roksbi, Filippa, "Yak riatuiut vid viiny khvorykh na rak ukrainskykh ditei" ("How Ukrainian Children with Cancer Are Being Saved from War"), *BBC News Ukraine*, 26 March 2022, https://www.bbc.com/ukrainian/features-60880184 [accessed: 31.07.2024].

Rozenko, Maksym, "'Rak – vin, yak "druha armiya svitu": strashnyi, poky nevidomyi', – Osadcha pro vlasnu bitvu z Onko" ("'Cancer Is Like the "Second Army of the World": Scary, Yet Unknown' – Osadcha about Her Own Battle with Cancer"), *Radio Trek* (*Radio Track*), 05 June 2023, https://radiotrek.rv.ua/news/rak-vin-yak-druga-armiya-svitu-strashniy-lishe-poki---nevidomiy---osadcha-pro-vlasnu-bitvu-z-onko_309310.html [accessed: 31.07.2024].

Sakhnik, Vita, "Koly u tebe dvi viiny. Iak onkokhvori znakhodiat prykhystok na Volyni" ("When You Have Two Wars: How Cancer Patients Find Refuge In Volyn"), *Pershii Kanal Sotsialnykh Novyn* (*First Social News Channel*), 12 March 2022, https://pershyj.com/p-koli-u-tebe-dvi-viini-yak-onkohvori-znahodyat-prihistok-na-volini-56128 [accessed: 31.07.2024].

Semakovska, Tetiana, "Yak likuyut rak v Nimechchyni: dosvid bakhmutyanky" ("How Cancer Is Treated in Germany: The Experience of a Bakhmut Woman"), *Bahmut.in.ua*, 13 February 2023, https://bahmut.in.ua/62-korysnee/4287-yak-likuyut-rak-v-nimechchini-dosvid-bakhmutyanki [accessed: 31.07.2024].

Slovo i Dilo (Word and Deed), "Reytyng najsylnishykh armiy svitu: yake mistse posilyi Ukrayina ta rosiya" ("Ranking of the World's Strongest Armies: Where Ukraine and Russia Stand"), 06 January 2023, https://www.slovoidilo.ua/2023/01/06/novyna/svit/rejtynh-najsylnishyx-armij-svitu-yake-misce-posily-ukrayina-ta-rosiya [accessed: 31.07.2024].

Slovo i dilo (Word and Deed), "Lyashko rozpoviv, yak viyna vplyne na zdorovya ukrayintsiv u dovhostrokoviy perspektyvi" ("Lyashko Explains How the War Will Affect the Health of Ukrainians in the Long Term"), 18 August 2022, https://www.slovoidilo.ua/2022/08/18/novyna/suspilstvo/lyashko-rozpoviv-yak-vijna-vplyne-zdorovya-ukrayinicziv-dovhostrokovij-perspektyvi [accessed: 31.07.2024].

Stepanenko, Maryna, "Dumaty pro maibutnie zaraz: ekspert MOZ Ukrainy pro zapobihannia epidemii raku psilia viyny" ("Thinking about the Future Now: Expert of the Ministry of Health of Ukraine on Preventing the Epidemic of Brain Cancer"), *RFI-Ukraina*, 30 March 2023, https://www.rfi.fr/uk/%D1%83%D0%BA%D1%80%80% D0%B0%D1%97%D0%BD% 0%B0/20230330 [accessed: 15.04.2024].

Sullivan, Richard, "What impact does war have on Ukrainian cancer care?", *King's College London*, 29 April 2022, https://www.kcl.ac.uk/what-impact-does-war-have-on-ukrainian-cancer-care [accessed: 31.07.2024].

Surh, Young-Joon, "The 50-Year War on Cancer Revisited: Should We Continue to Fight the Enemy Within?", *Journal of Cancer Prevention* 26(4), 2021, 219–223, doi: 10.15430/JCP.2021.26.4.219. https://www.ncbi.nlm.nih.gov/pmc/articles/PMC8749321/ [accessed 31.07. 2024].

Ukrainian Ministry of Health, "Shist bezoplatnykh doslidzhen dlia rannoho vyiavlennia onkolohii" ("Six Free Tests for Early Detection of Cancer"),08 June 2022, https://moz.gov.ua/article/news/shist-bezoplatnih-doslidzhen-dlja-rannogo-vijavlennja-onkologii [accessed: 31.07.2024].

UNIAN: Informatsiine ahenstvo (UNIAN: Information Agency), "'Velyke budivnytstvo': u Kharkovi ziavytsia novyi onkotsentr na pivtysiachi lizhok" ("'Big Construction': A New Oncology Centre with Five Hundred Beds to Be Built in Kharkiv"), 07 February 2022, https://www.unian.ua/health/velike-budivnictvo-u-harkovi-z-yavitsya-noviy-onkocentr-na-piv-tisyachi-lizhok-novini-harkova-11696071.html [accessed: 31.07.2024].

Uzlova, Anna, "Fond pidtrymki doroslykh onkopatsiyentiv Inspiration family: dosvid medychnoyi evakuatsiyi ukrayinskykh onkopatsiyentiv" ("Inspiration Family Foundation to Support Adult Cancer Patients: The Experience of the Medical Evacuation of Ukrainian Cancer Patients"), *Health.ua.com*, 03 March 2023, https://health-ua.com/article/72140-fond-pdtrimki-doroslih-onkopatcntv-Inspiration-family-dosvd-medichno-evakua [accessed: 31.07.2024].

Venglinska, Tetyana, "Fighting Disease During the War: A Story of a Cancer Patient", *UkraineWorld*, 12 September 2022, https://ukraineworld.org/articles/stories/story-cancer-patient [accessed: 31.07.2024].

Vladimirovna, Darya, (Facebook profile), "U mene pytannya hto likuyetsya v Germaniyi..." ("I have a question about treatment in Germany..."), post in the Facebook group "Athena. Women against cancer – a group of mutual support for cancer patients", 12 June 2023, https://www.facebook.com/groups/247646882376950/search/?q=%D0%91%D1%96%D0%B6%D0%B5%D0%BD%D1%86%D1%96 [accessed: 15.04.2024].

Yaremenko, Oleksiy et al., "Naymasshtabnisha podiya vitchyznyanoyi onkolohiyi – UpToDate 3.0. Congress" ("The Largest Event in National Oncology – Uptodate 3.0 Congress"), *Health.ua.com*, 13 January 2023, https://health-ua.com/article/71478-najmasshtabnsha-podya-vtchiznyano-onkolog-kongres-UpToDate30 [accessed: 31.07.2024].

Zozulynskyj, Taras, "Yak voyuyut ukrayinski onkologhy" ("How Ukrainian Oncologists are Fighting"), *Detectives. Byuro zhurnalistskih rozsliduvan* (*Detectives: Office of Journalistic Investigations*), 11 November 2022, EUROSaccessed: 31.07.2024].

Authors

Biographies

Denys Brylov is head of the European Center for Strategic Analytics. He is a psychologist and an anthropologist of religion and holds a PhD in Religious Studies and Theology. He is associate professor in the Department of Theology and Religious Studies at the National Pedagogical Dragomanov University (Kyiv, Ukraine). His main academic interests are Islam, political activism in Islam and transnational Islamic movements, religious factors in conflicts, and religion and nationalism. Located in Kyiv, Denys Brylov was a 2022/2023 non-resident Prisma Ukraïna fellow at the Forum Transregionale Studien. (https://orcid.org/0000-0001-6214-2782)

Ihor Dvorkin is associate professor in the Department of Ukrainian Studies, Cultural Studies and History of Science at the National Technical University "Kharkiv Polytechnic Institute" (Kharkiv, Ukraine). He received his PhD (Candidate of Science in History) from Volodymyr Dahl East Ukrainian University (Luhansk, Ukraine). His research interests include memorialisation of the Second World War in Ukraine, history of Ukraine, museum studies, and contemporary Ukrainian historiography. (https://orcid.org/0000-0001-9190-8265)

Olha Haidamachuk has been working in the Department of Ukrainian Studies, Cultural Studies, and History of Science at the National Technical University "Kharkiv Polytechnic Institute" (Kharkiv, Ukraine). Since 2019, she has been a member of the Kharkiv Historical and Philological Society. She received her PhD in Philosophy from the V. N. Karazin Kharkiv National University. Her research interests include philosophy of culture, philosophical anthropology, Ukrainian studies, Ukrainian and European culture, philosophy of language, history of philosophy, ethics, and aesthetics. Since 2022, Olha Haidamachuk has been a member of the Prisma Ukraïna *War, Migration, Memory* research group. She is a 2024–2025 fellow of the Gerda Henkel Foundation at the Forum Transregionale Studien in Berlin. (https://orcid.org/0000-0002-0005-1380)

Roman Holyk is a doctor of historical sciences and a senior researcher at the Department of Modern History of Ukraine in the I. Krypiakevych Institute of Ukrainian Studies of the National Academy of Sciences of Ukraine (Lviv, Ukraine). His main fields of scientific research include the secular and religious mentality of Ukrainian society, history and culture of Lviv and Galicia, history of Ukrainian literature and culture, history of writing and reading, history of ideas, theoretical issues of semiotics of culture, literary studies, as well as history and methodology of humanitarian sciences. (http://orcid.org/0000-0003-3123-1920)

Mykola Homanyuk is associate professor in the Department of Geography and Ecology at Kherson State University, chairperson of the NGO Kherson Entity of the Sociological Association of Ukraine, and runs the independent theater company Totem Theatre Lab. He holds a PhD in sociology from the V. N. Karazin Kharkiv National University. In 2018, he won the ADAMI Media Prize for Cultural Diversity in Eastern Europe. His current research is dedicated to ethnic minorities, the transformation of war memorials, modern toponymic practices, and problems of social representation in contemporary documentary theater. He has been a non-resident fellow and member of the Prisma Ukraïna *War, Migration, Memory* research group since 2022 and is a 2024–2025 Prisma Ukraïna fellow of the Gerda Henkel Foundation. (https://orcid.org/0000-0002-9625-1968)

Tetiana Kalenychenko is the executive director of the European Center for Strategic Analytics. She holds a PhD in Sociology of Religion from the National Pedagogical Dragomanov University (Kyiv, Ukraine). Her research includes the topics of religion and conflict, and religion and peace. Tetiana Kalenychenko, located in Bucha, was a 2022/2023 non-resident Prisma Ukraïna fellow at the Forum Transregionale Studien. (https://orcid.org/0000-0003-4025-6820)

Ivan Kozachenko holds a researcher position that is attached both to the Centre of Migration Research and to the Centre of Excellence in Social Sciences, University of Warsaw (Poland). He received his PhD in Sociology from the University of Aberdeen (UK). His research interests include migration and diaspora studies, national and ethnic identities in post-Soviet states, and the role of social media in social movements and cultural representations. His current research project explores the relationships between identity, new media use, and the integration of Ukrainian temporary protected persons in Poland. He was a 2020/2021 Prisma Ukraïna fellow. (https://orcid.org/0000-0002-0346-1967)

Lidia Kuzemska is a sociologist with an interdisciplinary interest in forced migration, internal displacement, borders, and citizenship. She received her PhD from Lancaster University (UK) in 2022. She also holds an MA in Economy and Society from Lancaster University (UK), an MA in European Studies from the College of Europe (Belgium and Poland), and an MA in Sociology from the Ivan Franko National University of Lviv (Ukraine). Kuzemska is a 2024–25 Prisma Ukraïna fellow of the Gerda Henkel Foundation at the Forum Transregionale Studien. Since 2022, she has been a member and, since September 2023, academic coordinator of the research group *War, Migration, Memory.* (https://orcid.org/0000-0003-4829-4362)

Olha Labur (†) worked as an associate professor in the Department of History of the Igor Sikorsky Kyiv Polytechnic Institute (Kyiv, Ukraine) and obtained her PhD (Candidate of Science in History) in 1999. She was member of the Ukrainian Association for Researchers in Women's History. As a historian, she focused on women's experiences in the 20th century. Since 2022, Olha Labur had been a member of the Prisma Ukraïna *War, Migration, Memory* research group. In 2024/2025, she was a fellow of the Gerda Henkel Foundation at the Forum Transregionale Studien in Berlin.

Alina Mozolevska is professor in the Faculty of Philology at Petro Mohyla Black Sea National University (Mykolaiv, Ukraine). She holds a PhD in Linguistics with a major in Roman languages from Taras Shevchenko National University (Kyiv, Ukraine). Her research interests include media studies, discourse analysis, and border studies, and she has published on borders and identity in literary and political discourses. In 2024, she is a ZOiS Ukraine-based fellow and has been a member of the Prisma Ukraïna *War, Migration, Memory* research group since 2022. (https://orcid.org/0000-0002-1550-8734)

Janush Panchenko is a PhD student at Zaporizhzhia National University and fellow of the non-residential programme at Indiana University (USA). He is a Ukrainian ethnographer, specialising in the study of the culture and language of Roma in Ukraine. Born in the city of Kakhovka, he comes from a family of settled Roma in the second generation and became the first Roma in his city to receive a university education. His contribution to the development of Roma culture was recognised with the Ronald Lee Award. (https://orcid.org/0000-0001-9974-3266)

Olha Polishchuk is an associate professor at the Faculty of Philology at Petro Mohyla Black Sea National University (Mykolaiv, Ukraine). She holds a PhD in Theory of Literature. Currently, she collaborates with the UniGR-Center for Border Studies and the Chair of North American Literary and Cultural Studies at Saarland University (Germany). (https://orcid.org/0000-0001-8133-2813)

Andrii Portnov is co-director of the Viadrina Center for Polish and Ukrainian Studies, professor of Entangled History of Ukraine at the European University Viadrina (Frankfurt/Oder, Germany). He defended his PhD thesis on the Ukrainian emigration in interwar Poland at the Ivan Krypiakevych Institute of Ukrainian Studies in Lviv. His publications deal with intellectual history, historiography, genocide, and memory studies in Central and Eastern Europe. He came to Berlin in 2012 as a fellow of the Institute for Advanced Study (Wissenschaftskolleg zu Berlin). In 2015, he initiated and co-founded the Berlin-Brandenburg Ukraine Initiative, which became the Prisma Ukraïna Research Network Eastern Europe at the Forum Transregionale Studien Berlin in 2016. (https://orcid.org/0000-0003-1913-8811)

Taisiia Ratushna is associate professor at the Department of Sociology at Zaporizhzhia National University. She received her PhD in Sociology from the Classical Private University (Zaporizhzhia, Ukraine). Since then, she has been working at the Department of Sociology at Zaporizhzhia National University and has been researching communication processes in urban spaces and virtual environments. In 2020, she received a master's degree in psychology. Her current research interests are digitalisation and the impact of the Internet and social media on modern society. Taisiia Ratushna has been a member of the *War, Migration, Memory* research group at the Forum Transregionale Studien since 2022. In 2024–2025, she is a Prisma Ukraïna fellow of the Gerda Henkel Foundation. (https://orcid.org/0000-0001-7351-6647)

Viktoriya Sereda is a sociologist, head coordinator of the Virtual Ukraine Institute for Advanced Study, member of and senior advisor to the Prisma Ukraïna *War, Migration, Memory* research group that she initiated and directed at the Forum Transregionale Studien in 2022/23. Since 2020, she has also been a senior research fellow at the Institute of Ethnology of the National Academy of Sciences of Ukraine and professor in the department of Sociology at the Ukrainian Catholic University (Lviv, Ukraine). Her main areas of research include nationalism, migration and identity studies, memory studies, civil society, and urban sociology. (https://orcid.org/0000-0002-9474-8209)

Denys Shatalov obtained his PhD in History from Oles Honchar Dnipro National University (Dnipro, Ukraine). Since January 2015, he has been a Research Fellow at the "Tkuma" Ukrainian Institute for Holocaust Studies. His main research interests are everyday notions about the past, their shaping and functioning in society. In his work, he concentrates on issues of WWII and Holocaust memorialisation and commemoration, and its representations in the USSR and Ukraine; and the history of the "Cossack Myth" as a crucial part of the modern Ukrainian national identity. He was a Prisma Ukraïna visiting fellow in 2019/2020 and a 2022/2023 non-resident Prisma Ukraïna fellow at the Forum Transregionale Studien. He is a member of the *War, Migration, Memory* research group since 2022, and a 2024–25 Prisma Ukraïna fellow of the Gerda Henkel Foundation.

Tetiana Shestopalova is professor at Petro Mohyla Black Sea National University (Mykolaiv, Ukraine) and visiting scholar at Saarland University (Saarbrücken, Germany). She is a researcher and member of research teams in a number of international and Ukrainian research projects financed by the governments of Ukraine, the USA, and Germany. Her research has focused on modern Ukrainian literary criticism and the legacy of Ukrainian literary emigration after the Second World War. Current research interests also include the contemporary Ukrainian literary process against the background of Russian invasion. (http://orcid.org/0000-0002-0687-5225)

Olena Strelnyk obtained her PhD in Sociology in 2018 at Taras Shevchenko Kyiv National University (Ukraine). As a gender expert and researcher, Olena cooperated with UN Women, OSCE, the World Bank, USAID, the Heinrich Böll Foundation, and many think tanks and NGOs in Ukraine. Currently, she studies various aspects of the impact of the war on gender ideas and discourses, and on the situation and rights of women in Ukraine. (https://orcid.org/0000-0001-9027-4758)

Yuliia Soroka is Professor of Sociology at the N.V. Karazin Kharkiv National University (Ukraine) and a senior researcher in the Human Geography Unit of the Department of Geosciences at the University of Fribourg (Switzerland). Her research considers symbolic spaces of Ukrainian society in different empirical fields. Currently, she focuses on the role of culture in reproducing societal power relationships. Located in Fribourg, Switzerland, Yuliia Soroka has been a member of the *War, Migration, Memory* research group since 2022. In 2024/2025, she is a Prisma Ukraïna fellow of the Gerda Henkel Foundation. (https://orcid.org/0000-0002-4158-1636)

Yuliya Yurchuk is a senior lecturer in the History of Ideas at Södertörn University (Huddinge, Sweden). She specialises in memory studies, history of religion, and the study of nationalism in East European countries. Her recent work focuses on memory and religion. She also translates Swedish literature into Ukrainian and is currently working on projects in the field of transnational intellectual history. She was a Prisma Ukraïna visiting fellow in 2017/2018. (https://orcid.org/0000-0002-6835-0862)

Oleksandr Zabirko serves as a senior researcher at the Slavic Department of the University of Regensburg (Germany) and is a member of the editorial boards of the Journal of European Studies. He holds a PhD in Slavic Literature and Cultures from the University of Münster (Germany). His primary areas of interest encompass literary models of spatial and political order, contemporary literature from Russia and Ukraine, and fantastic literature as a whole. (https://orcid.org/0000-0002-2141-7636)

Natalia Zaitseva-Chipak is a sociologist and professor in the Department of Sociology at the Ukrainian Catholic University (Lviv, Ukraine). Prior to this position, she was a professor in the Department of Sociology at the Ivan Franko National University of Lviv. She completed her PhD in Sociology from the Classic Private University (Ukraine). Her scientific interests focus on problems of modern Ukrainian society and individual social groups, such as youths or internally displaced persons (IDPs). Natalia Zaitseva-Chipak has been a non-resident Prisma Ukraïna fellow and member of the *War, Migration, Memory* research group since 2022. She is a 2024/2025 fellow of the Gerda Henkel Foundation at the Forum Transregionale Studien. (https://orcid.org/0000-0002-5351-3040)

Emine Ziyatdinova is a Crimean Tatar documentary photographer and independent consultant currently working in the non-profit and media development spheres. The desire to advocate for people who are often silenced to voice their concerns brought her to the career paths of sociology and documentary photography. She holds an MA degree in Sociology from Ivan Franko National University of Lviv and an MA degree in photojournalism from Ohio University's School of Visual Communication (USA). In 2017, she left Ukraine and relocated to the UK, where she has been working in the non-profit sector. Her photography projects were exhibited in Ukraine as well as internationally.